Atlas of Urinary Cytopathology

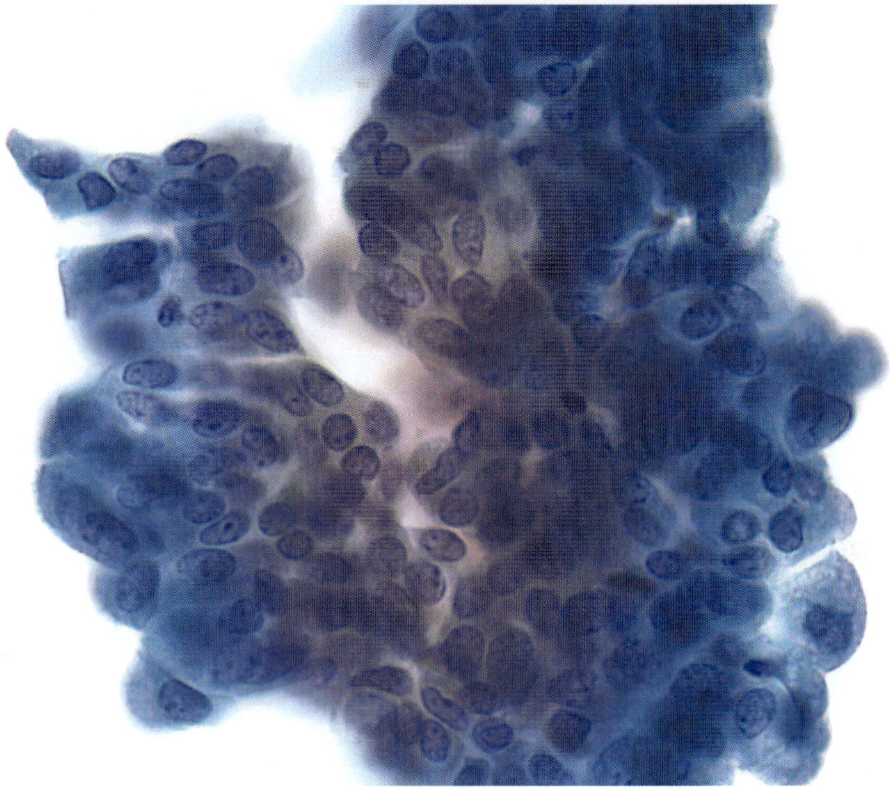

Syed Z. Ali, MD
Associate Professor of Pathology and Radiology
The Johns Hopkins Hospital
Baltimore, Maryland

Tehmina Z. Ali, MD
Assistant Professor of Pathology
University of Maryland Medical Center
Baltimore, Maryland

Dorothy L. Rosenthal, MD
Professor of Pathology, Oncology, and Gynecology and Obstetrics
The Johns Hopkins Hospital
Baltimore, Maryland

Jonathan I. Epstein, MD
Professor of Pathology, Oncology, and Urology
The Johns Hopkins Hospital
Baltimore, Maryland

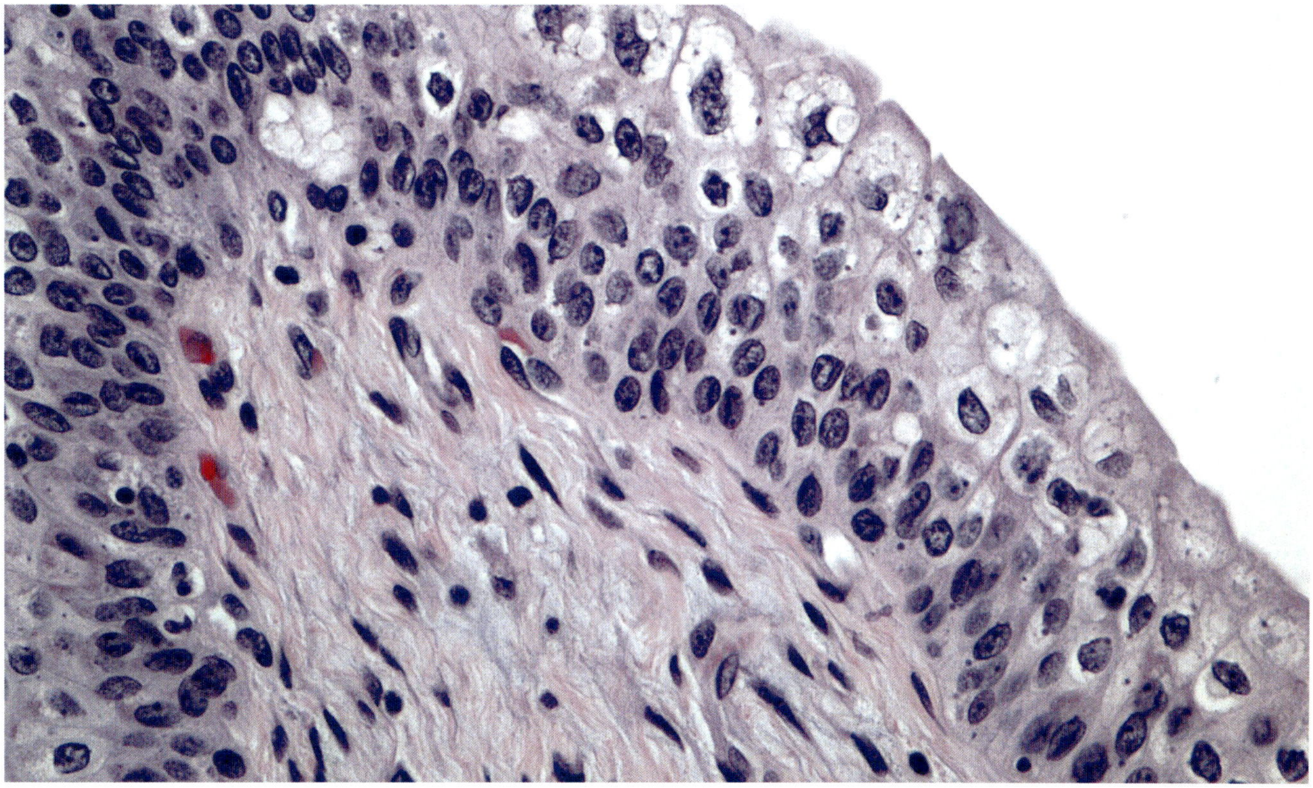

Atlas of Urinary Cytopathology

with Histopathologic Correlations

demosMEDICAL

Acquisitions Editor: *Richard Winters*
Cover Design: *Steve Pisano*
Compositor: *Publication Services Inc.*
Printer: *Bang Printing*

Visit our website at www.demosmedpub.com

Library of Congress Cataloging-in-Publication Data
Atlas of urinary cytopathology with histopathologic correlations / Syed Z. Ali ... [et al.].
p. ; cm.
Includes bibliographical references and index.
ISBN 978-1-933864-66-2 (hardcover : alk. paper) 1. Urinary organs—Cytopathology—Atlases. 2. Urinary organs—Histopathology—Atlases. I. Ali, Syed Z.
[DNLM: 1. Urologic Neoplasms—pathology—Atlases. 2. Cytodiagnosis—methods—Atlases. 3. Histological Techniques—Atlases. 4. Urinary Tract—cytology—Atlases. 5. Urologic Neoplasms—diagnosis—Atlases.
WJ 17 U88179 2010]
RC900.9.A85 2010
616.6'0700223—dc22 2009044204

Special discounts on bulk quantities of Demos Medical Publishing books are available to corporations, professional associations, pharmaceutical companies, health care organizations, and other qualifying groups. For details, please contact:
Special Sales Department
Demos Medical Publishing
11 W. 42nd Street, 15th Floor
New York, NY 10036
Phone: 800–532–8663 or 212–683–0072
Fax: 212–941–7842
E-mail: rsantana@demosmedpub.com

Made in the United States of America
14 15 16 5 4 3

Contents

Foreword

Dr. John K. Frost was the founder of the Cytopathology Laboratory at Johns Hopkins Hospital in Baltimore, Maryland. He was one of the most decent people I have ever had the privilege of knowing and a wonderful friend. His premature death from lung cancer (he never smoked) was a shock to all of us.

I am so glad that at least a part of his extensive archives will be published as an, *Atlas of Urinary Cytopathology with Histopathologic Correlations* by his successor, Dr. Dorothy Rosenthal, and her colleagues. The competence of the contributors virtually guarantees the outstanding scientific and visual value of the volume that honors the memory of Dr. Frost.

Leopold Koss, MD
New York, New York

Preface

Among the more diagnostically challenging human cancers is that affecting the bladder, not because the cytologic changes are so difficult to appreciate, but because the implications of those changes are so misunderstood by pathologists and urologists. Leopold Koss expresses that misunderstanding in the fifth edition of his seminal work, *Diagnostic Cytology and its Histopathologic Bases.* "The problem with cytology of the urinary tract is the lack of basic understanding of the accomplishments and limitations of the method and of the pathologic processes accounting for it." [p. 739]

While this volume cannot begin to match Koss's expansive treatise, the authors hope by the sheer number of illustrations in this atlas to clear some of the misunderstandings of this cancer that afflicts some 70,000 new patients per year and kills another 14,000 in the United States. A noteworthy statistic: more that 500,000 people in the US are survivors of this cancer!

In addition to the skills of the authors, this volume would not have been possible without the dedicated efforts of Frances Burroughs, SCT (ASCP), who caringly selected the cytologic examples from the extensive archives of the John K. Frost Cytopathology Laboratory at The Johns Hopkins Hospital.

The authors hope that this volume will serve as a guide to pathologists in selecting appropriate samples when our diagnostic menu is amplified by molecular and genetic markers of prediction and prognosis for those patients unfortunately afflicted with urothelial carcinoma. Until then, may it continue to guide those involved in traditional morphologic diagnosis of urothelial cancer and other malignancies of the bladder and upper urinary tracts.

Syed Z. Ali
Dorothy L. Rosenthal
Tehmina Z. Ali
Jonathan I. Epstein

Baltimore, Maryland

*Technical Note: The predominant method used to prepare the illustrated specimens is SurePath® technology.

1

Normal Urothelium, Other Cells, and Contaminants

- Urothelial Cells
- Glandular and Squamous Cells
- Gynecologic and Male Genital Tract Contamination
- Renal Tubular and Other Cells
- Urinary Crystals
- Lubricant and Other Contaminants

Figure 1.1 — Normal urothelium, histologic section. Typically, the urinary bladder urothelium is composed of six to seven layers of epithelial cells in the nondistended state. The basal cells rest on the basement membrane and are responsible for replenishing the superficial cell layers. The rest of the urothelial cells making up the intermediate layer have somewhat ovoid nuclei, frequently with a longitudinal groove, and are arranged perpendicular to the basement membrane. The cell has a moderate amount of cytoplasm, which is eosinophilic to clear in appearance. The most superficial cells are called the umbrella cells. These are larger cells arranged horizontally, with each umbrella cell covering two to three urothelial cells. The umbrella cells can have ample eosinophilic to vacuolated cytoplasm with large nuclei, sometimes binucleated (H&E, low power).

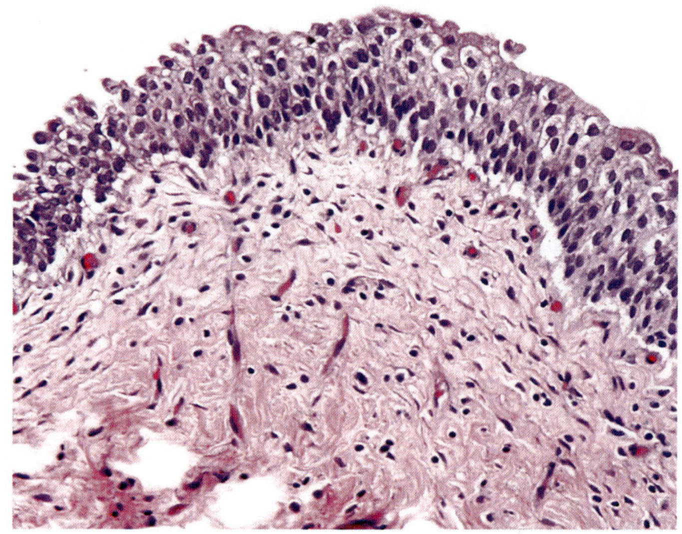

Figure 1.2 — Normal urothelium, histologic section. Multilayered cells are arranged parallel to each other and perpendicular to the basement membrane, topped by umbrella cells. Size of the cells and nuclei is uniform. Nuclear membrane outlines are smooth. A good reference is the ever-present stromal lymphocyte, compared to which, the benign urothelial nuclei are up to two to three times the size. The basement membrane separates the urothelial cells from the underlying lamina propria. The lamina propria has abundant connective tissue and contains a rich vascular and lymphatic network (H&E, low power).

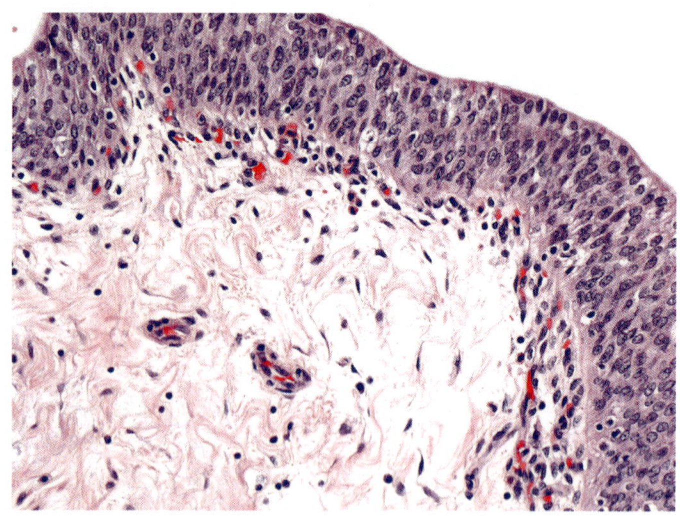

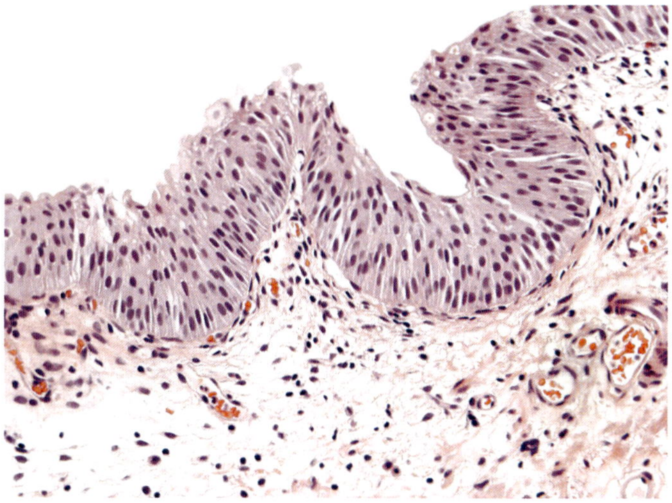

Figure 1.3 — Normal urothelium, histologic section. Benign bladder epithelium is thrown into folds. Notice the uniform size of the nuclei and polarity to each other. Some umbrella cells are also visible on the surface, which are larger with vacuolated cytoplasm and span two to three underlying intermediate cells. Underlying lamina propria contains stromal lymphocytes and small blood vessels (H&E, low power).

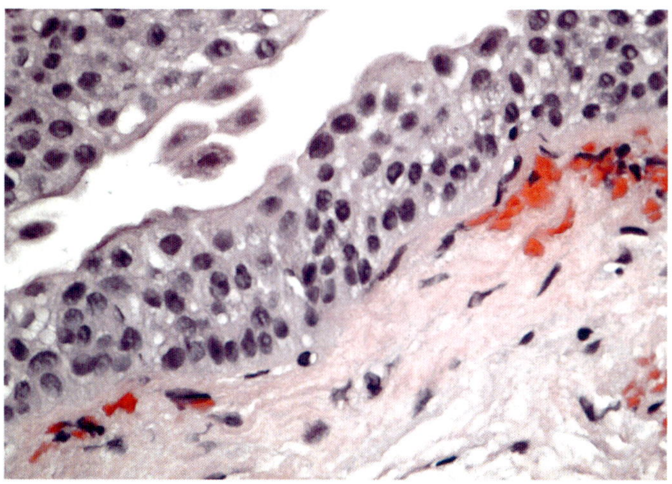

Figure 1.4 — Normal urothelium, histologic section. Close-up view of normal urothelium with the nuclei showing a uniform appearance and polarity. Occasional small nucleoli and nuclear grooves are visible. Luminal surface displays umbrella cells. This urothelium has mild reactive features and some small submucosal hemorrhaging. The nuclear membranes are smooth, and compared to the stromal lymphocytes, the nuclei are within the normal size range (H&E, high power).

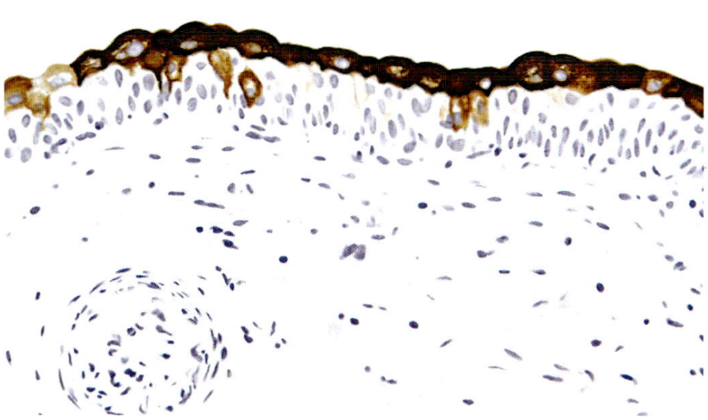

Figure 1.5 — Normal urothelium, histologic section. Benign urothelium immunostained with cytokeratin 20 (CK20) selectively highlights the umbrella cells. The underlying intermediate urothelial cells do not stain; however, in the presence of urothelial carcinoma in situ, the malignant cells also stain with CK20. Thus, CK20 is a useful marker in difficult cases where inflammation or other injury makes the urothelial cells appear hyperchromatic and enlarged. Reactive urothelial cells do not stain with CK20 (immunostain CK20, low power).

Figure 1.6 — Normal urothelium, voided urine. Benign urothelial cells in cytologic samples come in essentially two sizes, larger umbrella cells and smaller basal cells, each with the same size nucleus, providing an internal control for the rest of the sample. Umbrella cells are essentially the same size as mature squamous epithelial cells and may be confused with them in voided urine from a female. Males also can have intermediate squamous epithelial cells in bladder samples. The distinguishing characteristic is the texture of the urothelial umbrella cell, which is finely vacuolated, whereas squamous epithelial cells have homogeneous opaque cytoplasm. Umbrella cell nuclei are usually larger than intermediate squamous nuclei, in the range of 15–20 microns in diameter. Umbrella cells are also frequently multinucleated. The basal cells have the same finely vacuolated cytoplasm (Papanicolaou stain, medium power).

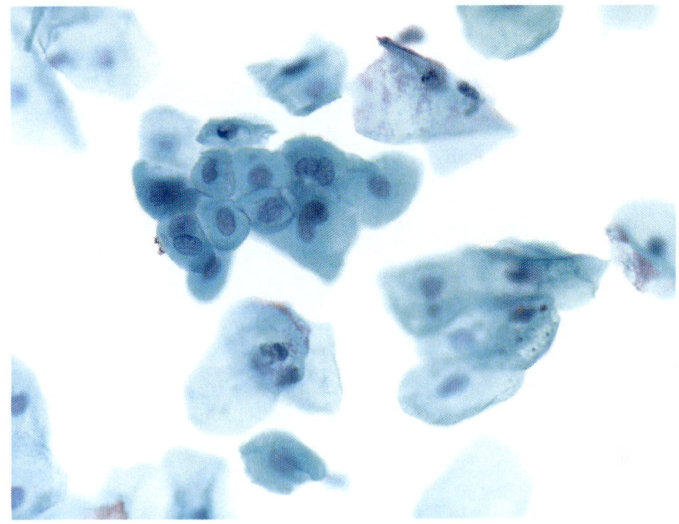

Figure 1.7 — Normal urothelium, voided urine. Umbrella cells frequently display a thickened outer cuff of cytoplasm compared to the central, more vacuolated and textured area close to the nucleus. This change should not be mistaken as viral induced, i.e., a koilocyte. Instead, it is a reflection of the asymmetric unit membrane, which is unique to the umbrella cell (Papanicolaou stain, high power).

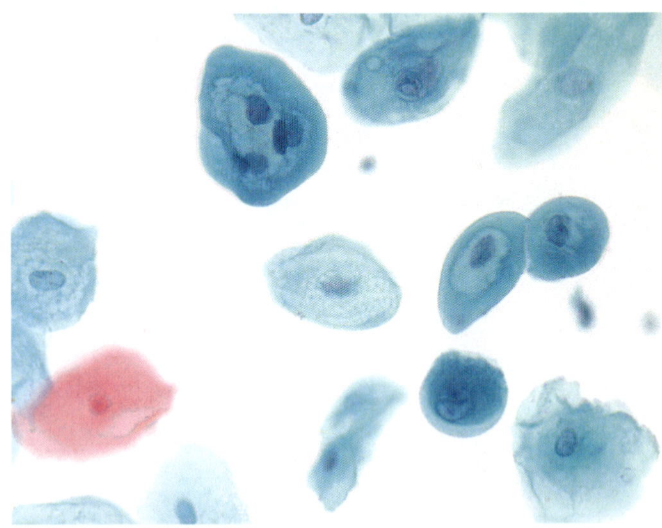

Figure 1.8 — Normal urothelium, voided urine. Five basal urothelial cells in a group are distinct from the two squamous cells in the left half of the photograph. Farthest left is a mature squamous intermediate cell, alongside of a metaplastic squamous cell. The smaller size of the nucleus can be appreciated in these squamous cells when compared to those of the basal cells. Also, the quality of the cytoplasm of the squamous epithelial cells is more opaque than the finely vacuolated cytoplasm of the basal urothelial cells (Papanicolaou stain, high power).

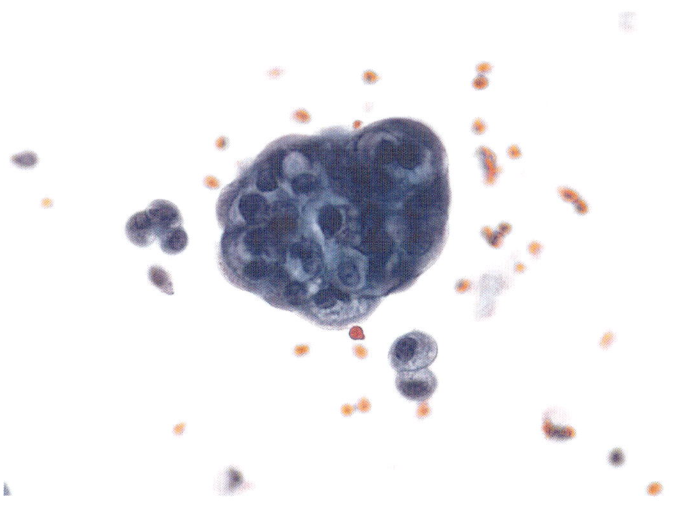

Figure 1.9 — Normal urothelium, instrumented urine. A large group of umbrella cells is centered in the photo and surrounded by red blood cells and several smaller basal urothelial cells. The thickened asymmetric unit membranes of the umbrella cells can be seen bordering the group. The finely vacuolated perinuclear cytoplasm is also characteristic of urothelial cells and can be appreciated in both the basal and umbrella cells in the picture. The group of umbrella cells should not be interpreted as having come from a papillary lesion, but rather having been exfoliated due to instrumentation. The round nuclei, finely vacuolated cytoplasm, and low nuclear to cytoplasmic (N/C) ratio are features of benign cells in a group, not a neoplastic transformation (Papanicolaou stain, high power).

Figure 1.10 — Normal urothelium, instrumented urine. A group of normal umbrella cells prominently displays the luminal asymmetric unit membrane in the cytoplasm, which is thicker and more opaque than the perinuclear, finely vacuolated cytoplasm. The small basal cell to the left of the group displays the vacuolated cytoplasm but not the thickened asymmetric unit membrane since it does not abut the bladder lumen in the normal urothelium (Papanicolaou stain, high power).

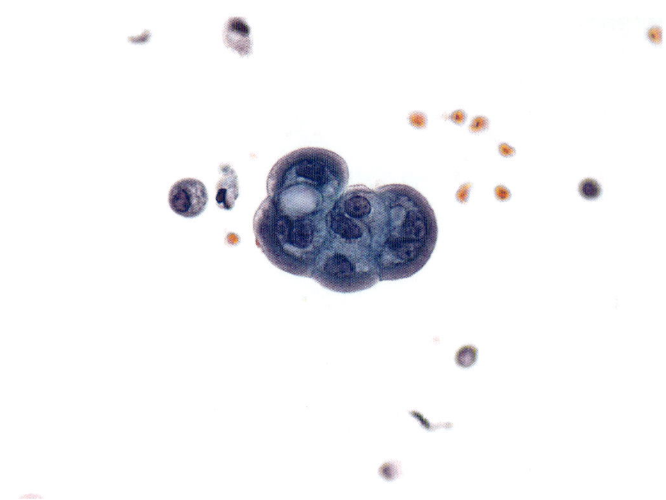

Figure 1.11 — Normal urothelium, voided urine. Normal umbrella cells do not always demonstrate the asymmetric unit membrane and may be difficult to distinguish from normal squamous epithelial cells. The quality of the cytoplasm in the umbrella cells is more transparent and textured than the squamous epithelial cells that can be seen in this image in the lower left hand corner and in the center of the photograph (arrows). The nuclei of the umbrella cells are also larger than those of the intermediate squamous epithelial cells and normally have at least one prominent small nucleolus (Papanicolaou stain, high power).

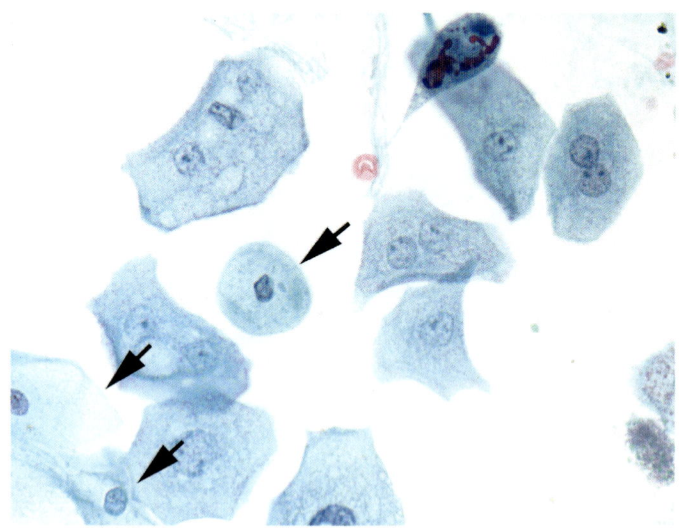

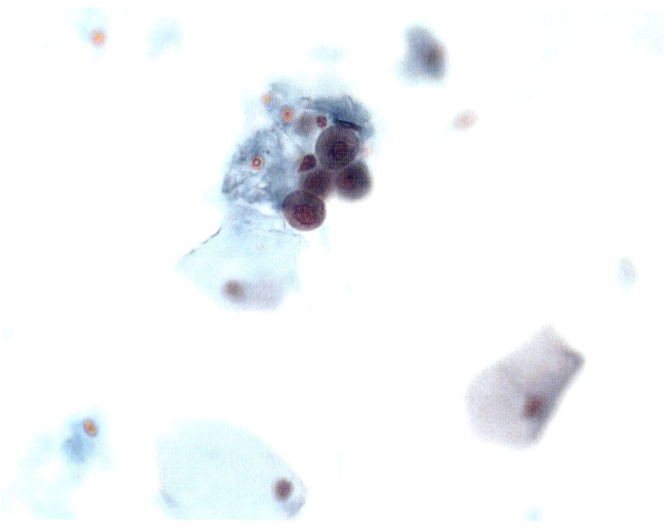

Figure 1.12 — Normal urothelium, voided urine. Small metaplastic-type cells could be from the bladder but they also could be from the female genital tract. The opacity of cytoplasm distinguishes them from typical basal urothelial cells, and the nuclei are slightly smaller than basal cells from the bladder. The surrounding squamous epithelial cells attest to the probable lower gynecological tract origin of these metaplastic cells (Papanicolaou stain, high power).

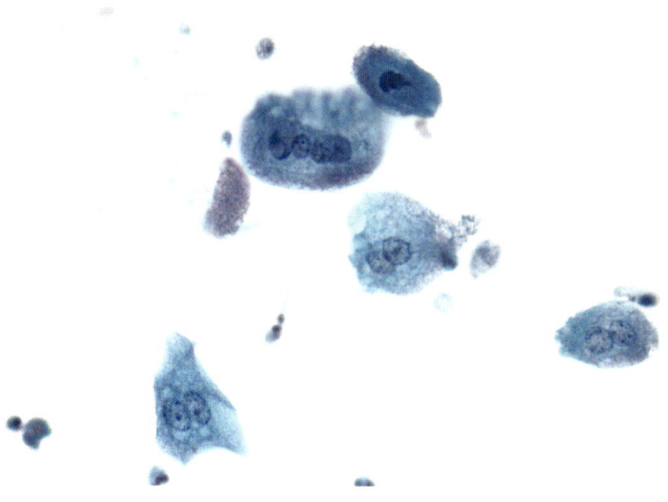

Figure 1.13 — Normal urothelium, voided urine. Multiple nuclei in urothelial umbrella cells are common as are nucleoli and should not be construed as a neoplastic or reactive change. The asymmetric unit membrane is quite obvious in the cells (Papanicolaou stain, high power).

Figure 1.14 — Normal urothelium, voided urine. The finely textured cytoplasm of the urothelial cells distinguishes them from the opaque cytoplasm of the squamous epithelial cells in the same sample. Squamous cells can originate in the trigone of the bladder and should not be interpreted necessarily as "contamination" from the external genitalia or the female vaginal tract. The staining quality and color of the urothelial nuclei is more delicate than the hyperchromatic nuclei of the squamous epithelium (Papanicolaou stain, high power).

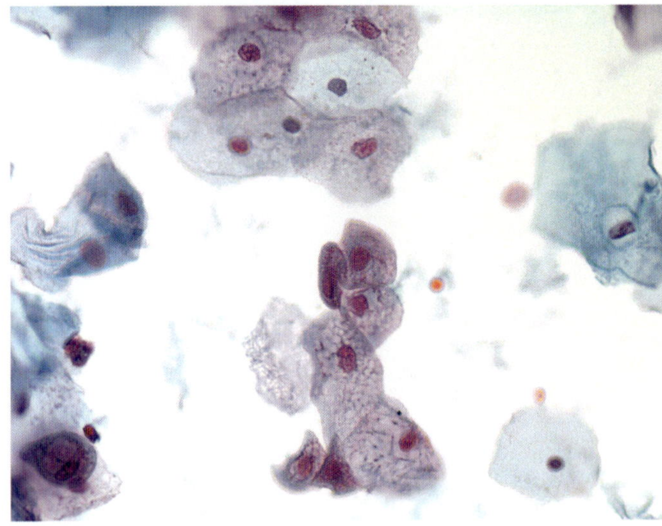

Figure 1.15 — Normal urothelium, voided urine. The superficial squamous epithelial cell (arrow) has an opaque and uniform cytoplasmic texture when compared to the finely vacuolated cytoplasm of the umbrella cells below. These umbrella cells appear slightly smaller than the squamous epithelial cells but display the thickened asymmetric unit membrane so characteristic of the umbrella urothelial cells (Papanicolaou stain, high power).

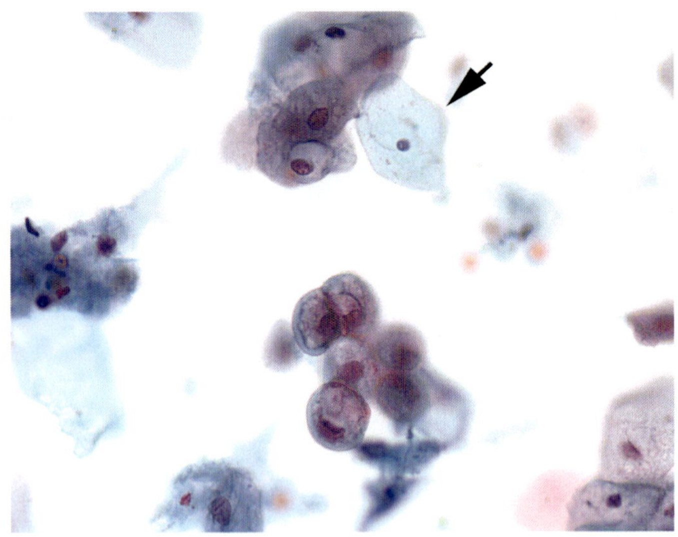

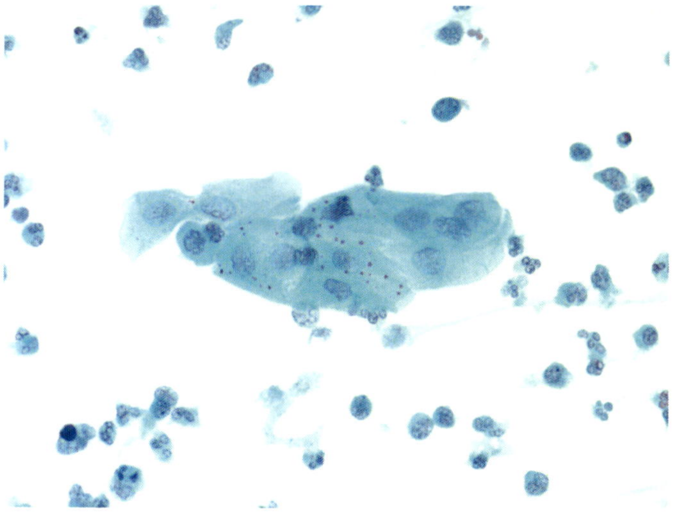

Figure 1.16 — Normal urothelium, voided urine. Sometimes urothelial cells are difficult to distinguish from squamous epithelial cells, as in this photograph. The cytoplasmic texture is homogenous as in a squamous cell, but regardless of the origin of the cells, they appear benign (Papanicolaou stain, high power).

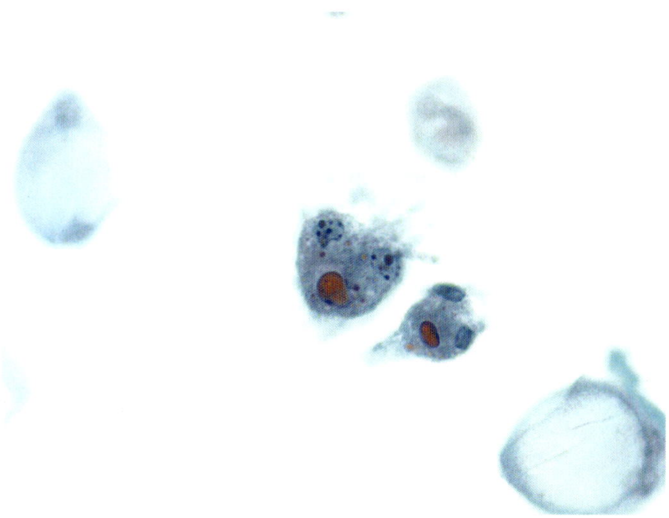

Figure 1.17 — Benign urothelium, voided urine. Cellular degeneration is not uncommon in exfoliated urothelial cells and may range from subtle nuclear and cytoplasmic changes to marked nuclear pyknosis, cytoplasmic vacuolization and globoid eosinophilic or orangeophilic cytoplasmic inclusions (Papanicolaou stain, high power).

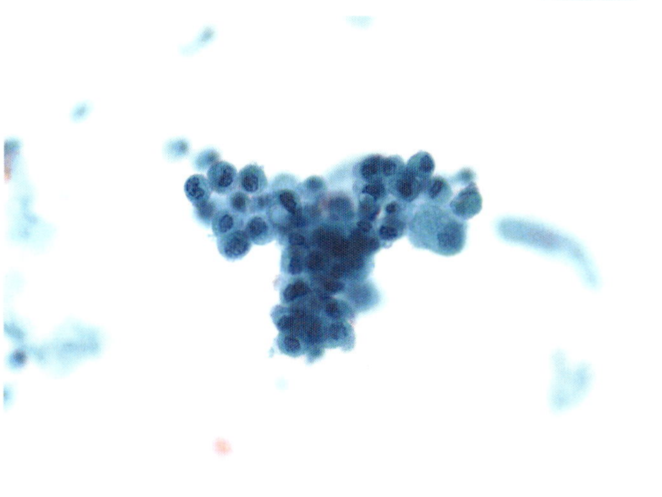

Figure 1.18 — Normal voided urine. Renal tubular epithelial cells are extremely small, and usually occur singly or in small groups. This photograph is unusual in the number of tubular epithelial cells that are present. Their crenated nuclei and vacuolated cytoplasm are different from the basal cells of the urothelium. The resemblance of these cells to histiocytes is a further characteristic of renal tubular epithelial cells (Papanicolaou stain, high power).

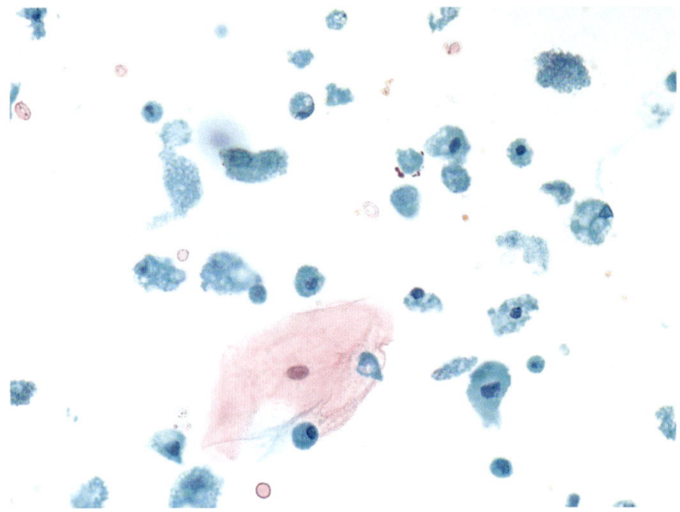

Figure 1.19 — Normal voided urine. Degenerated renal tubular epithelial cells usually occur singly, and are considerably smaller than the squamous epithelial cell in the photograph. Cytoplasmic fragments have lost their nuclei due to marked cellular degeneration (Papanicolaou stain, high power).

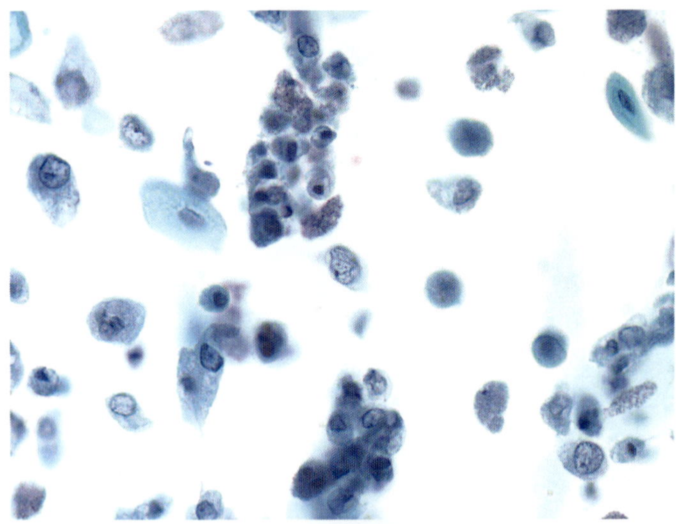

Figure 1.20 — Normal voided urine. Renal tubular epithelial cells come in varying sizes depending upon whether they are from the proximal tubule or the distal tubule. Note the small, dark, pyknotic nucleus and prominently granular cytoplasm (Papanicolaou stain, high power).

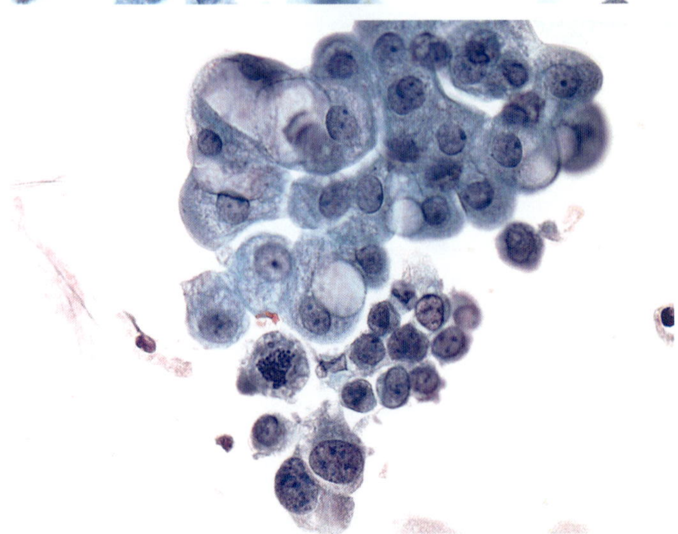

Figure 1.21 — High-grade urothelial carcinoma and benign urothelial cells, voided urine. Compare and contrast the benign superficial urothelial cells with relatively abundant and vacuolated cytoplasm, well defined cell borders, and uniform nuclei with small nucleoli (upper half of the image) to urothelial carcinoma cells with high N/C ratios, pleomorphic nuclei, prominent single or multiple nucleoli, and mitosis (lower half of the image; Papanicolaou stain, high power).

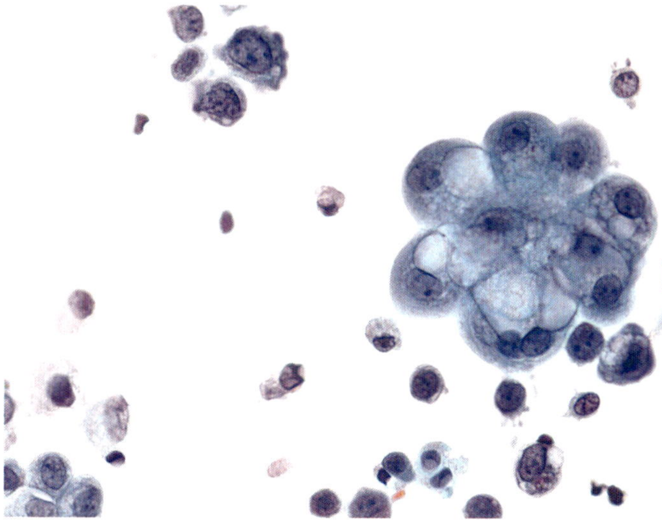

Figure 1.22 — High-grade urothelial carcinoma and benign urothelial cells, voided urine. Single high-grade urothelial carcinoma cells are the usual way in which these tumor cells exfoliate, making them easy to spot even on low power. However, if they are scarce, they may be overlooked. A small fragment of benign urothelium is present (center right) for comparison (Papanicolaou stain, high power).

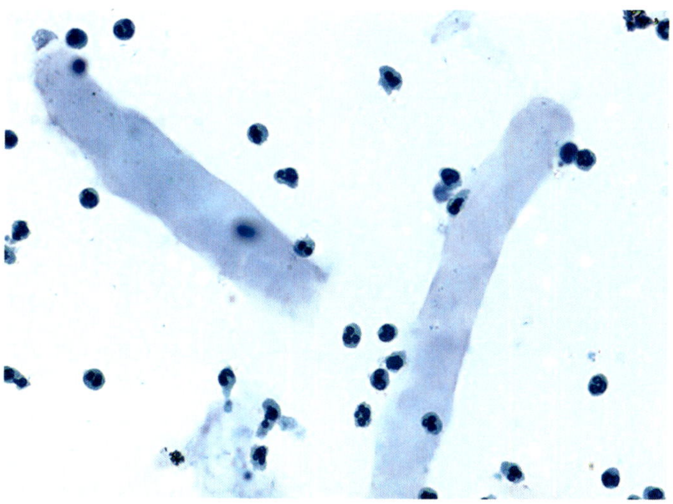

Figure 1.23 — Casts, voided urine. Waxy casts are characterized by a homogeneous appearance without adherent cells. The acute inflammation surrounding these casts is not invariable as these casts do not always accompany an inflammatory process (Papanicolaou stain, high power).

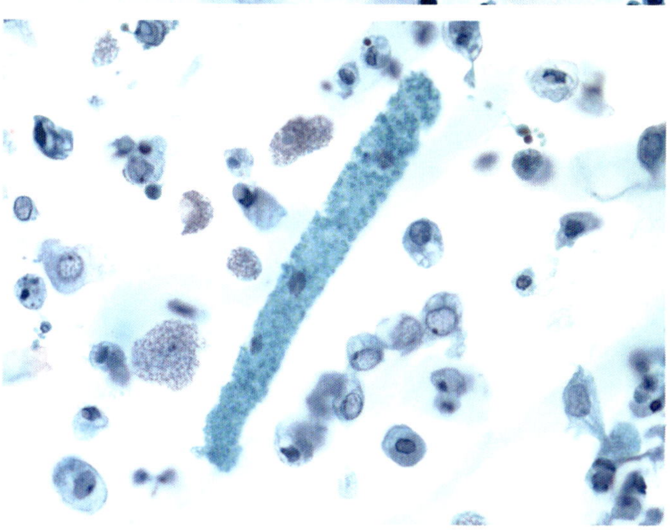

Figure 1.24 — Casts, voided urine. Granular casts can be of any length as illustrated in this photograph. Most characteristic is the textured contents, hence the name granular cast. Numerous degenerated urothelial and renal tubular cells are also seen here in the background (Papanicolaou stain, high power).

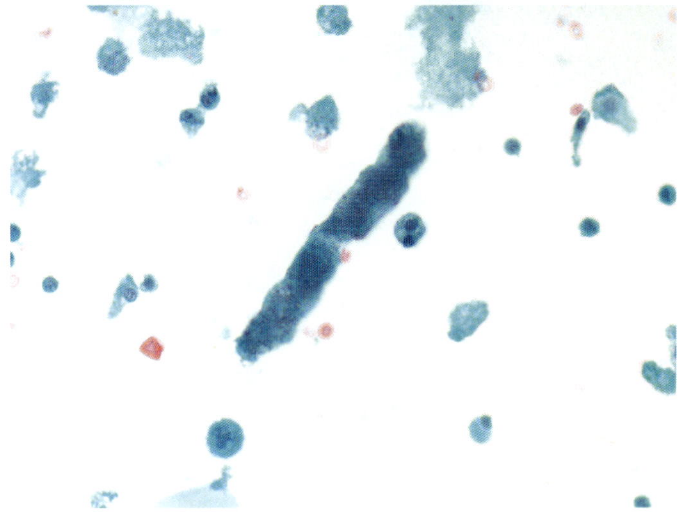

Figure 1.25 — Casts, voided urine. Another granular cast with granular material in the background. This patient may be suffering from a protein-losing nephropathy. However, granular casts are the most frequently seen of all tubular casts in urinary cytology, including patients with no renal disease. Clinical correlation is important (Papanicolaou stain, high power).

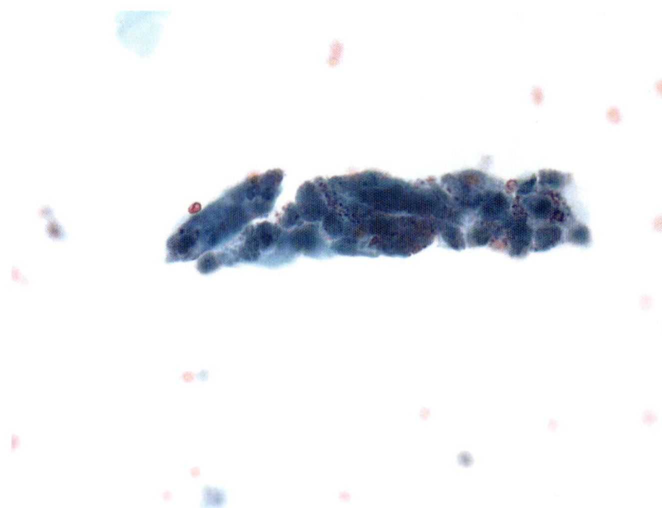

Figure 1.26 — Casts, voided urine. When neutrophils are collected in a cast, the diagnosis of pyelonephritis is most likely. In this particular cast, red blood cells are also included along with the neutrophils, implying glomerular permeability (Papanicolaou stain, high power).

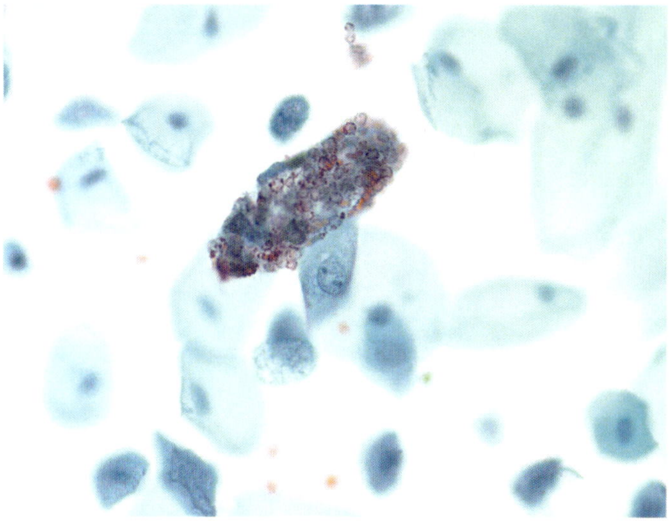

Figure 1.27 — Casts, voided urine. A red blood cell cast is easily appreciated, and includes a few neutrophils. These do not necessarily imply pyelonephritis, but may be part of the blood entering the renal tubules (Papanicolaou stain, high power).

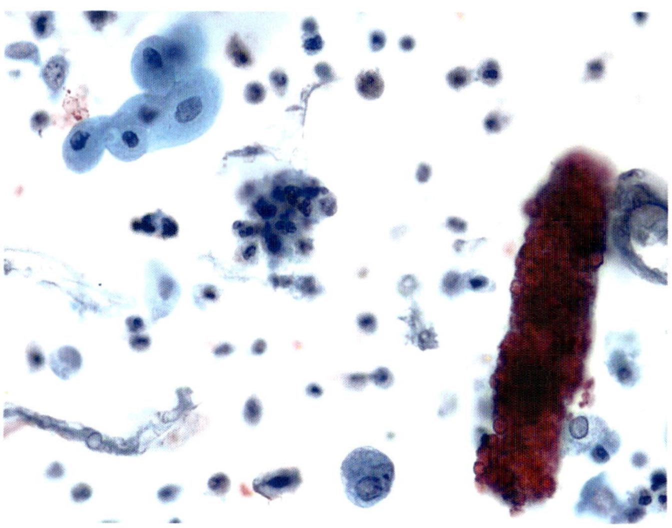

Figure 1.28 — Casts, voided urine. This large red blood cell cast accompanies scattered neutrophils as well as atypical urothelial cells. Each entity needs to be clearly described, as this patient has multiple diseases affecting the urinary tract (Papanicolaou stain, high power).

Figure 1.29 — Casts, voided urine. Red blood cell cast accompanied by acute inflammation and benign-appearing urothelial cells. The patient's hematuria is no doubt arising in the kidney and not in the bladder, removing a urothelial lesion from the potential list of cytologic diagnoses (Papanicolaou stain, high power).

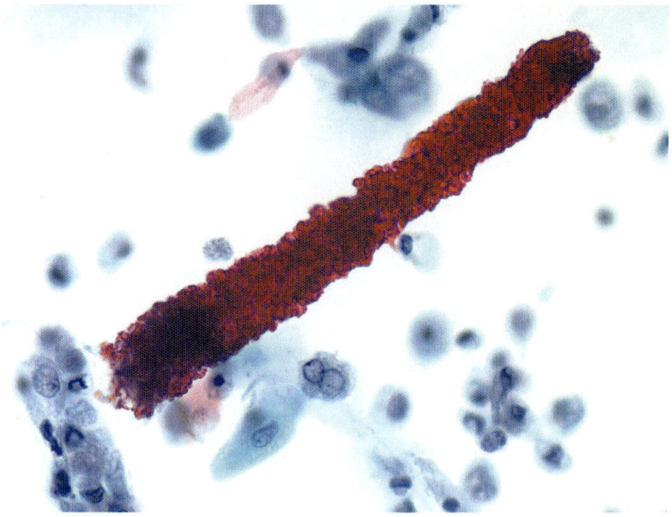

Figure 1.30 — Casts, voided urine. Renal tubular epithelial cells are best seen when encased in the protein of these tubular epithelial casts. Scattered single tubular epithelial cells are seen in the background. The patient's diagnosis is most likely lower nephron nephrosis (Papanicolaou stain, medium power).

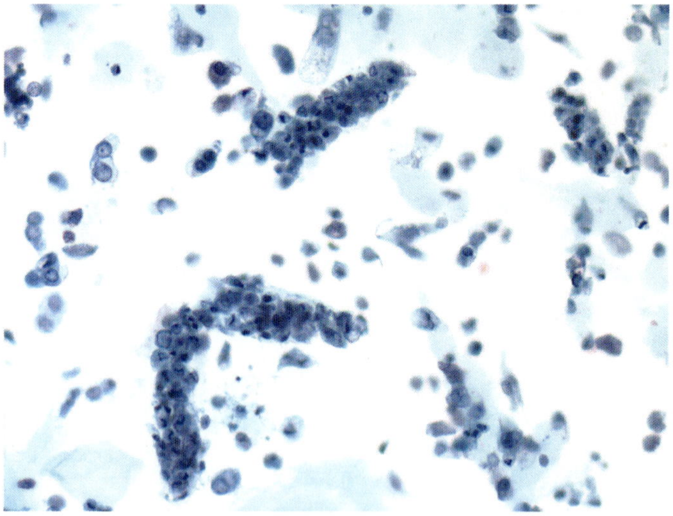

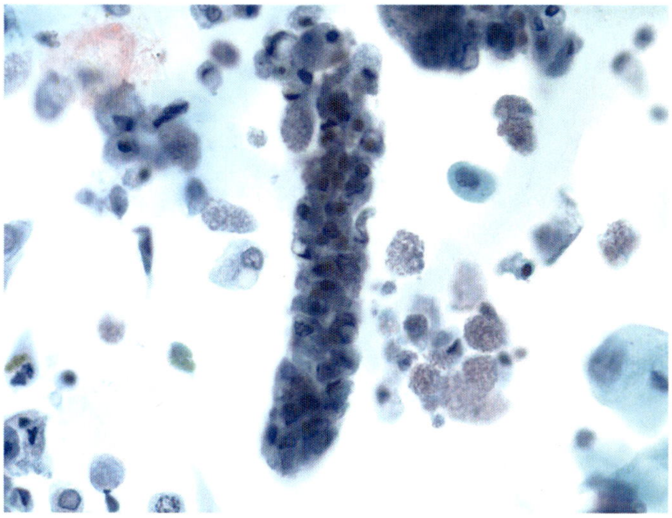

Figure 1.31 — Casts, voided urine. This is a mixed cast, both granular and tubular epithelial cell casts accompanied by scattered renal tubular epithelial cells and small granular casts (Papanicolaou stain, high power).

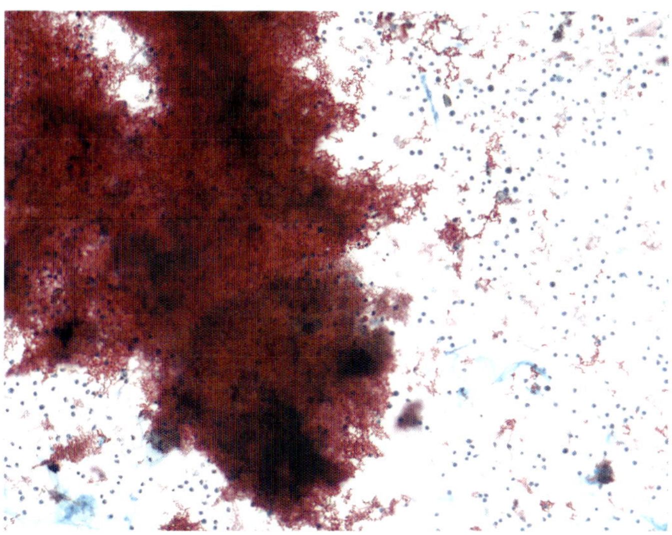

Figure 1.32 — Hematuria, voided urine. Since hematuria is the most common presenting symptom for patients with urothelial neoplasia, the exact source of blood must be determined when at all possible. This specimen is no doubt grossly bloody, with abundant lysed red blood cells and neutrophils in the background. Careful screening for malignant cells is mandatory. If the patient is a woman and the specimen is voided, not catheterized, the recommendation for a repeat catheterized specimen is imperative to establish the source of the bleeding (Papanicolaou stain, low power).

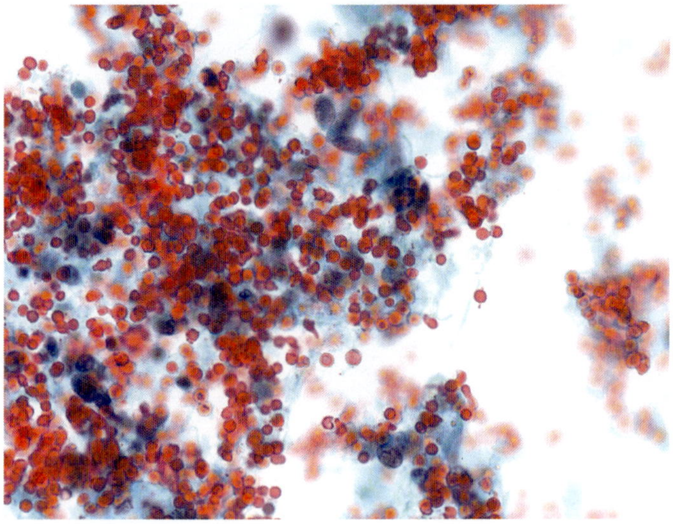

Figure 1.33 — Hematuria, voided urine. High power of a bloody specimen discloses intact red blood cells as opposed to lysed red cells, indicating acute bleeding. If the patient is a woman, menstrual blood may be the source of this blood if the specimen has been voided; in any other case, a papillary lesion should be suspected, as the vascular stalk of the papillary tumor can break off causing blood to escape into the urine (Papanicolaou stain, high power).

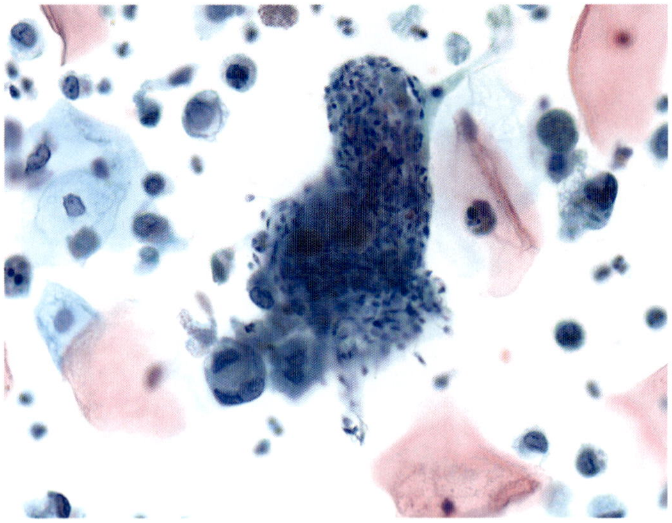

Figure 1.34 — Spermuria, voided urine. An accumulation of spermatozoa in a protein cast, most likely from ejaculate in the urine. Retrograde ejaculation can be seen when patients have had a transurethral resection of the bladder or prostate (TURB or TURP) and one of the ducts from the testicles has been nicked. One may also see seminal vesicle cells in such a specimen, which can be confused with high-grade urothelial carcinoma cells. Seminal vesicle cells are usually infrequent, and cytoplasmic pigment may confirm the diagnosis (Papanicolaou stain, high power).

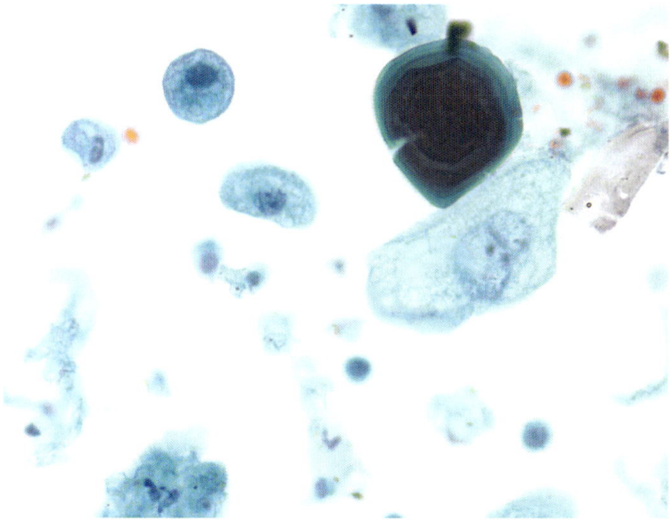

Figure 1.35 — Corpora amylacea, voided urine. Corpora amylacea are found in urine specimens from men, usually older and with some degree of prostatic hypertrophy. Their identification is confirmed by the concentric rings within the corpora (Papanicolaou stain, high power).

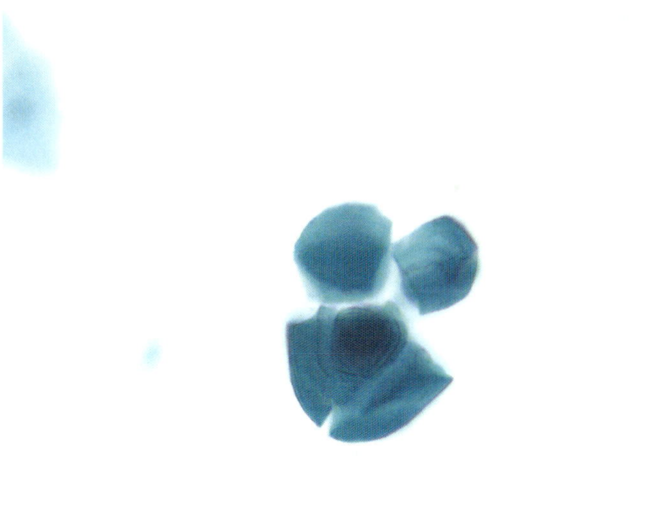

Figure 1.36 — Corpora amylacea, voided urine. Corpora amylacea with fracturing of one of the bodies might suggest that this is instead a calcific body and not a corpora amylacea. Any uncertainties should be communicated to the clinician, especially if the patient has a history of renal calculus (Papanicolaou stain, high power).

Figure 1.37 — Crystalluria, voided urine. Crystals are frequently seen in urine depending upon the pH of the fluid. Most urinary crystals are clinically insignificant or may indicate metabolic disorders. With routine stains and conventional Köhler illumination, crystals frequently have no color and are difficult to appreciate. Polarization is the best way to appreciate the character of the crystals and enable identification. Generally, clinically significant crystals are present in freshly voided urines. The oval-shaped crystals seen here possibly represent calcium oxalate monohydrate (Papanicolaou stain, medium power).

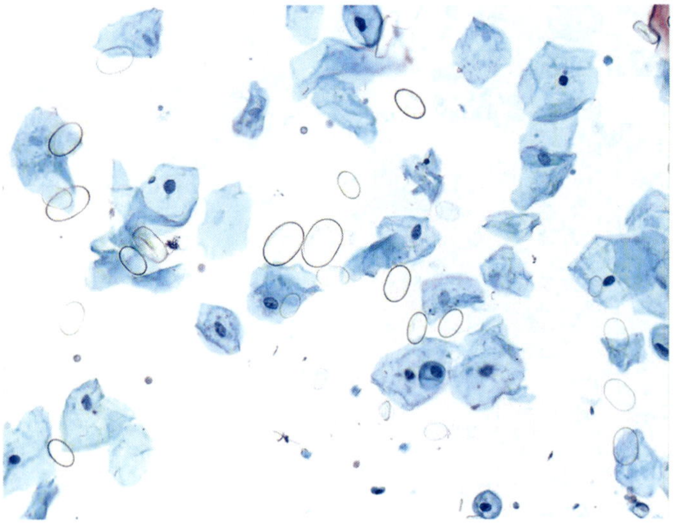

Figure 1.38 — Crystalluria, voided urine. Even without polarizing lenses, the shape of uric acid crystals is quite characteristic. Uric acid crystals are the most common type seen in urine, typically at a pH of less than 6.0. However, they can be confused with schistosomal ova if one is not careful. The eggs of parasites will not polarize, whereas uric acid crystals are brilliantly colored. In this particular case, a single malignant cell from a high-grade urothelial carcinoma is also noted in the middle of the field. Uric acid crystals, when accompanied by increased serum uric acid levels, may be associated with clinical gout (Papanicolaou stain, high power).

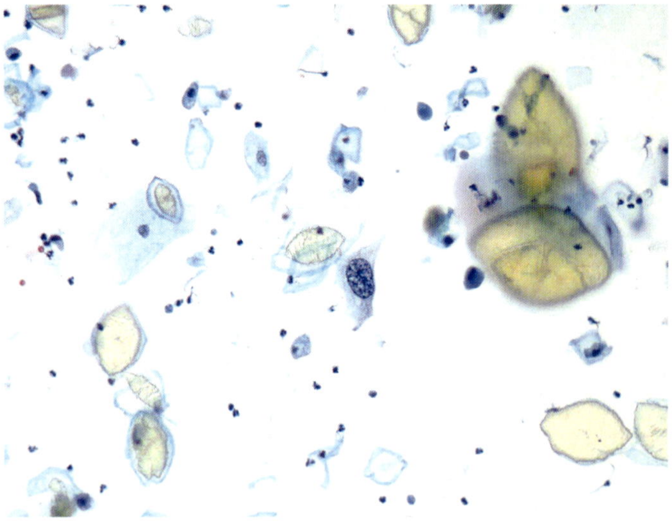

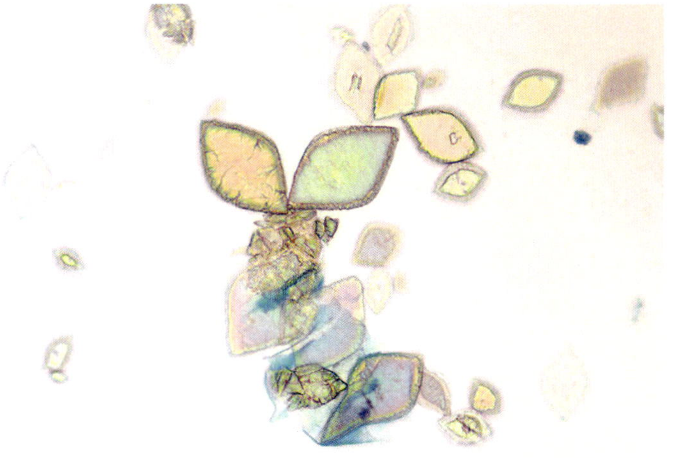

Figure 1.39 — Crystalluria, voided urine. Uric acid crystals come in various sizes, and although many are the shape of schistosomal eggs, the latter are of uniform size and quantitatively fewer in number, often accompanied by intense inflammatory reaction. Crystal composition may imply the presence of urinary calculi. Crystals precipitate out in urine when the concentration in the liquid is greater than the solubility threshold for that solute. Uric acid crystals are typically yellow or reddish brown and quite polymorphous in appearance. They can be prisms, four-sided flat plates, irregular plates, pointed-ended ovals, wedges, or rosettes (Papanicolaou stain, high power).

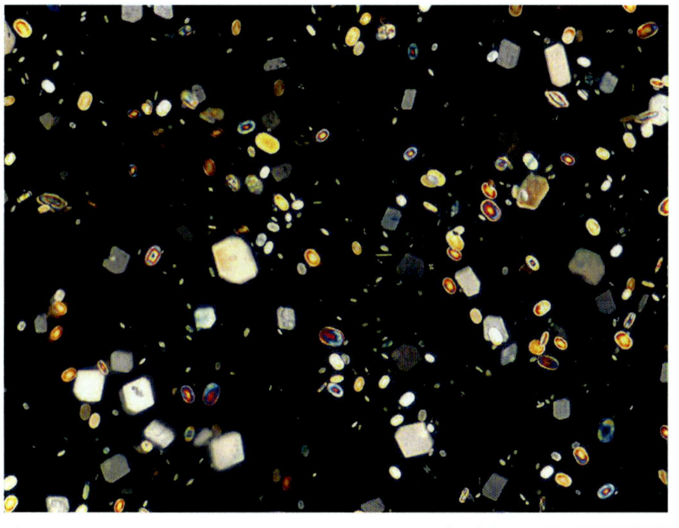

Figure 1.40 — Crystalluria, voided urine. This assortment of crystals is best appreciated with polarized illumination. The most brilliantly colored are from uric acid, whereas the rhomboid shaped crystals are triple phosphate. The larger, pale-yellow crystals are also of urate type (Papanicolaou stain, polarized microscopy, low power).

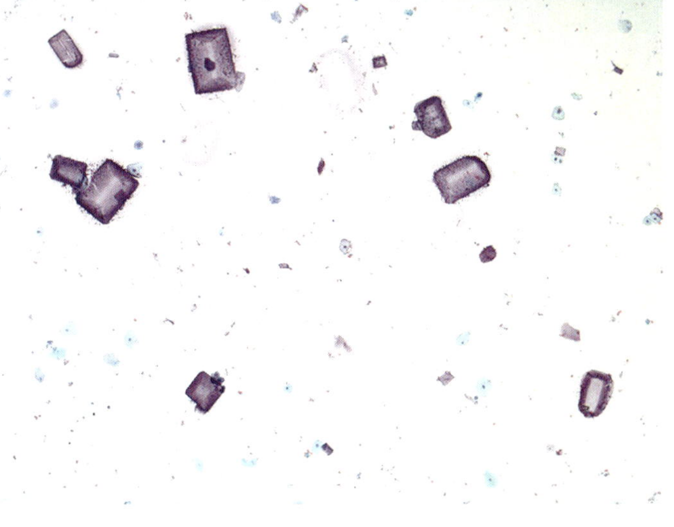

Figure 1.41 — Crystalluria, voided urine. Triple phosphate (ammonium magnesium phosphate) crystals, also called "struvite," have the characteristic rectangular, rhomboid, or the so-called "coffin lid" appearance. These crystals form in neutral or alkaline urine and display three to six sides and oblique ends (Papanicolaou stain, low power).

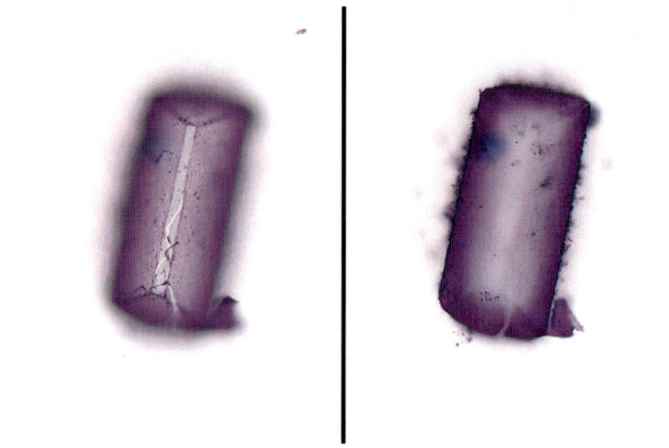

Figure 1.42 — Crystalluria, voided urine. Triple phosphate (ammonium magnesium phosphate) crystals with the classic "coffin lid" appearance. Although these crystals are often seen in urines of clinically normal individuals, triple phosphate crystals can form urinary calculi, especially in the setting of pyelonephritis caused by the Proteus species (Papanicolaou stain, high power).

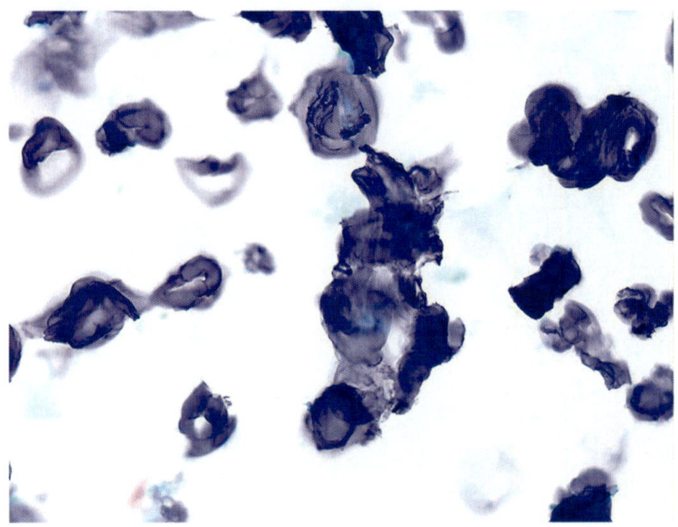

Figure 1.43 — Instrumented urine. Abundant lubricant material as a result of instrumentation is seen in this urine. This should not be confused with corpora amylacea, psammoma bodies, parasite eggs, or other foreign body material. Abundant lubricant, as seen here, may obscure cells, hampering cytologic evaluation (Papanicolaou stain, low power).

Cystoscopic Characteristics of Urinary Tract Lesions

2

Toby C. Chai, MD

John D. Young Professor of Surgery
Division of Urology
University of Maryland Medical Center
Baltimore, Maryland

- Normal Urinary Tract
- Bladder Diverticula
- Calculus Disease
- Cystitis
- Schistosomiasis
- Cystitis Cystica
- Papillary Lesions
- Upper Urinary Tract Disease
- Other Lesions

Introduction to Cystoscopy

There is an art to cystoscopy, because the cystoscopic appearances within the bladder can vary widely between individuals. Multiple images of normal bladder urothelium are shown in the first series of figures to give the reader a better appreciation of variations. Cystoscopy is performed in a systematic fashion to visualize the entire urothelial surface within the bladder. Assessment of the ureteral orifices is also required. With rigid cystoscopes, different degrees of lenses allow the urologist to have different fields of view so that no area of the bladder are missed. With the advent of flexible cystoscopes, retroflexion of the flexible scope, in which the visual field (at tip of the scope) is deflected back on itself (as if one had "eyes on the back of the head"), allows visualization of the bladder neck in an "antegrade" (following flow of urine stream) fashion. Also, the urethra, both in the male and female, is assessed during cystoscopy.

In **Figure 2.1**, the bladder is partially distended as evidenced by the presence of urothelial folds in the floor of the bladder. As the bladder fills, these folds will flatten and disappear. However, the prominence of folds varies greatly, and some bladders do not have folds, even in a decompressed state. In order to see "behind" these folds, one must make sure that the bladder is adequately distended as not to miss any tumors or other abnormalities. The range of blood vessel (capillary) pattern ranges from what is seen in **Figure 2.2** (more dense) to that seen in **Figure 2.3** (less dense). **Figure 2.10** shows a very fine capillary pattern. In a male bladder, retroflexion of a flexible cystoscope can reveal the presence of a median prostatic lobe intruding through the bladder neck into the bladder lumen proper (**Figure 2.4**). One can appreciate how the median lobe can behave as a "ball valve" and block urinary flow through the bladder neck. The orientation of **Figure 2.4** is such that the anterior is to the right (the anterior bladder wall is in the right upper portion of this cystoscopic image). The presence of a median lobe of the prostate cannot be detected on a transrectal prostate ultrasound and retroflexion of a flexible cystoscope is the best technique to determine presence of a prostatic median lobe.

Various images of ureteral orifices are shown in **Figures 2.5–2.8**. Visualization of the upper urinary tracts (ureter, renal pelvis, calyces) involves insertion of a pyeloureteroscope (now usually a flexible design) through the orifice. When cystoscopy is done for the indication of gross hematuria, sometimes one can be fortunate enough to localize upper urinary tract bleeding by observing efflux of grossly bloody urine from one of the ureteral orifices (**Figure 2.11**, arrow).

A scar from previous urothelial biopsy is shown in **Figure 2.9**. There is a typical stellate, whitish appearance to the scar.

Papillary Urothelial Tumors

The next series of Figures show appearances of papillary urothelial carcinoma tumors.

In **Figure 2.12**, one can see a cauliflower-like mass extending from urothelial surface into lumen of bladder. Just to the right side of this cystoscopic image, one can just see the appearance of another papillary tumor. **Figure 2.13** shows a very small papillary tumor that has been biopsied by a cystoscopic biopsy forceps (post-biopsy picture in **Figure 2.14**). **Figure 2.15** shows a larger papillary tumor that fills the entire cystoscopic field. One should appreciate that this tumor has more of a smooth appearance rather than papillary. **Figure 2.16** shows a broad, velvety micropapillary erythematous patch on the left side of the cystoscopic image. **Figure 2.17** also showed papillary patches (on left side of image). The histopathology from both **Figures 2.16** and **2.17** shows superficial urothelial carcinomas. The erythematous patchy appearance is just another way these urothelial carcinomas can appear. **Figure 2.18** depicts a small papillary tumor about to be biopsied.

Figure 2.19 shows the typical papillary tumor on a stalk. The top left panel shows that the tumor covers the left ureteral orifice. The top right panel shows that when the cystoscopic irrigation is turned on, the tumor is turned upwards and the left ureteral orifice is uncovered (arrow). The bottom panels show more images of the tumor lifted upwards on its stalk revealing the ureteral orifice (arrow).

In **Figure 2.20**, the top left panel shows how it can be difficult determining whether this periureteric area (black arrow) is a papillary urothelial carcinoma or normal periureteric folds (compare to **Figure 2.6**). The contralateral ureteric orifice on the right is normal (top right panel). This patient also had an extremely small papillary lesion shown in the bottom panels. All of these lesions were superficial urothelial carcinomas.

Figure 2.21 shows a distal left ureteral tumor extruding out of the ureteral meatus with surrounding periureteral erythema (top right and bottom right panels). This patient had left hydroureteronephrosis. The right ureteral orifice is normal (top left panel). The bottom left panel shows a normal right bladder wall.

Figure 2.22 shows multiple papillary tumors in the bladder wall (top left panel, arrows) and papillary tumors over the right lateral bladder wall (bottom right panel, arrows). The two ureteral orifices are normal (top right and bottom left panels). The papillary tumors were all superficial urothelial carcinomas.

Figure 2.23 shows a sessile, smooth tumor emanating from a Hutch diverticulum (paraureteric diverticulum). This tumor was a small-cell carcinoma. Because bladder diverticula are only lined with urothelium and no detrusor muscle, a carcinoma arising within a diverticulum has much less tissue to traverse before becoming non-organ confined.

Cystoscopic Imaging of the Urethra

Evaluation of the urethra can reveal papillary tumors as well. **Figures 2.24a** and **2.24b** show a papillary tumor in a male urethra at the level of the bulbous urethra just distal to the external urethral sphincter (or membranous urethra) as seen in **Figure 2.25**. The lumen at the membranous urethra is delineated by the arrow. As can be seen, the membranous urethra forms a sphincteric appearance. In the female, the urethra is on average 30 mm in length and the evaluation using a cystoscope is more difficult. The most common pathology visualized in a female urethra is a urethral diverticulum. This is seen in **Figure 2.26**. The diverticular neck in this patient is wide mouthed and the lining of the diverticulum is easily seen.

Nonneoplastic Lesions Seen on Cystoscopy

Figure 2.27 shows a patient with a neurogenic bladder (bladder function affected by a neurologic lesion, which in this case is from multiple sclerosis). There are the typical prominent detrusor fascicles that would be called *trabeculations*. The pseudodiverticula formed by the trabeculations are called *cellules*. These cellules are not true diverticula, because they are still lined with all layers of the bladder including urothelium, muscularis propria, and serosa, whereas true diverticula would have only urothelium and serosa.

Various foreign bodies can be detected during cystoscopy. **Figure 2.28** shows a small stone in the bladder. **Figure 2.29** shows a four-panel composite of a much larger bladder stone. This bladder stone has been "chipped away" with cystoscopic guided laser lithotripsy as shown in the lower right panel. **Figure 2.30** shows an encrusted blue (polypropylene) suture in the upper lateral wall of the bladder. This suture was from a suburethral sling placement. It is probable that the suture was passed into the bladder during the sling surgery and was not detected at the primary surgery.

Different inflammatory lesions can be seen. **Figure 2.31** shows the typical appearance of bullous edema. The most typical cause of bullous edema is from chronic presence of a foreign body such as a Foley catheter or a double-J ureteral stent. **Figure 2.32** shows the appearance of cystitis glandularis. Diffuse inflammatory changes in the bladder are seen in **Figures 2.33** and **2.34**. The cause of diffuse inflammation cannot be always determined. As a general rule, the most common cause of diffuse bladder inflammation would be bacterial cystitis, but this would not be the most common cause of inflammation seen cystoscopically because the presence of bacterial infection is a contraindication to performing cystoscopy. Nonspecific focal areas of chronic inflammation are shown in **Figure 2.35**. Biopsies of these areas showed vascular congestion and chronic inflammatory changes (with lymphocytes). These focal areas of chronic inflammation can cause severe bladder symptoms including dysuria, stranguria, urinary urgency, and frequency. Treatment of these focal inflammatory lesions is laser fulguration as shown in the right panel of **Figure 2.35**. The laser used is a YAG (yttrium aluminium garnet) beam that, when used with the typical laser probe, leaves small rounded pitted areas after obliteration of the lesion. After laser fulguration, patients improve quickly, but these inflammatory lesions will reoccur (along with symptoms). The pathophysiology of these focal inflammatory lesions is unknown.

Colovesical fistula, most commonly secondary to colonic diverticular disease, can also be seen **(Figure 2.36a)**. Around the fistulous tract, there is edema and inflammation. The classic symptom of pneumaturia is present. **Figure 2.36b** shows the colovesical fistulous tract excised.

One of the purported diagnostic procedures for interstitial cystitis is bladder hydrodistention under anesthesia. Appearance of glomerulations or micropetechiae, seen in the urothelium immediately after release of intravesical fluid, is supposedly pathognomonic for interstitial cystitis. **Figure 37**, top left panel, shows a bladder maximally distended under anesthesia with appearance of capillary interruptions and smooth muscle. In the other three panels, the glomerulations are seen throughout the bladder.

Figure 2.38 shows a typical lesion of schistosomiasis (reddened lesion). A normal right ureteral orifice is seen in the bottom left panel. **Figure 2.39** shows a wire placed into a vesicovaginal fistulous tract with the other end of the wire coming through the anterior/apical vaginal wall. There is surrounding bullous edema around the fistulous tract. In the United States, the most common cause of a vesicovaginal fistula is iatrogenic secondary to hysterectomy. In **Figure 2.40**, this patient has a vesicouterine fistula with a wire in the tract (the other end of the wire comes out of the uterine cervix). The cause of this fistula was due to obstetrical Caesarean section). **Figure 2.41** shows a vesicovaginal fistula (arrows in the two panels on the left and wire through fistulous tract in rightmost panel) in the right wall of the bladder posterior to the right ureteral orifice (yellow ureteral catheter entering the orifice). The cause of this fistula was an overly aggressive bladder tumor resection at the right posterior wall that perforated into the vagina. This is an uncommon cause.

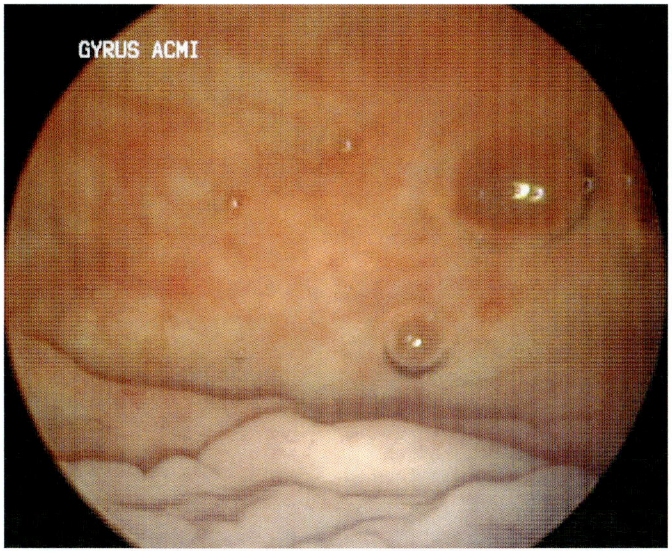

Figure 2.1 — Normal urinary bladder displaying air bubble in most independent portion of the bladder (anterior wall).

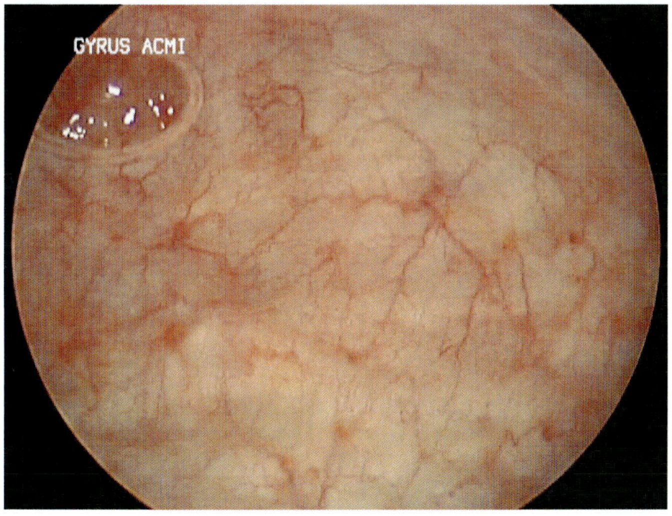

Figure 2.2 — Normal bladder, another view.

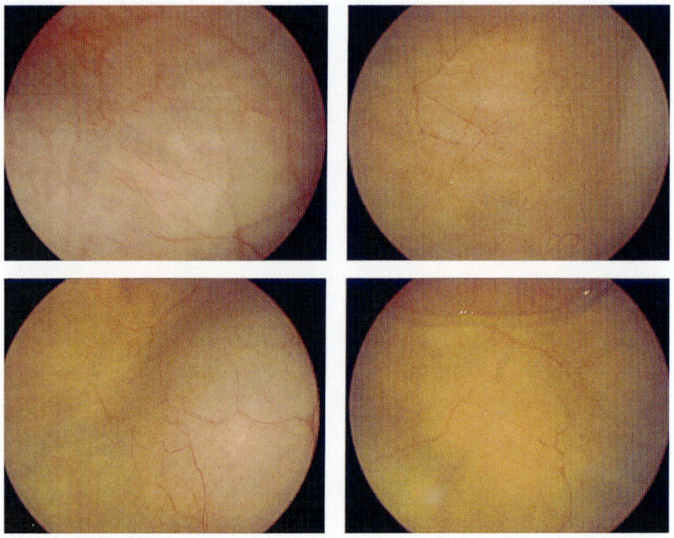

Figure 2.3 — Normal bladder in four different sections.

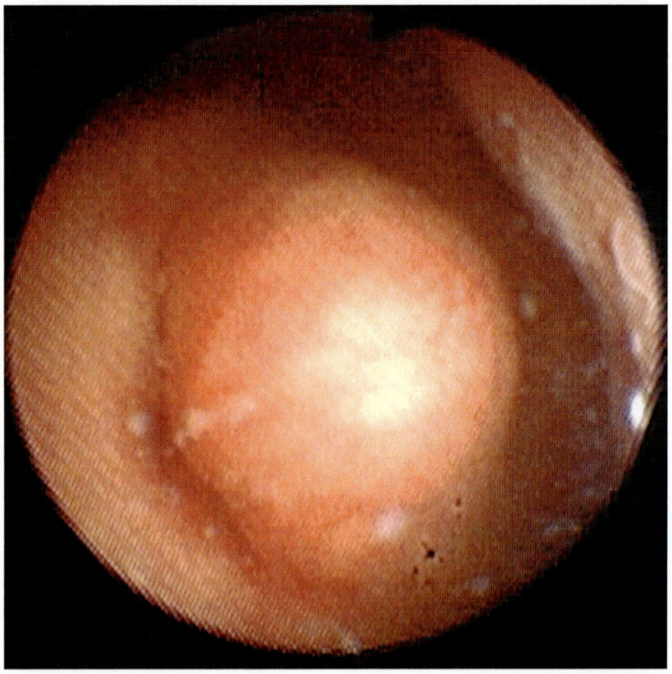

Figure 2.4 — Median lobe of prostate seen on retroflexion of a flexible cystoscope.

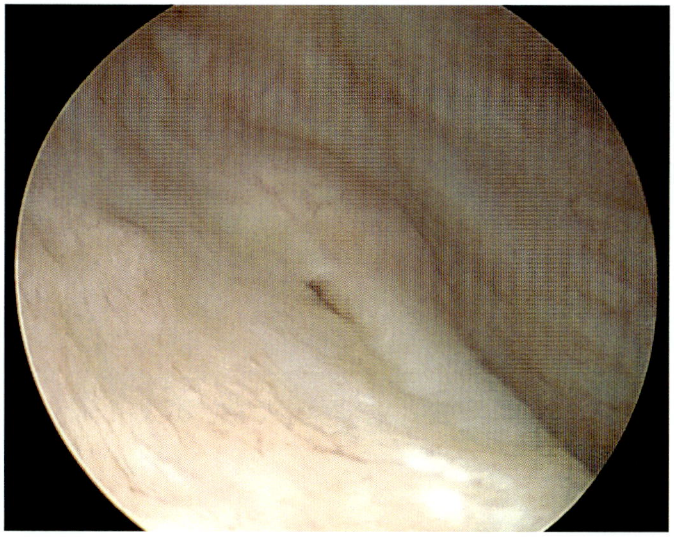

Figure 2.5 — Right ureteral orifice. This is one typical ureteral meatal appearance. By placing a ureteroscope through this orifice, one can visually image the upper urinary tract.

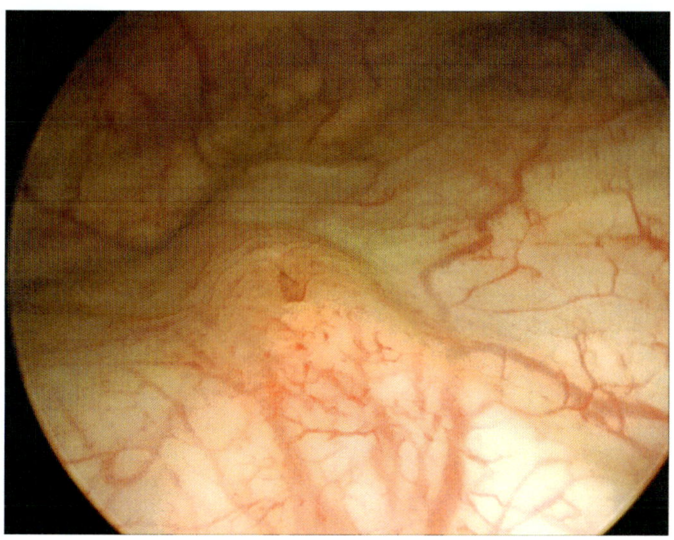

Figure 2.6 — Right ureteral orifice with normal urothelial folds at ureteral meatus. Sometimes these periureteral folds can be difficult to distinguish from a papillary urothelial carcinoma especially if the folds are prominent and results in a heaped appearance.

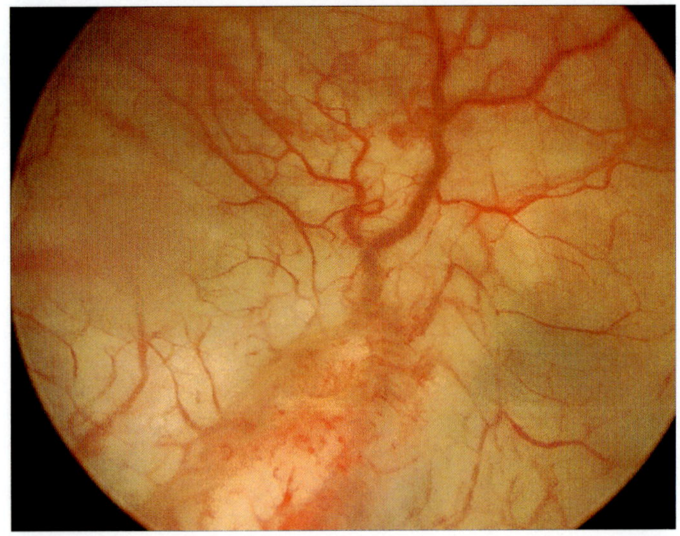

Figure 2.7 — Left ureteral orifice. The trigonal ridge is the raised ridge of bladder going down away from the left ureteral orifice.

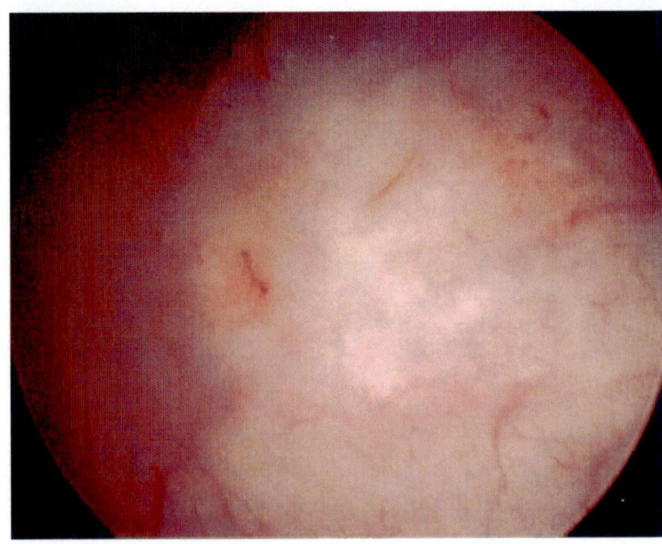

Figure 2.8 — Complete duplication of the upper urinary tract (two ureteral orifices on one side).

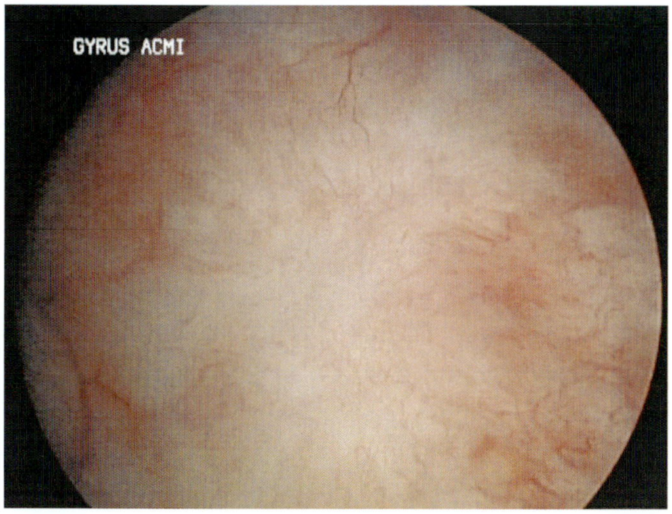

Figure 2.9 — Scar from a previous bladder biopsy (stellate scar).

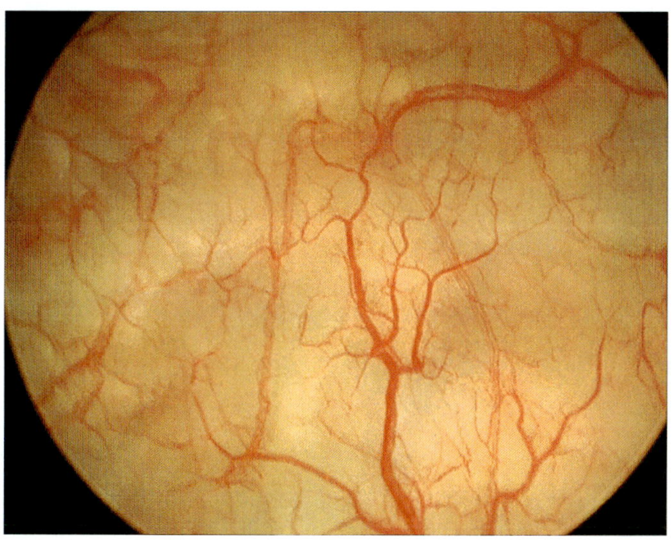

Figure 2.10 — Capillary network in suburothelium.

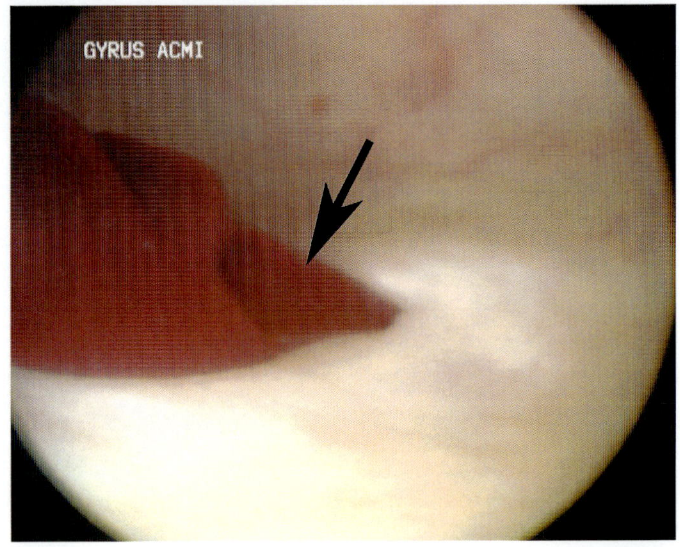

Figure 2.11 — Blood streaming from the left ureteral orifice (indicated by arrow), indicative of upper urinary tract bleeding.

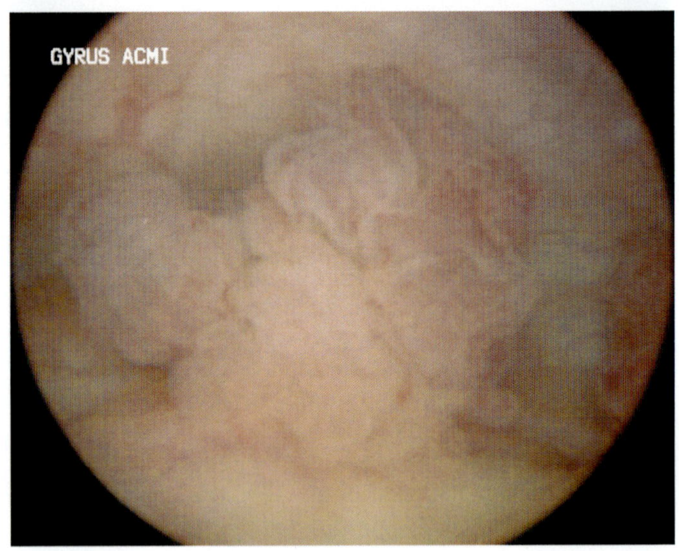

Figure 2.12 — Papillary urothelial tumor.

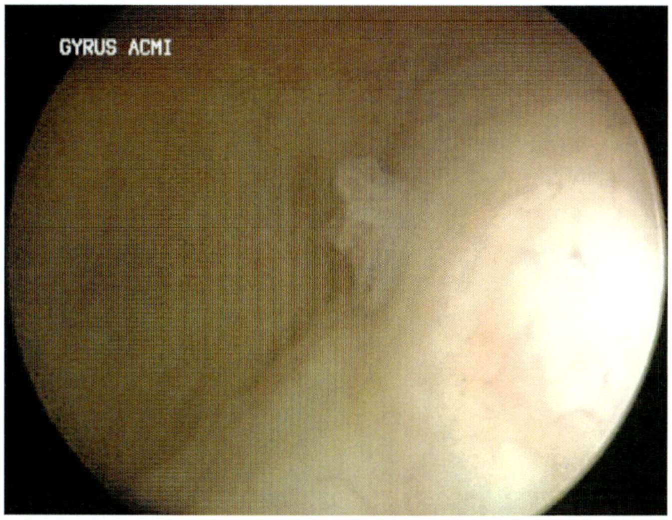

Figure 2.13 — Small papillary urothelial tumor.

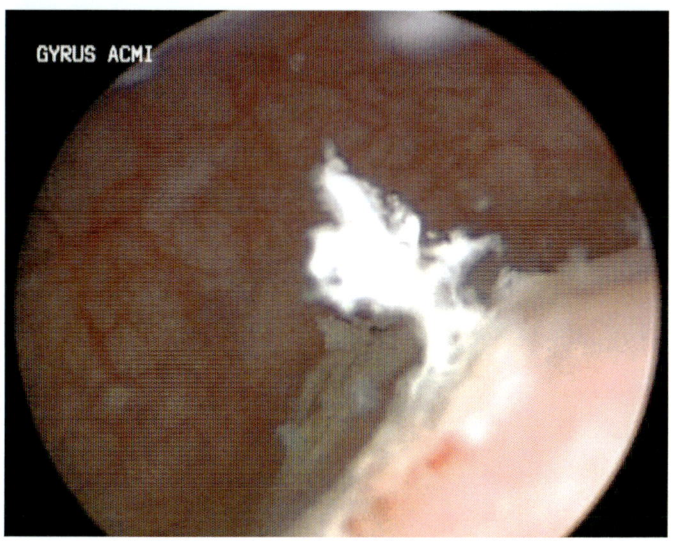

Figure 2.14 — Small papillary urothelial tumor after cold-cup (forceps) biopsy.

Figure 2.15 — Papillary urothelial tumor.

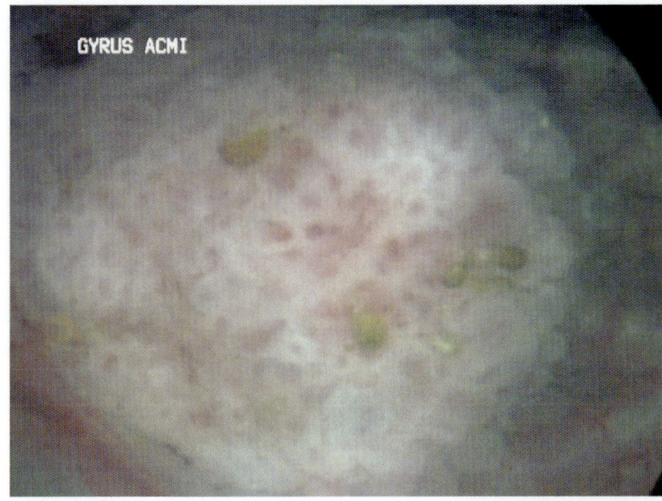

Figure 2.16 — Large patch of velvety papillary frondular area with sharp demarcation at normal urothelium (on the right side).

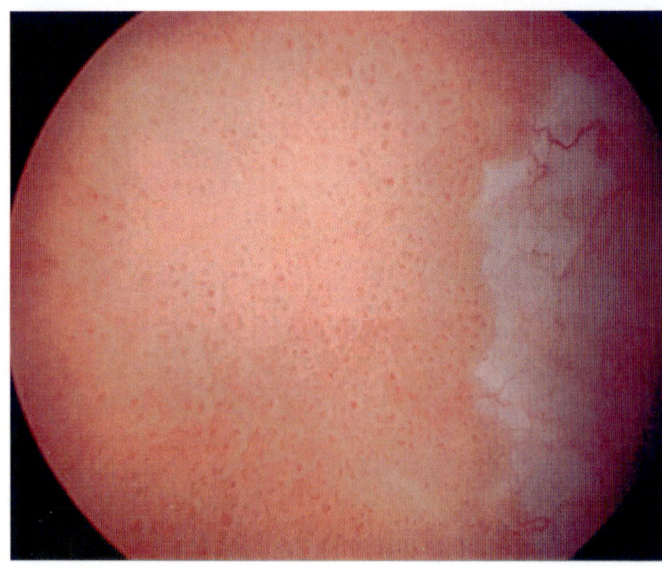

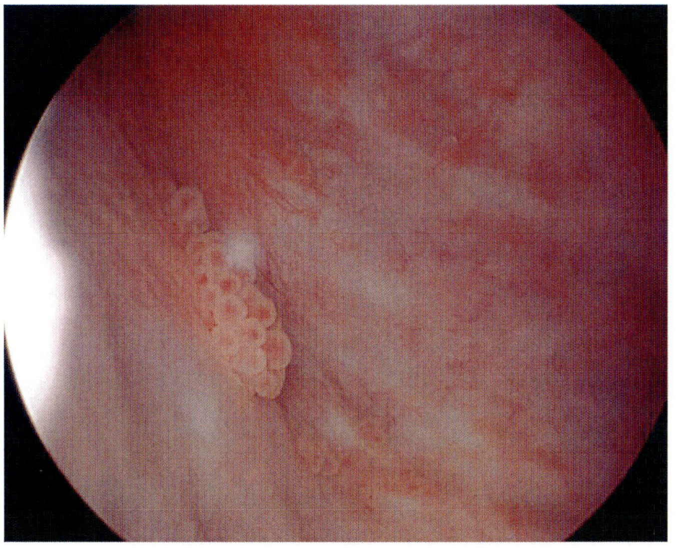

Figure 2.17 — Patch of papillary frondular area over right lateral wall of bladder.

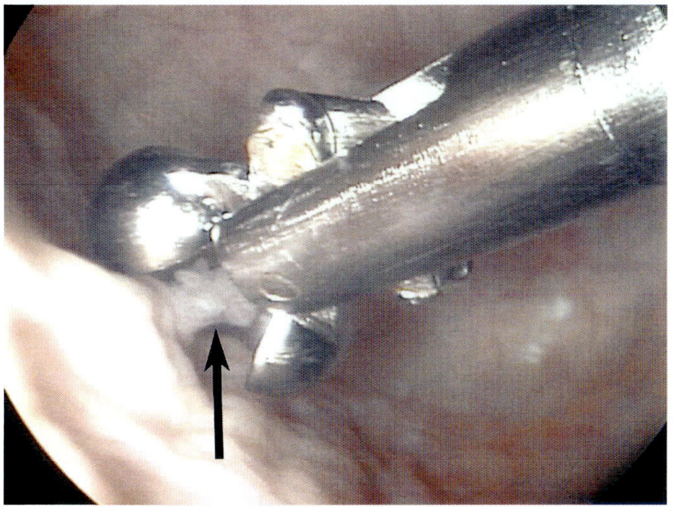

Figure 2.18 — Small papillary urothelial tumor (arrow) about to be biopsied with cold-cup biopsy forceps.

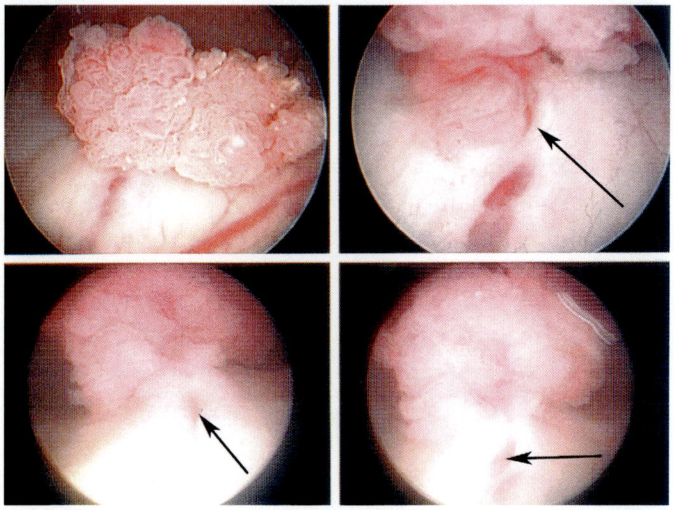

Figure 2.19 — Four panels from the same bladder. Top left—papillary urothelial tumor that covers left ureteral orifice. Top right—when cystoscopic irrigation is turned on, the papillary tumor is turned upwards and the left ureteral orifice is uncovered (arrow). Bottom left and bottom right—more images of papillary tumor reflected upwards exposing left ureteral orifices (arrows point out left ureteral orifice).

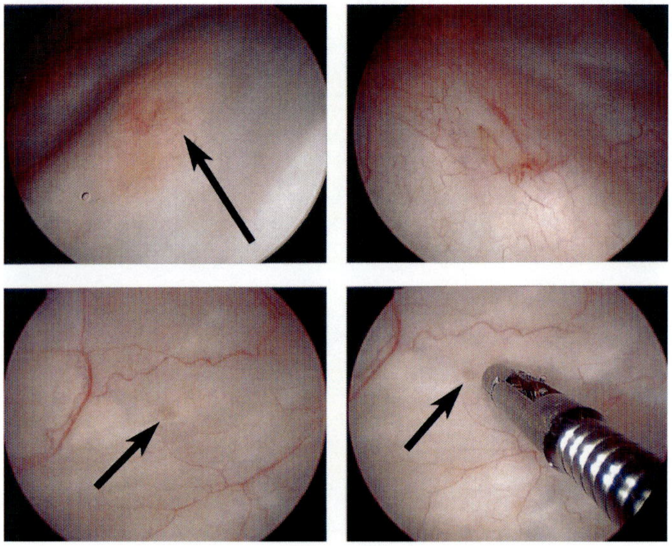

Figure 2.20 — Four panels from the same bladder. Top left—velvety patch over left ureteral orifice (arrow). Top right—right ureteral orifice which is different in appearance to left ureteral orifice. Bottom left—minute papillary tumor (arrow). Bottom right—cold-cup biopsy forceps next to the tumor.

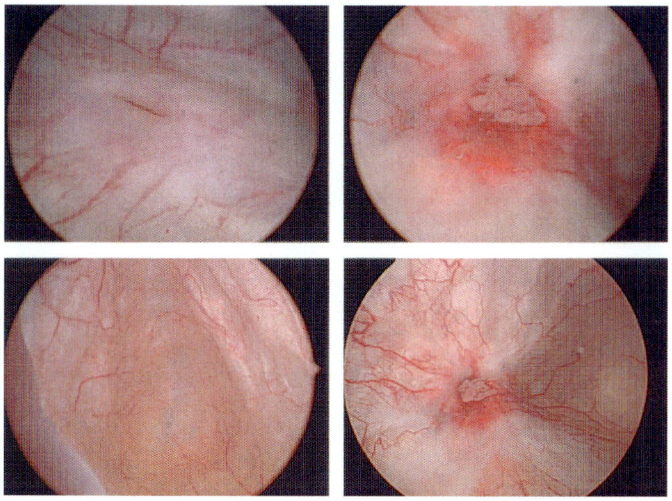

Figure 2.21 — Four panels from the same bladder. Top left—normal right ureteral orifice. Top right—papillary urothelial tumor in distal left ureter exiting left ureteral orifice. Bottom left—normal area of bladder. Bottom right—further view of the neoplasm exiting left ureteral orifice.

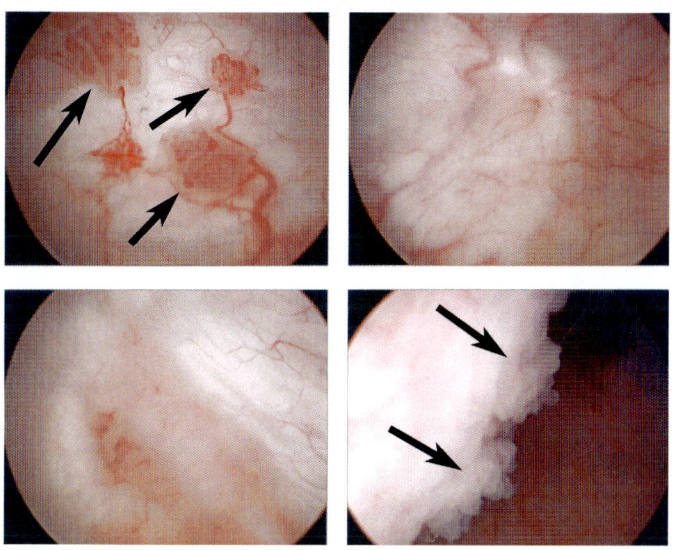

Figure 2.22 — Four panels from the same bladder. Top left—multiple papillary tumors (arrows). Top right—normal left ureteral orifice. Bottom left—normal right ureteral orifice. Bottom right—papillary tumor at left bladder neck (arrows).

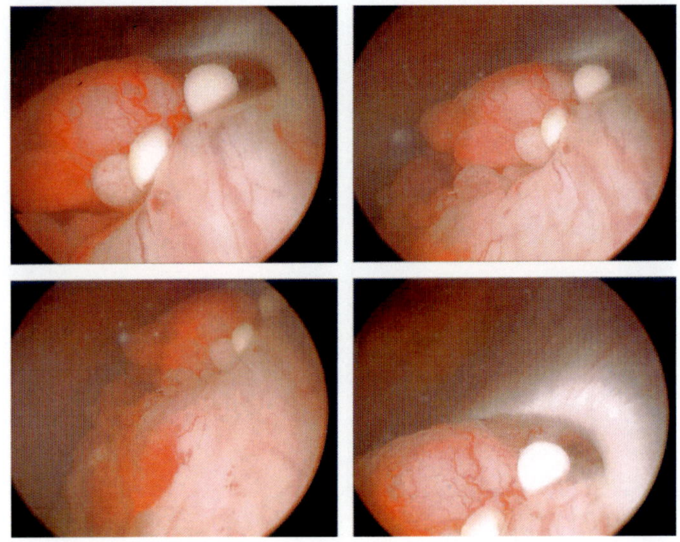

Figure 2.23 — Four panels from the same bladder. All panels show a smooth walled tumor emanating from Hutch bladder diverticulum (paraureteric diverticulum). This tumor turned out to be a primary small-cell carcinoma of the bladder.

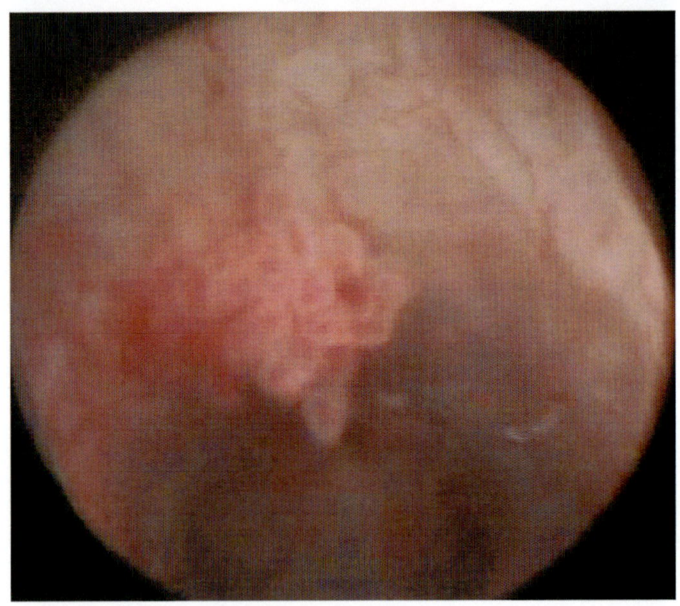

Figure 2.24a — Papillary tumor within male urethral lumen.

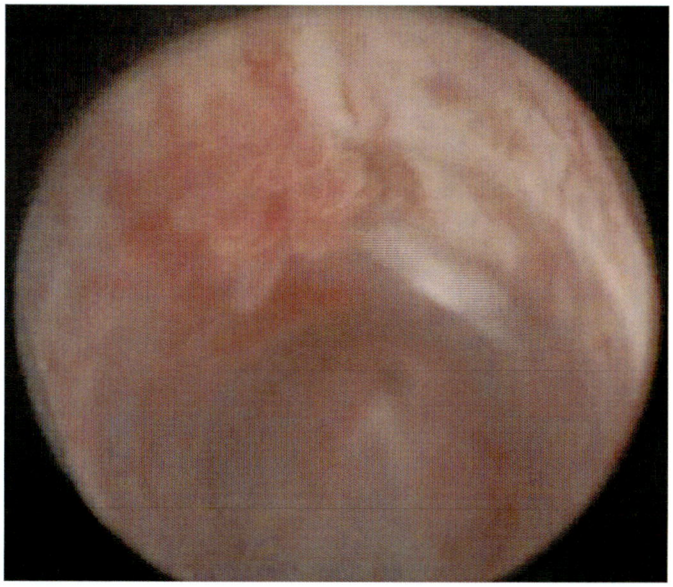

Figure 2.24b — Another view of the urethral papillary tumor showing the opening to the bulbomembranous urethra in the background (more proximal).

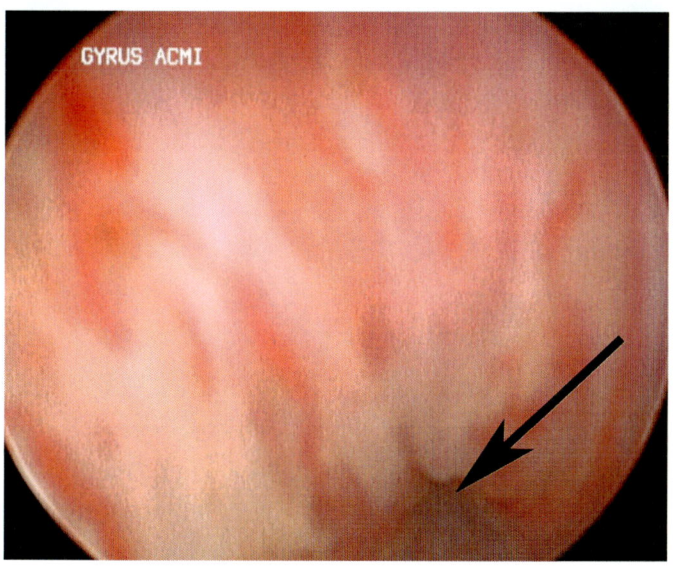

Figure 2.25 — Opening to the bulbomembranous urethra (arrow) in a male urethra.

Figure 2.26 — Urethral diverticulum (arrows) in a female urethra.

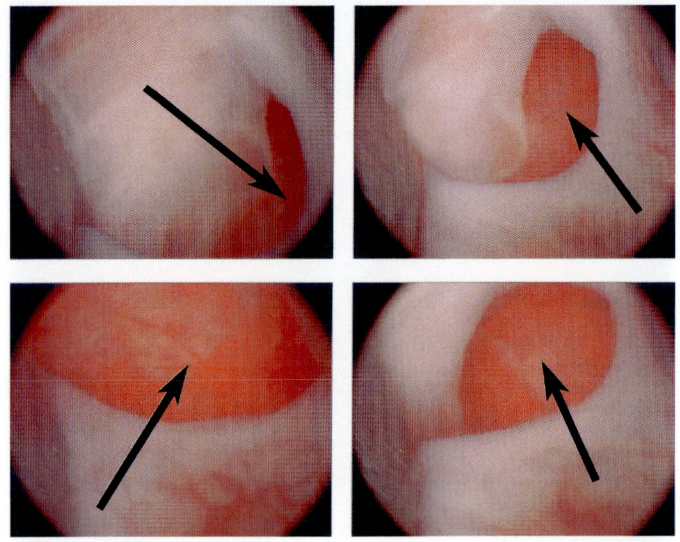

Figure 2.27 — Trabeculated bladder in a patient with neurogenic bladder (compare to Figures 2.1–2.3).

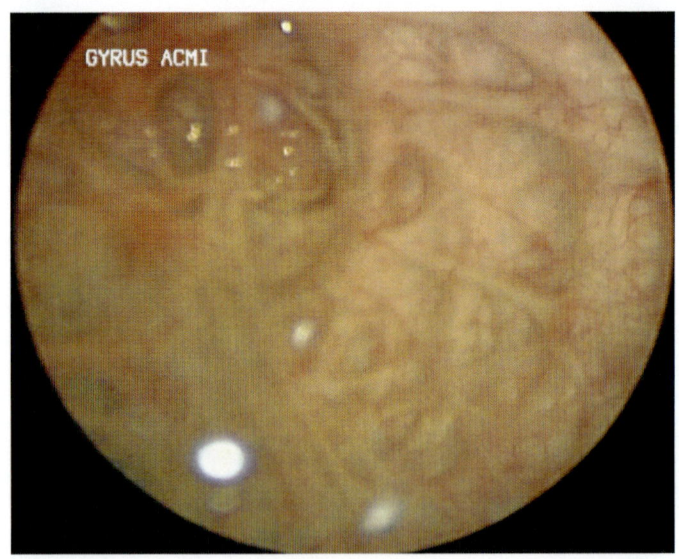

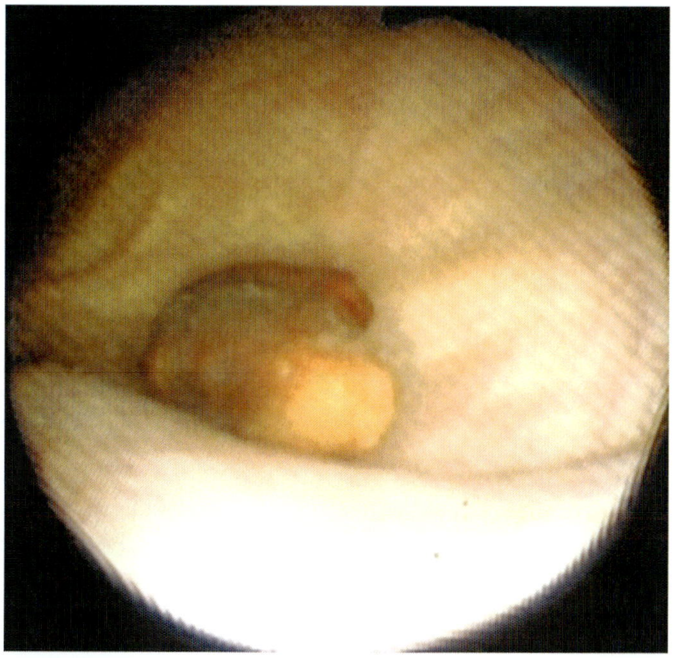

Figure 2.28 — Foreign body (stone) in the bladder.

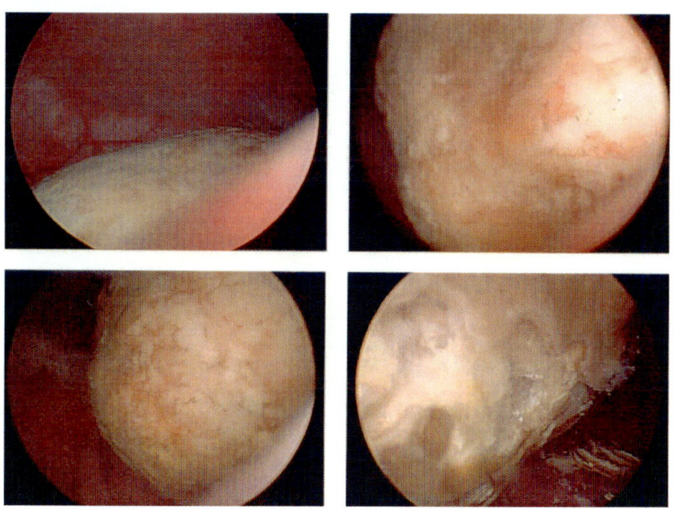

Figure 2.29 — Larger stone in the bladder, lower right panel shows several "divots" in stone from laser fragmentation.

Figure 2.30 — Suture material in the bladder with stone encrustation; suture was from a suburethral sling surgery performed for stress urinary incontinence.

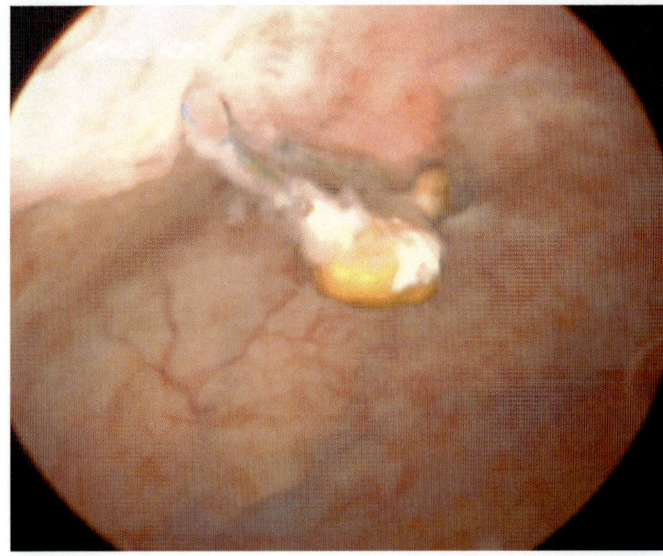

Figure 2.31 — Bullous edema of the bladder.

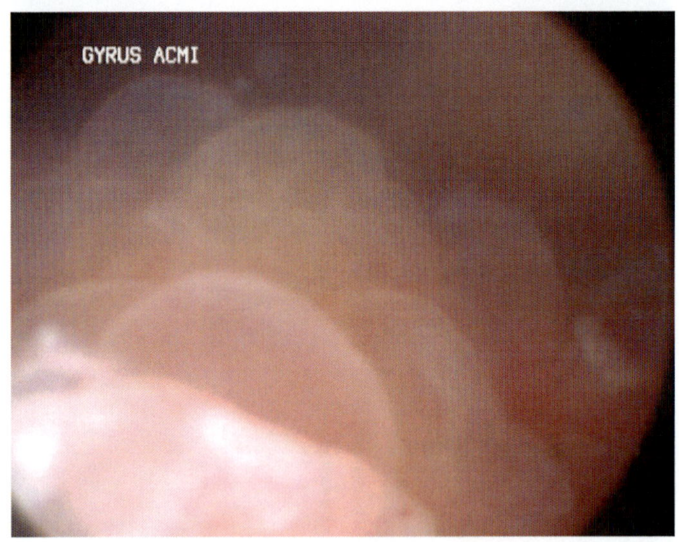

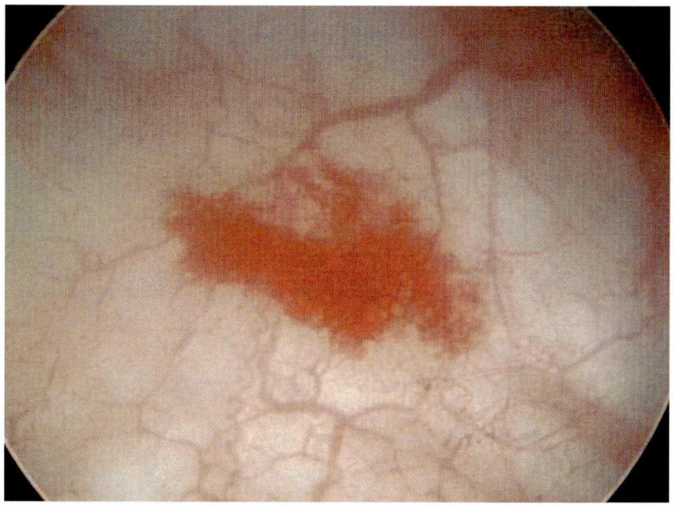

Figure 2.32 — Cystitis glandularis of the bladder.

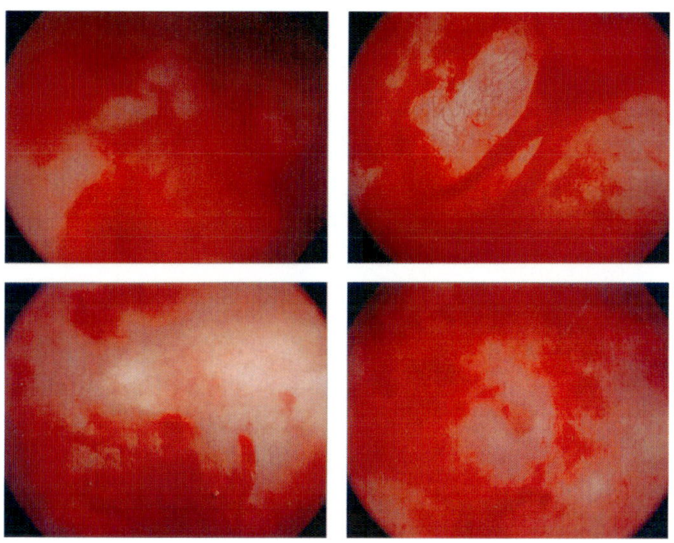

Figure 2.33 — Chronic cystitis with friable urothelium and bleeding.

Figure 2.34 — Four panels from the same bladder. Arrows depict areas of focal inflammatory changes with hyperemia.

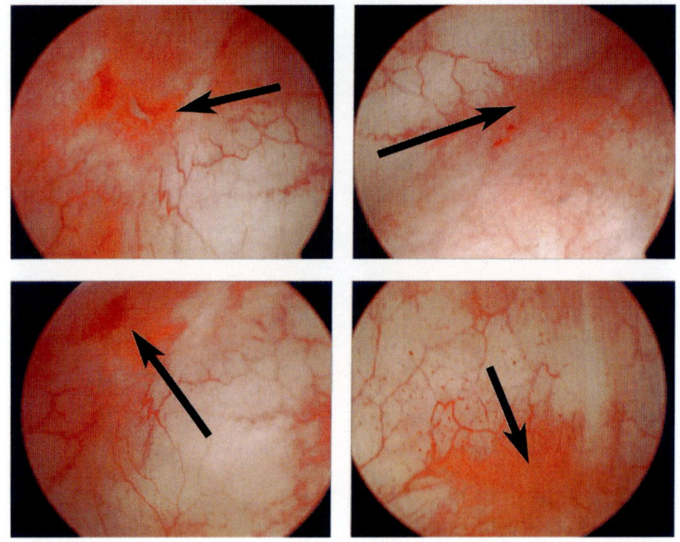

Figure 2.35 — Two panels from the same bladder. Left panel shows focal area of inflammation and hyperemia, right panel shows same area after YAG-laser fulguration. These lesions typically cause bladder pain and increased voiding frequency.

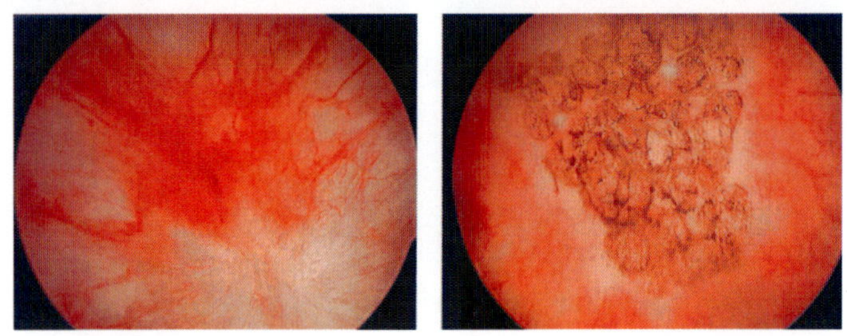

Figure 2.36a — Colovesical fistula seen cystoscopically with surrounding inflammation.

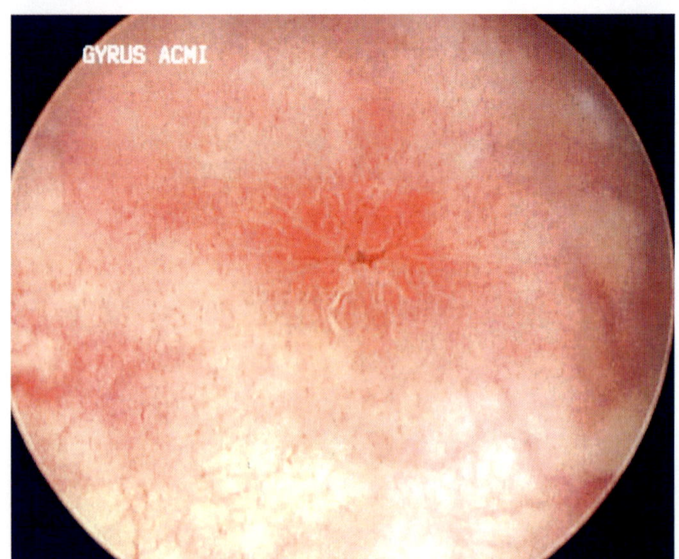

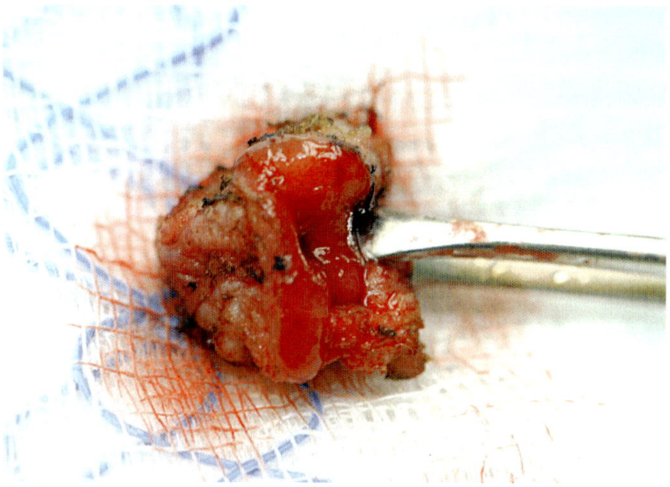

Figure 2.36b — Same colovesical fistula seen grossly after open excision.

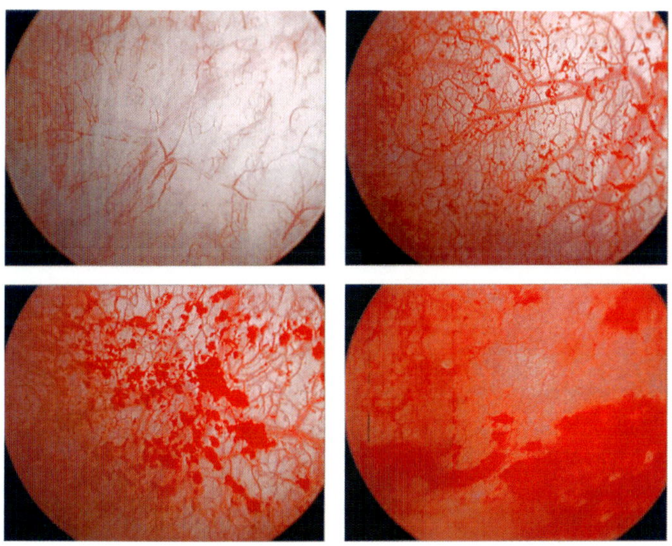

Figure 2.37 — Four panels from the same bladder. Top left shows a maximally distended bladder (pressure limited to 80 cm water) of a patient under general anesthesia (there is 900 cc of fluid in the bladder in this image). Note the appearance of detrusor muscle bundles (appears as crisscrossing fibrils) in this image. The rest of the panels are images in different areas of the bladder during the release of the 900 cc of fluid showing appearance of pinpoint petechial hemorrhages (glomerulations). The findings of glomerulations are thought by some to be indicative of interstitial cystitis, although this remains controversial.

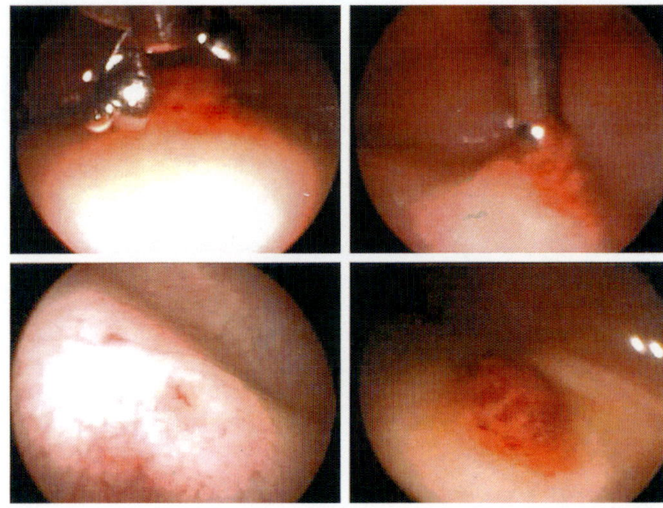

Figure 2.38 — Four panels from the same bladder. This patient had schistosomiasis. The top left, top right, and bottom right panels show the appearance of schistosomal bladder infection from egg deposits (reddened area). The bottom left panel shows a normal right ureteral orifice.

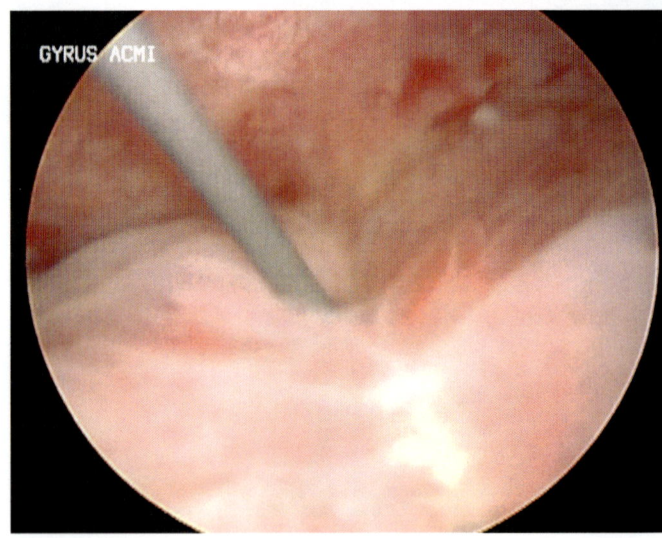

Figure 2.39 — A vesicovaginal fistula (after hysterectomy) seen in the floor of the bladder with a wire traversing the fistula. Note the surrounding inflammation and edema. The other end of the wire exits out of the vaginal introitus.

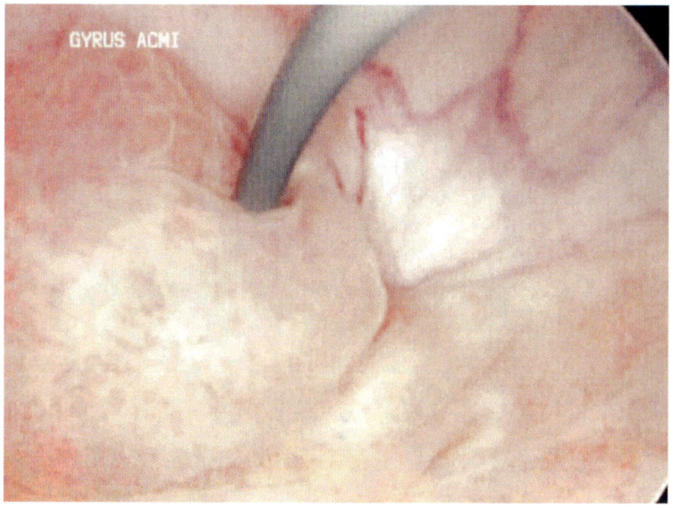

Figure 2.40 — A vesicouterine fistula (after Caesarean section delivery) seen in posterior wall of the bladder. A wire is traversing the fistula (with surrounding inflammation and edema) with the other end exiting the cervical os and then the vaginal introitus.

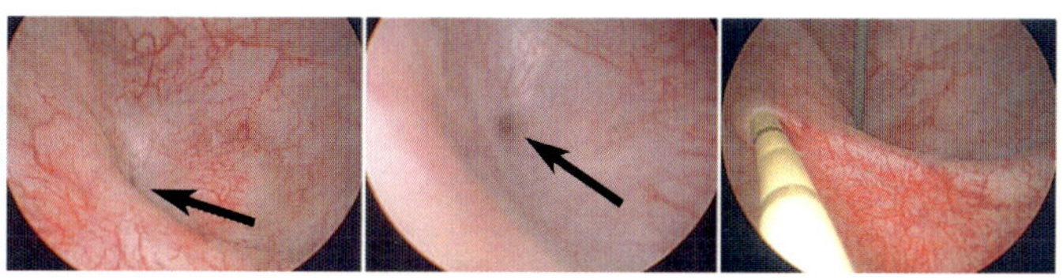

Figure 2.41 — A vesicovaginal fistula (after a transurethral resection of a bladder tumor). The two panels on the left show the fistulous tract (arrows). The rightmost panel shows the position of the fistula relative to the right ureteral orifice (which has been cannulated with a yellow 5-French ureteral catheter).

3

Nonneoplastic Lesions—Reactive Conditions

- Acute and Chronic Cystitis, Follicular Cystitis, Interstitial Cystitis
- Von Brunn's Nests
- Cystitis Cystica
- Nephrogenic Adenoma
- Granulomatous Cystitis
- Ileal Loop (Neobladder) Urine
- Amyloidosis of the Bladder
- Xanthogranulomatous Pyelonephritis

Figure 3.1 — Inflammation of bladder, histologic section. Intense inflammation of the submucosa and urothelium is seen. The inflammatory infiltrate is mixed with lymphocytes, plasma cells, eosinophils, and neutrophils. Some neutrophils are seen within the urothelium. The urothelial cells appear reactive with slight enlargement of the nucleus and prominent nucleoli. The nuclei are vesicular with smooth nuclear membranes. This type of inflammation can be seen in many conditions and is considered nonspecific. There may be increased mitotic rate (H&E stain, medium power).

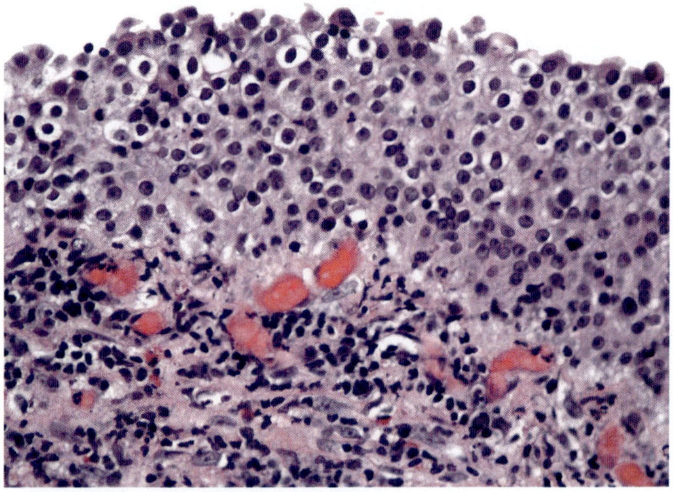

Figure 3.2 — Inflammation of bladder, histologic section. In chronic cystitis, the inflammatory infiltrates are mostly chronic with reactive nuclear changes. Presence of bladder calculi, indwelling catheters, other instrumentation, infections, bladder tumors, and so forth all predispose to chronic irritation of the bladder mucosa. The cytoplasm is slightly darker. With persistent or repeated inflammation, the lamina propria becomes fibrotic (H&E stain, medium power).

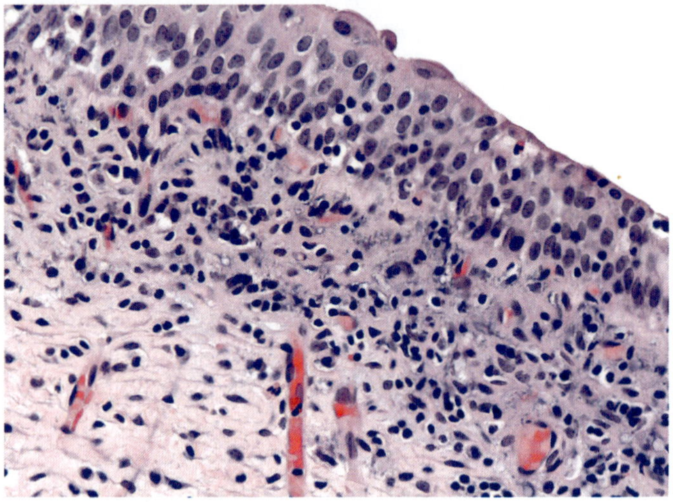

Figure 3.3 — Inflammation of bladder, histologic section. Inflammation of the bladder can frequently lead to denudation of the surface urothelium, with only a single layer of basal cells remaining. In this image, there is predominantly an eosinophilic infiltrate with surface denudation, and epithelial cells are seen within the von Brunn's nest. Predominantly eosinophilic infiltrates are seen in people with systemic allergies, with parasitic infections, (Schistosomiasis), or in response to adjacent malignancy; sometimes no specific cause can be elucidated (H&E stain, low power).

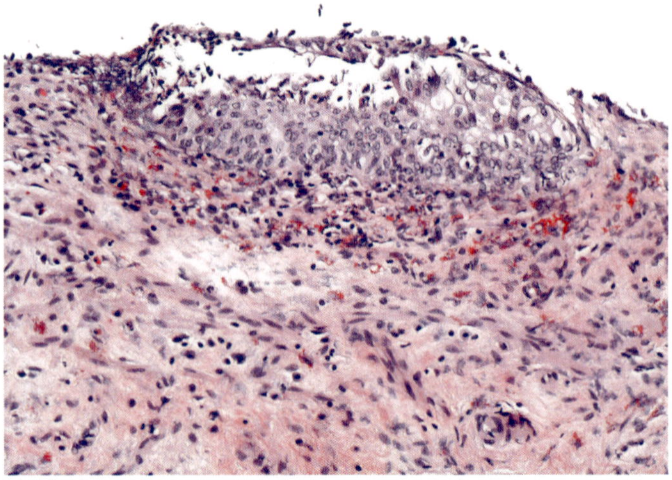

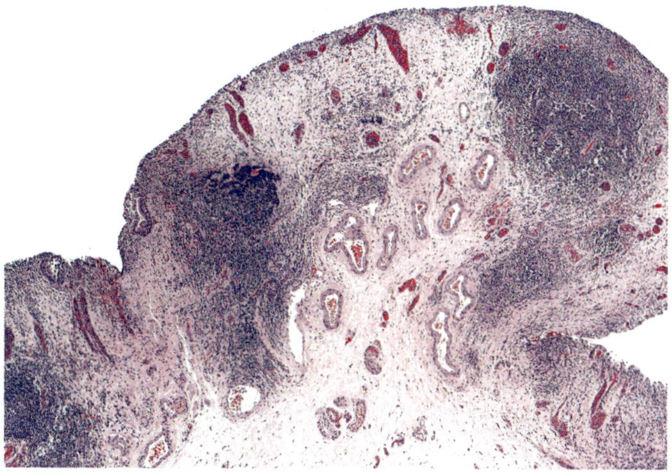

Figure 3.4 — Follicular cystitis, histologic section. This is a form of intense chronic inflammation of the bladder, where lymphoid follicles form in the lamina propria. Causes of follicular cystitis most commonly include viral infection in children and BCG treatment for superficial bladder cancer in adults. The lamina propria becomes fibrotic and the surface urothelium may be denuded (H&E stain, low power).

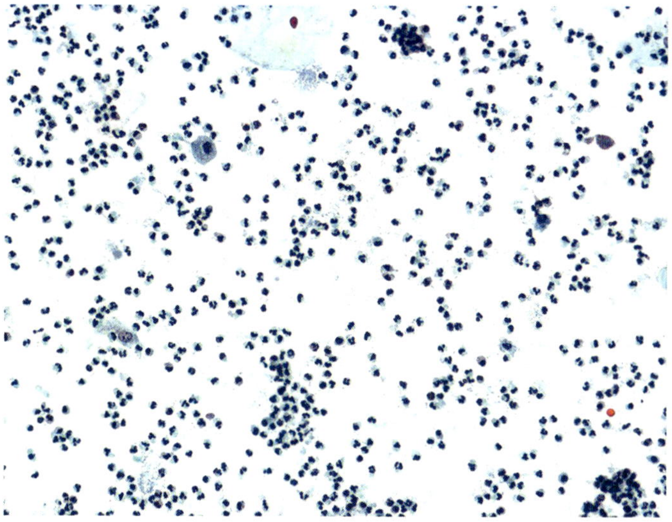

Figure 3.5 — Acute cystitis, voided urine. A sample from acute cystitis will predominantly include neutrophils with occasional macrophages and urothelial and squamous cells. Bacteria can frequently be found in the background, and while they may be the offending organism, they could simply be contamination of the sample. Preparing a culture is essential for identification of the infectious organism (Papanicolaou stain, low power).

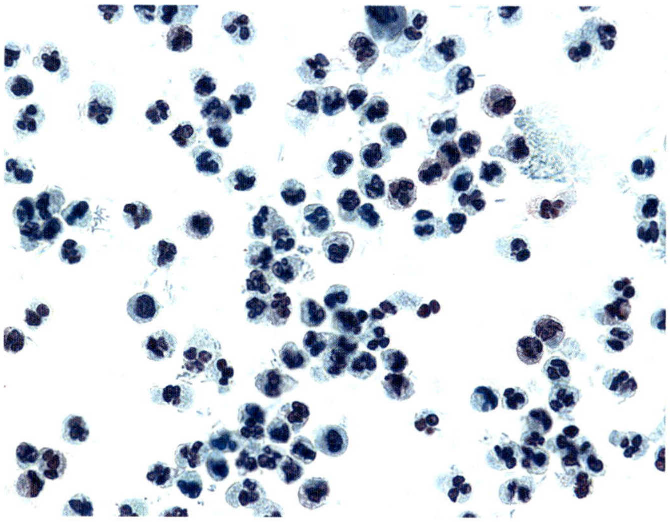

Figure 3.6 — Acute cystitis, voided urine. High-power image of the sample displays not only the abundant neutrophils, but occasional lymphocytes and numerous bacteria, short rods, probably E-coli. Here again, preparing a culture is necessary for proper identification (Papanicolaou stain, high power).

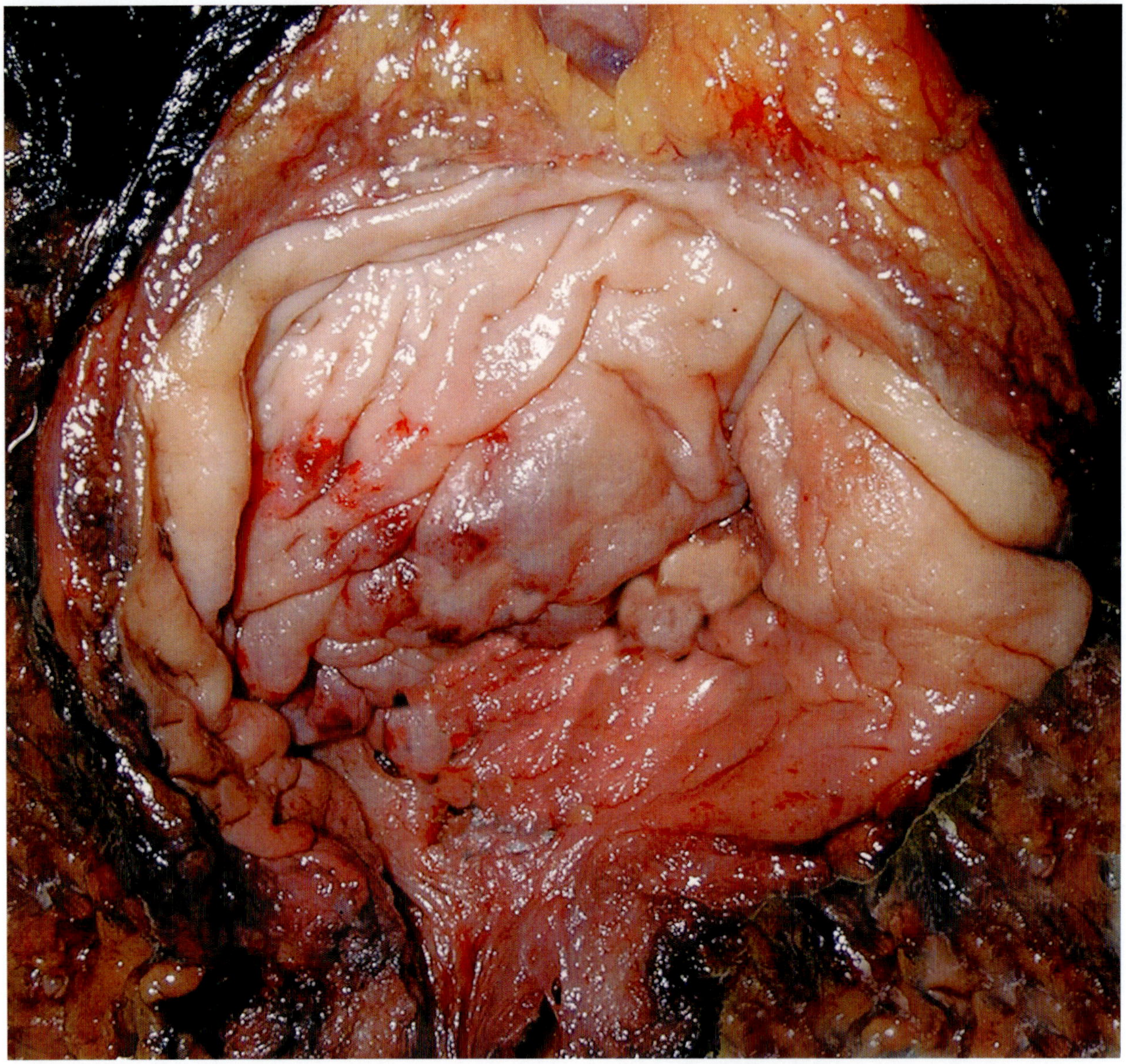

Figure 3.7 — Interstitial cystitis, gross image of urinary bladder, cystectomy specimen. Interstitial cystitis is a special form of cystitis that more commonly afflicts females. The patients suffer from frequency, dysuria, and suprapubic pain on filling of the bladder. Multiple urine cultures are typically negative. Submucosal hemorrhages are evident. The urothelium is benign. Eventually the bladder becomes contracted with fibrosis of the muscle layer. Due to the severity and relentless nature of the symptoms for some patients, cystectomy may be undertaken.

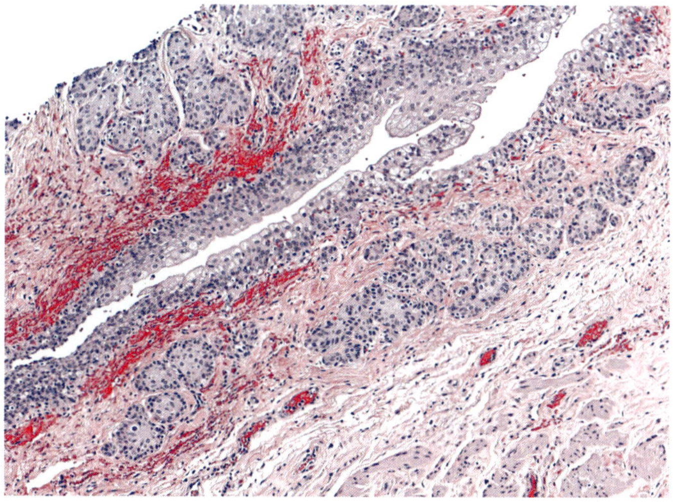

Figure 3.8 — Von Brunn's nests, histologic section. Invagination of the benign urothelium into the lamina propria can give rise to nests of urothelium within the lamina propria, which sometimes lose their connection to the surface urothelium. This is a common finding and is believed to occur secondary to a local inflammatory insult, recent or in the past, or it could be a normal morphologic variant. This image is from the renal pelvis and shows florid proliferation of von Brunn's nests, a process which mimics the nested variant of a urothelial carcinoma. Some of the features to look for are the nests composed of similar appearing cells as the surface, having a flat noninfiltrative base or lobular appearance (H&E stain, low power).

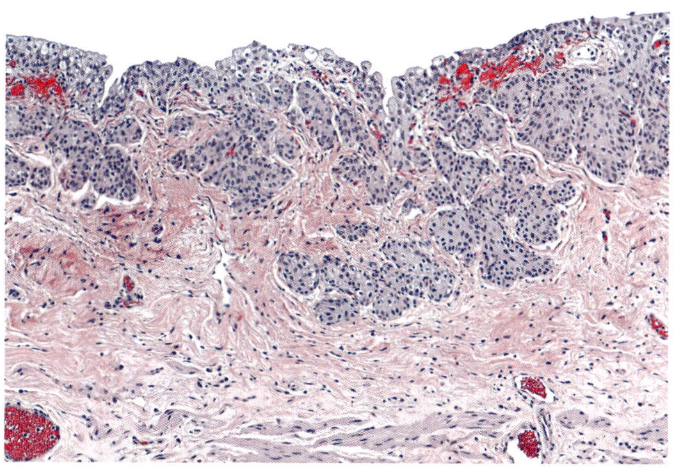

Figure 3.9 — Florid proliferation of von Brunn's nests, histologic section. A mimic of the nested variant of a urothelial carcinoma, when seen in a larger resection specimen, the lobular nature of the proliferating nests and a noninfiltrative base helps in coming to the right diagnosis. This image of the ureter shows the von Brunn's nests closely associated with the surface urothelium (H&E stain, low power).

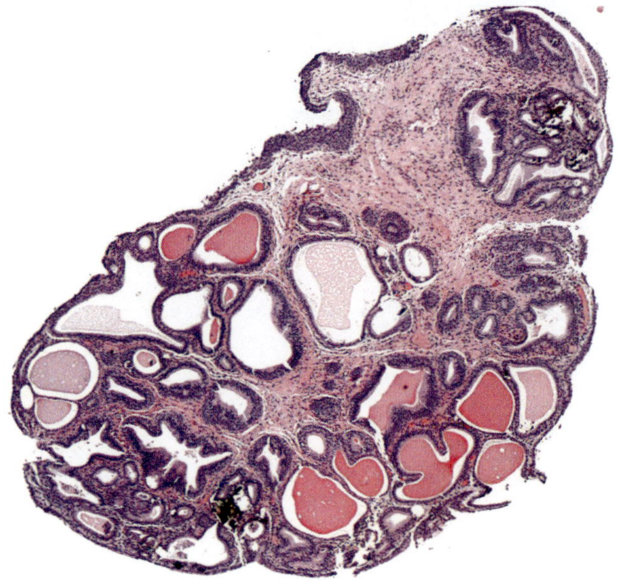

Figure 3.10 — Cystitis cystica et glandularis, histologic section. Benign bladder urothelium with cystic dilatation of von Brunn's nests, called cystitis cystica. Some cystic nests show acquisition of luminal cytoplasm; when that occurs, it is known as cystitis cystica et glandularis. Von Brunn's nests and cystitis cystica are benign conditions and are not known to undergo malignant transformation. These reactive conditions can occur secondary to a local insult, such as inflammation, urinary calculi, and so forth (H&E stain, very low power).

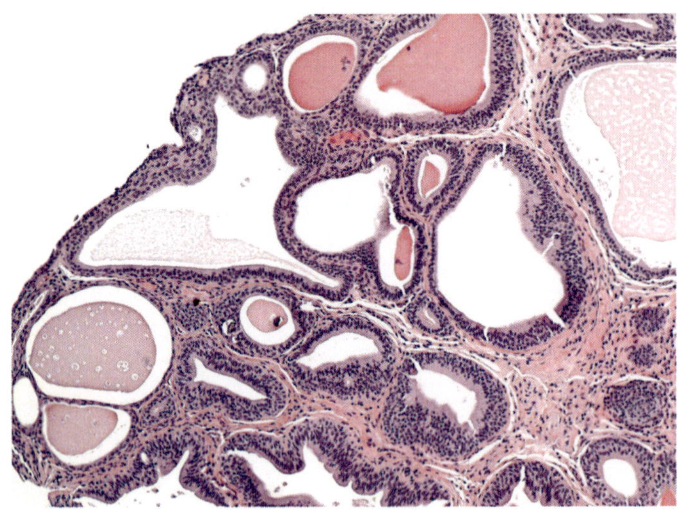

Figure 3.11 — Cystitis cystica et glandularis, histologic section. This image shows an example of cystitis cystica et glandularis nonintestinal type, with luminal acquisition of cytoplasm and appearance of glands. There is cystic dilatation of the spaces. There is no cytologic atypia present. This condition is frequently seen in normal bladders and is considered to have no neoplastic potential. It may be seen as a reactive response of the urothelium adjacent to a urothelial carcinoma secondary to injury caused by the malignant lesion rather than a precursor to such a lesion (H&E stain, low power).

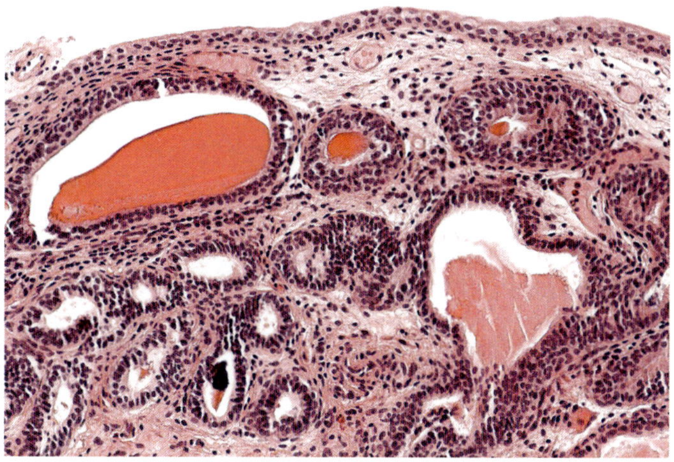

Figure 3.12 — Cystitis cystica, histologic section. Another example of cystitis cystica from the bladder is seen here. The surface urothelium appears benign, as do the cells lining the cystic spaces. Within some cystic spaces, the secretions have become inspissated and focally calcified (H&E stain, medium power).

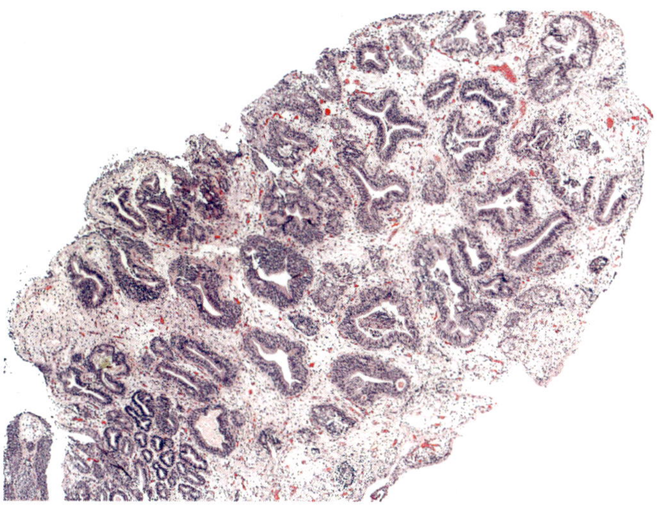

Figure 3.13 — Cystitis cystica (florid), histologic section. Benign bladder biopsy showing mildly inflamed lamina propria. The cystic nests display some infoldings, with some acquiring a cribriform appearance. There are oxalate crystals seen in the cystic spaces on the lower left side (H&E stain, very low power).

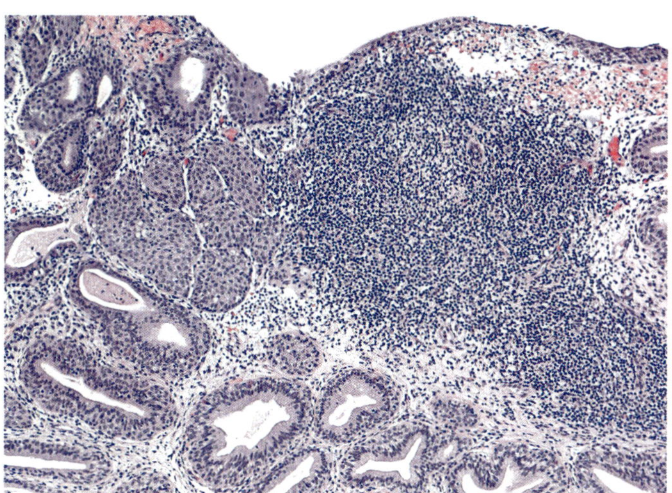

Figure 3.14 — Cystitis cystica et glandularis within an inflamed bladder, histologic section. This bladder biopsy shows benign urothelium with chronic inflammation and adjacent cystitis cystica et glandularis. Some von Brunn's nests without cystic spaces are also present (H&E stain, medium power).

Figure 3.15 — Cystitis cystica et glandularis with intestinal-type metaplasia, histologic section. This term is used when cystitis cystica acquires goblet cells. Lamina propria shows chronic lymphoplasmacytic inflammation. These goblet cells start to produce mucin. The presence of intestinal-type metaplasia is not associated with an increased risk of adenocarcinoma of the bladder, except in patients with bladder exstrophy (H&E stain, high power).

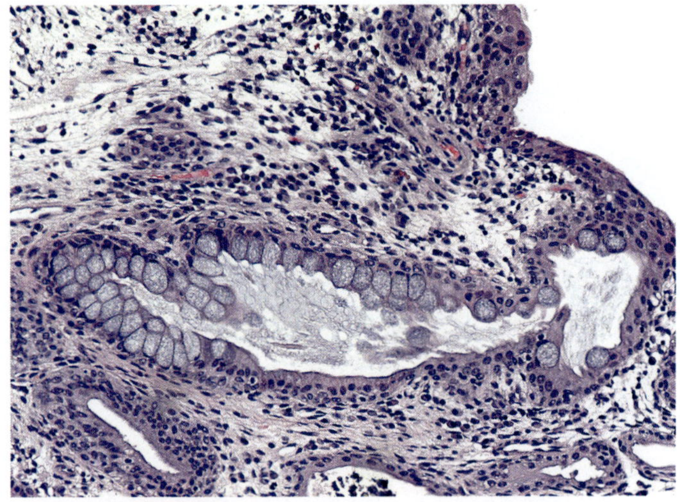

Figure 3.16 — Cystitis cystica et glandularis with florid intestinal-type metaplasia, histologic section. Cystitis cystica has completely become intestinal type, and extravasated mucin is visible on the top right-hand side of the image. In this case, no dysplasia is evident, which is often similar to dysplasia seen in the colonic adenomas. Additionally, this case had intestinal-type glands and mucin lakes adjacent to muscularis propria. Intestinal metaplasia can uncommonly be seen next to or within muscularis propria (detrusor muscle) without concerns of being malignant (H&E stain, medium power).

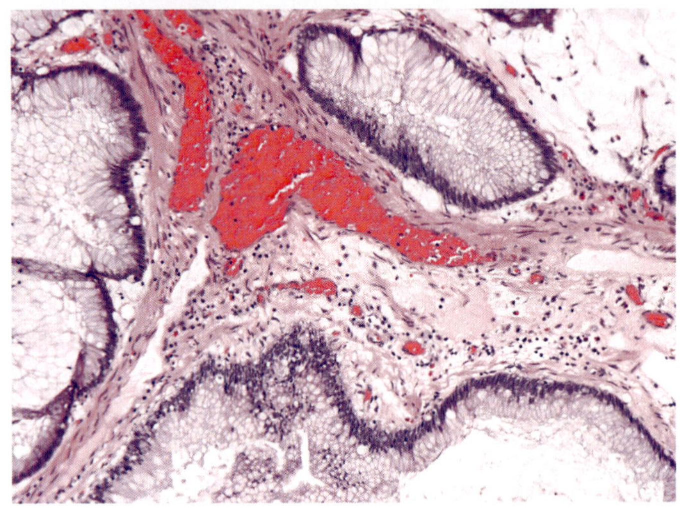

Figure 3.17 — Cystitis cystica, voided urine. Columnar cells in urine can originate in glandular rests in the dome of the bladder or the trigone or more commonly in the metaplasia of cystitis cystica et glandularis, a result of recurrent or continuous inflammation of the bladder. The usual characteristics of glandular epithelial cells may be seen, as well as reactive changes in them (Papanicolaou stain, medium power).

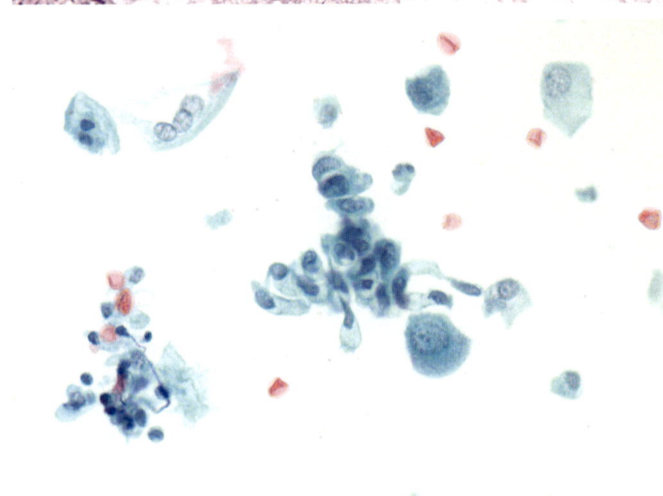

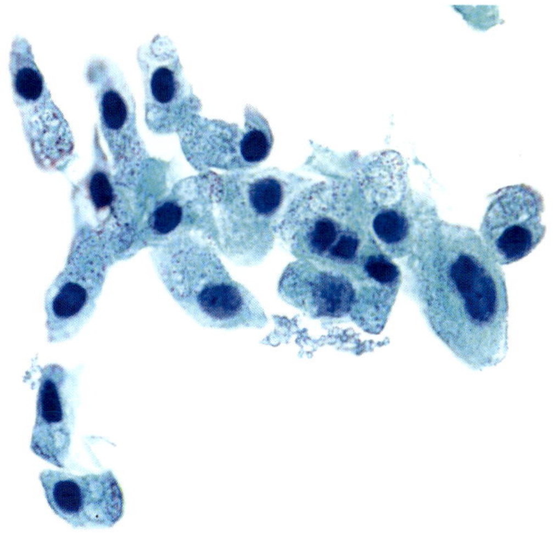

Figure 3.18 — Cystitis cystica, voided urine. Glandular cells from cystitis cystica are interpreted as benign using the same criteria as any other organ system. The nuclei are no larger than one-third of the total volume of the cytoplasm and are round and uniform in shape. Binucleation is to be expected in these replicating cells. Cytoplasm is delicate and usually vacuolated (Papanicolaou stain, high power).

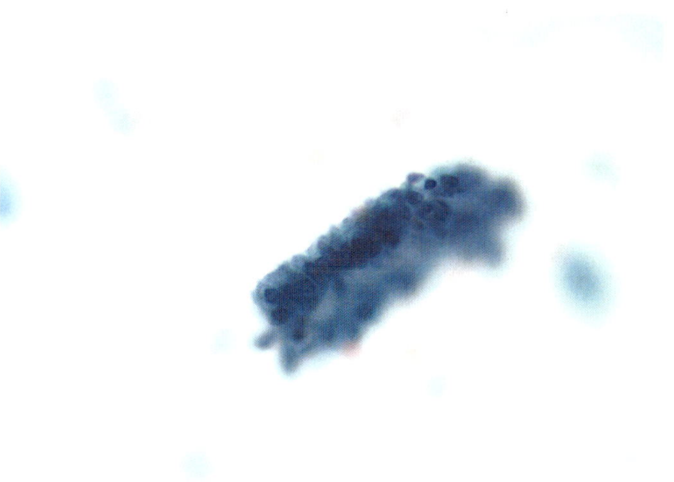

Figure 3.19 — Cystitis cystica, instrumented urine. A flat strip of glandular epithelium most likely was removed via catheterization and would not be expected to exfoliate spontaneously. The luminal edge is uniform, nuclei are the same general distance from the luminal edge, and their size is small (Papanicolaou stain, medium power).

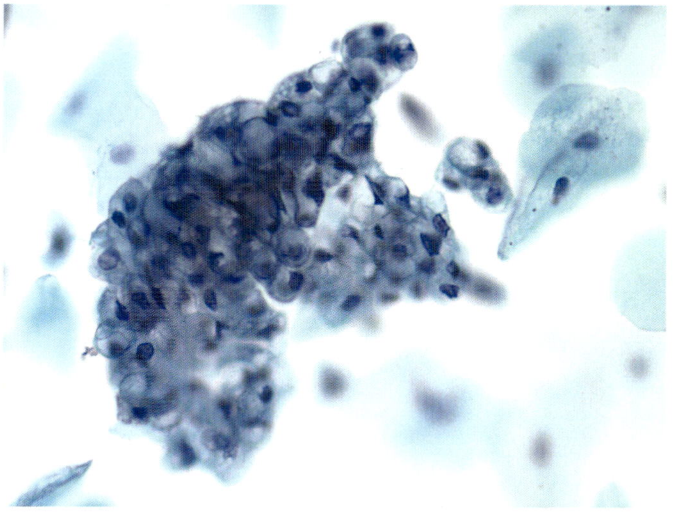

Figure 3.20 — Cystitis cystica, instrumented urine. A very large fragment of glandular epithelium needs careful inspection to assure that this is a benign change. The small size of the nuclei and generally benign nuclear characteristics are reassuring. Cytoplasmic vacuolization is characteristic of the lesion. Compare with the squamous cells in the background. (Papanicolaou stain, high power).

Figure 3.21 — Cystitis cystica, voided urine. A collection of small (compared to the background squamous cell), uniform cuboidal to low-columnar cells with round nuclei that appear to be basally placed. Cytoplasm is faintly granular and lacks the opacity of a urothelial or squamous cell. Just as in tissue biopsies, cystitis cystica and cystitis glandularis (referred to together as cystitis cystica et glandularis) are common incidental findings seen in association with long standing chronic cystitis (Papanicolaou stain, medium power).

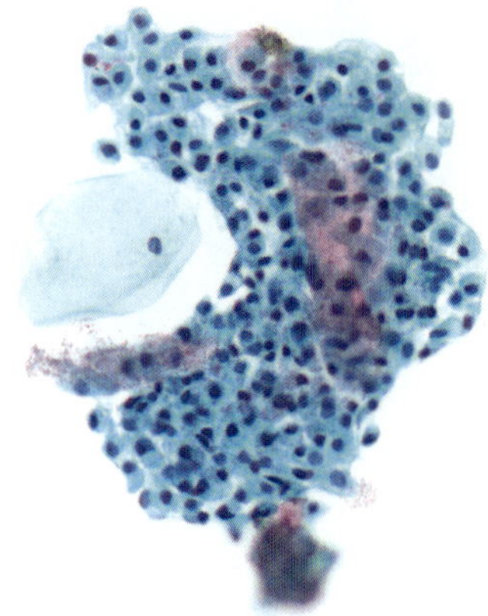

Figure 3.22 — Cystitis cystica, voided urine. A close-up view illustrating bland, extremely monotonous, cuboidal to short-columnar epithelial cells. These cells are said to arise via metaplasia or degenerative changes in von Brunn's nests and are seen in up to 60 percent of bladders on close inspection (Papanicolaou stain, high power).

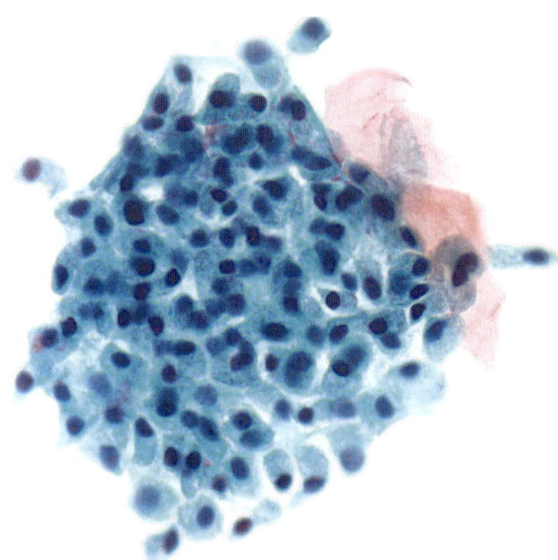

Figure 3.23 — Nephrogenic adenoma, histologic section. A nephrogenic adenoma develops in areas of injured urothelium. It can have varied architectural patterns, which include tubular structures, signet-ring cell-like appearance, and papillary architecture. This low power image shows the surface urothelium having been replaced by a single layer of cuboidal cells. The lamina propria is edematous, inflamed, congested, and is thrown into a papillary architecture. Underlying the papillae are small and mildly dilated tubular structures lined by flattened to cuboidal cells with a moderate amount of cytoplasm and ovoid nuclei. These nuclei display prominent nucleoli and have a hobnail appearance (H&E stain, low power).

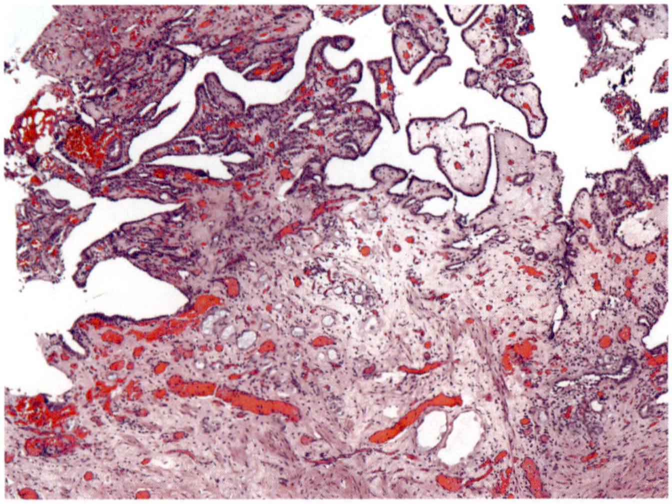

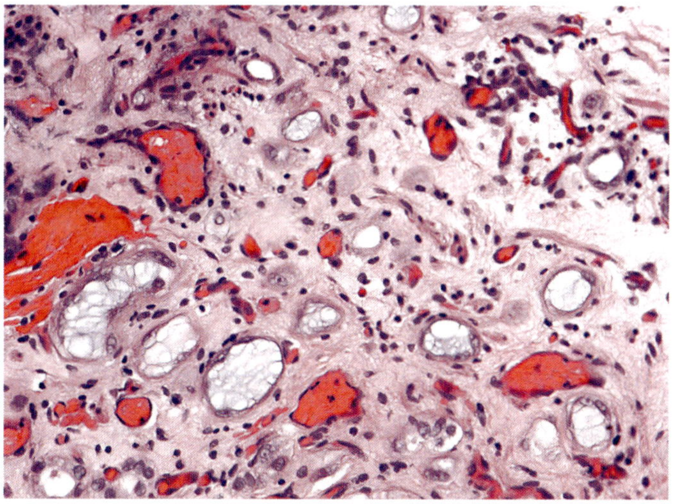

Figure 3.24 — Nephrogenic adenoma, histologic section. Higher magnification of the lamina propria tubules show flattened cells with a somewhat hobnailed appearance. Lumina of the tubules contain blue mucin, and there is peritubular hyalinization. The stroma is inflamed and congested from the preceding injury. These lesions are cytokeratin positive on immunoperoxidase labeling, in addition to expressing other renal tubular immunomarkers (e.g., AMACR, CD10, PAX 2); (H&E stain, high power).

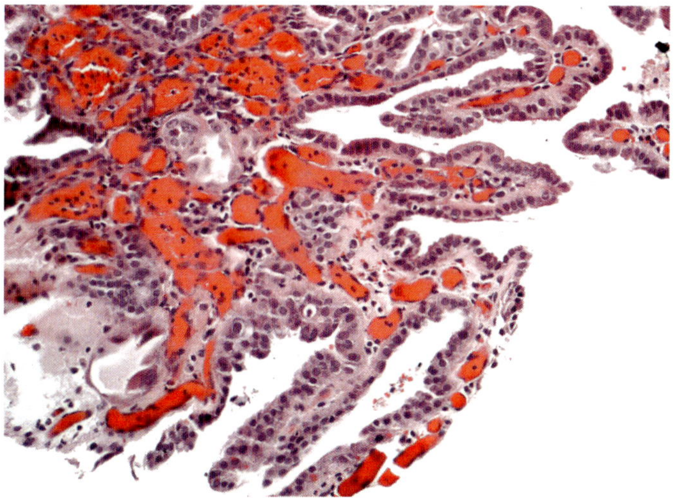

Figure 3.25 — Nephrogenic adenoma, histologic section. This example shows cuboidal cells lining the papillae. The cells are very uniform without cytologic atypia or mitoses. The papillae are broad based. Cystoscopically, these can mimic papillary urothelial tumors. The stroma is always inflamed and congested. Center of the lesion shows a tubular structure lined by hobnail cells with degenerative-type atypia (H&E stain, medium power).

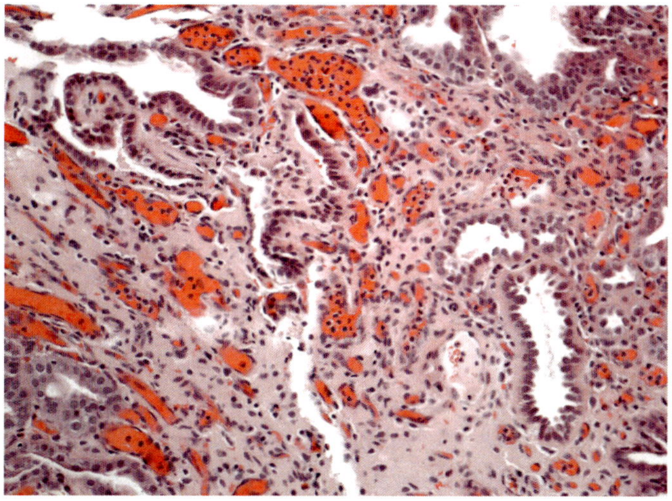

Figure 3.26 — Nephrogenic adenoma, histologic section. This example depicts the surface papillary architecture lined by uniform cuboidal cells without atypia and tubular structures formed by cuboidal hobnail cells. There is peritubular hyalinization. The stroma is inflamed and congested (H&E stain, medium power).

Figure 3.27 — Nephrogenic adenoma, instrumented urine. Tissue fragment in a cell block from a nephrogenic adenoma reveals monotonous population of epithelial cells with reactive changes, including occasional prominent nucleoli and abundant bubbly cytoplasm. A cytologic interpretation of this lesion is not possible on urine examination, and the diagnosis is only made on tissue biopsy (H&E stain, medium power).

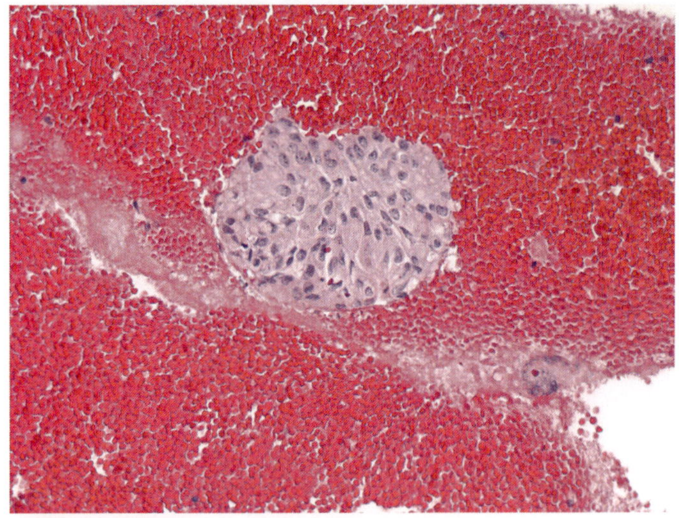

Figure 3.28 — Nephrogenic adenoma, instrumented urine. This diagnosis must be made solely on tissue biopsy. The cytologic interpretation of this urine sample (cell block section) should be limited to reactive cellular changes. Occasional cells have macronucleoli (arrows) and display marked nuclear atypia raising the suspicion of a significant urothelial lesion. Tissue biopsy is clearly indicated (H&E stain, high power).

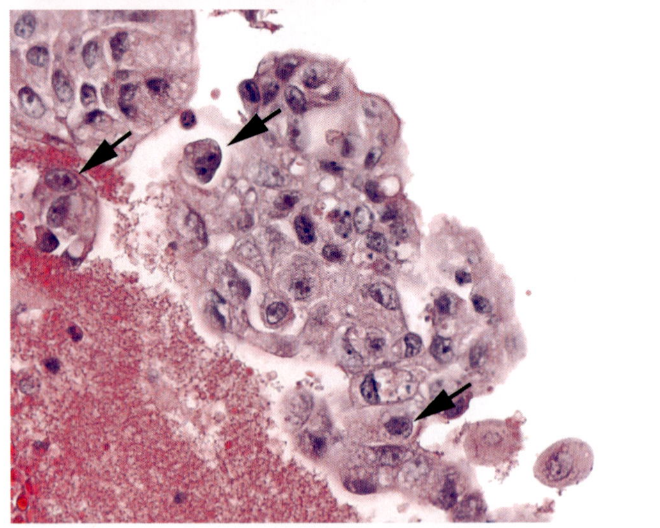

Figure 3.29 — Polypoid cystitis, histologic section. This is a reactive condition of the urothelium in response to injury, most often secondary to an indwelling catheter. The urothelium gets thrown into polypoid and papillary architecture due to the edema within the lamina propria. If the edema is intense, bullous cystitis is seen. As the lesion progresses, inflammation ensues and more nonarborizing, broad-based papillae are seen. This low power image of a bladder biopsy shows intense edema giving rise to bullous polypoid cystitis. Lamina propria is inflamed and congested (H&E stain, very low power).

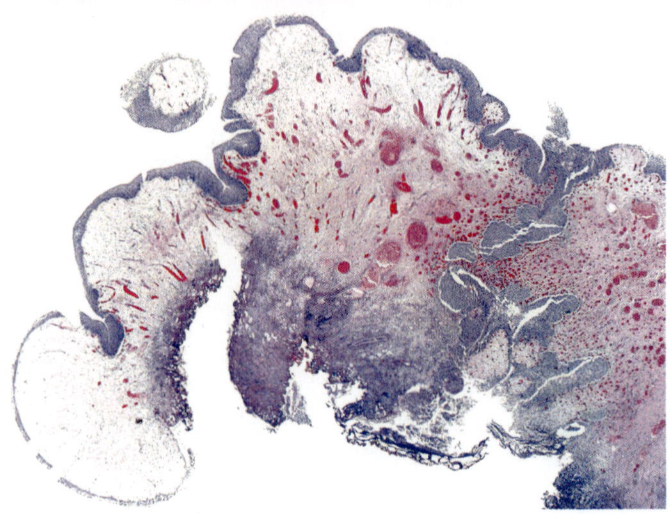

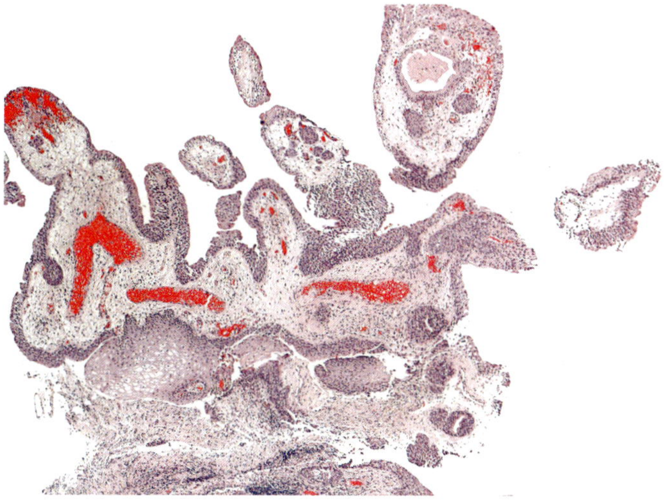

Figure 3.30 — Polypoid cystitis, histologic section. This example shows the urothelium with a papillary architecture and broad-based, nonarborizing papillae. The stroma is inflamed and becoming fibrotic. Cystitis cystica is also present within the papillae. There are no delicate fibrovascular cores as seen in papillary urothelial tumors. Since this is a reactive lesion occurring secondary to injury to the bladder lining, there is often squamous metaplasia of the urothelium that lines the papillae (H&E stain, very low power).

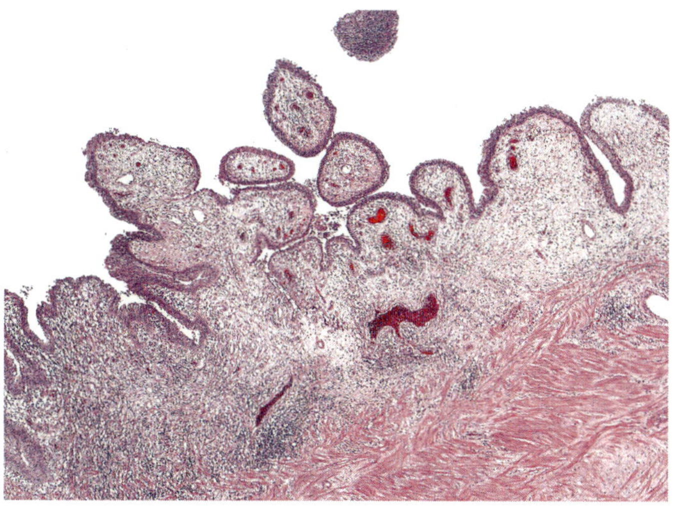

Figure 3.31 — Polypoid cystitis, histologic section. Low-power view of polypoid pyelitis of the renal pelvis. This patient had a stent causing chronic irritation to the pelvic urothelium. Note the broad based papillae with intense inflammation of the stroma (H&E stain, low power).

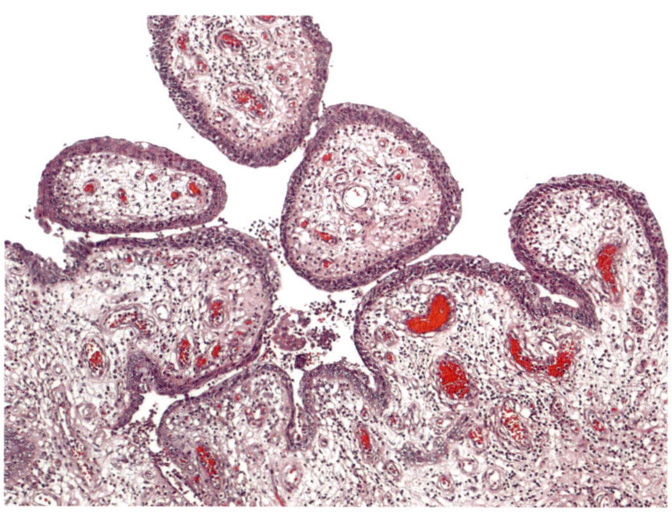

Figure 3.32 — Polypoid cystitis, histologic section. High magnification of the above case; squamous metaplasia of the urothelium lining the papillae is seen. There are no delicate fibrovascular cores as seen in papillary urothelial tumors. Stroma of the lamina propria is inflamed, edematous, and focally becoming fibrotic (H&E stain, medium power).

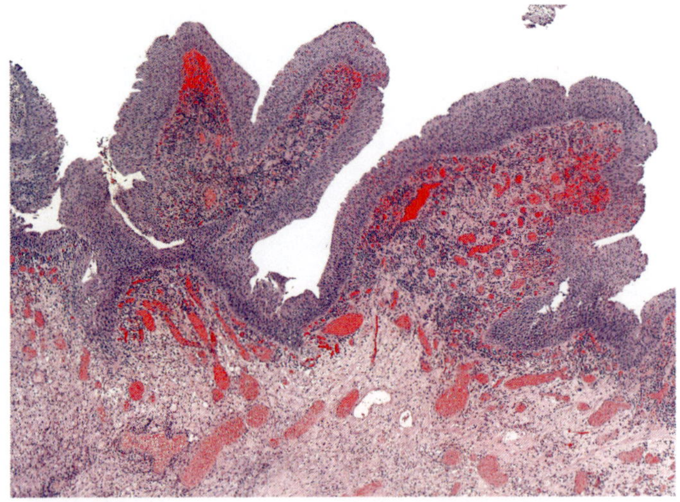

Figure 3.33 — Polypoid cystitis, histologic section. Polypoid cystitis passes through phases of polypoid to papillary cystitis, with inflammation and finally fibrosis predominating, respectively. This patient had a history of an indwelling catheter. Note the intense inflammation and edema with congestion of the lamina propria. The urothelium is intact with reactive changes (H&E stain, low power).

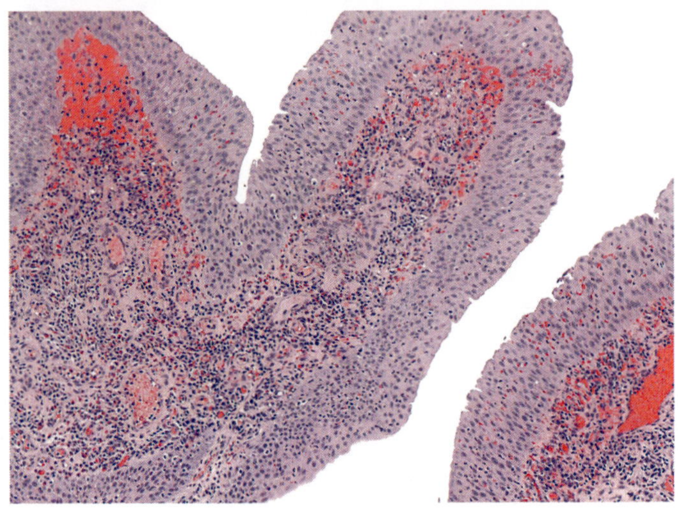

Figure 3.34 — Polypoid cystitis, histologic section. Slightly higher-power view of the same case depicts acute and chronic inflammatory infiltrates with neutrophils present within the urothelium. The urothelium, though intact, shows reactive atypia with slightly enlarged nuclei showing prominent nucleoli. The nuclear membranes are smooth, and cellular polarity is maintained (H&E stain, medium power).

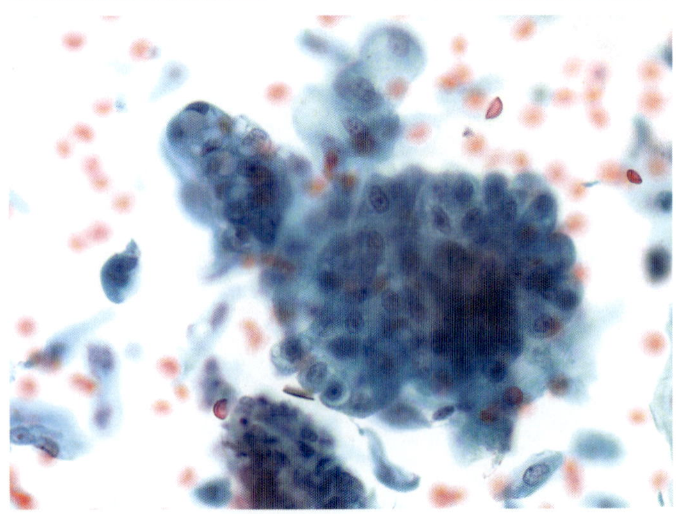

Figure 3.35 — Polypoid cystitis, instrumented urine. Polypoid cystitis is an uncommon reactive entity, usually not prospectively diagnosed. This specimen demonstrates the thick fragments of mildly atypical urothelium. A significant lesion must be considered, and a low-grade neoplasm should be included in the differential diagnosis. Distinguishing features of a benign lesion are present, that is, small nuclei, bland chromatin. Tissue biopsy is essential in such cases. Clinical history of a chronic indwelling catheter is often a helpful clue (Papanicolaou stain, high power).

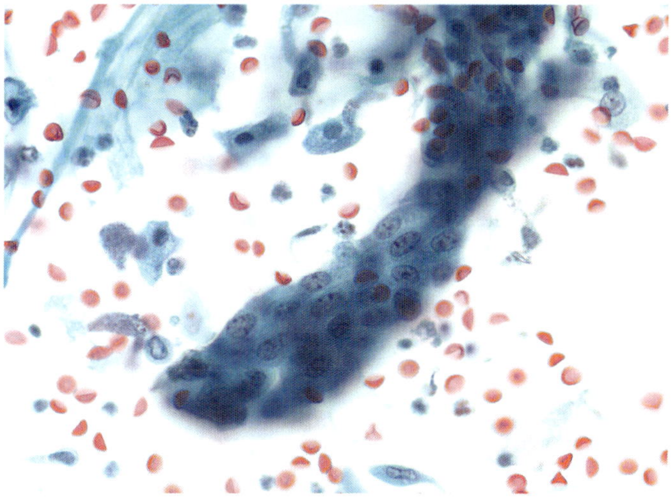

Figure 3.36 — Polypoid cystitis, instrumented urine. Polypoid cystitis, if symptomatic, will present with hematuria. The differential includes a low-grade papillary urothelial lesion or a well-differentiated adenocarcinoma. Tissue confirmation is essential, as is the search for any lesion coming from the surrounding structures. Abundant red blood cells are often present in the slide background with or without chronic inflammatory cells (Papanicolaou stain, high power).

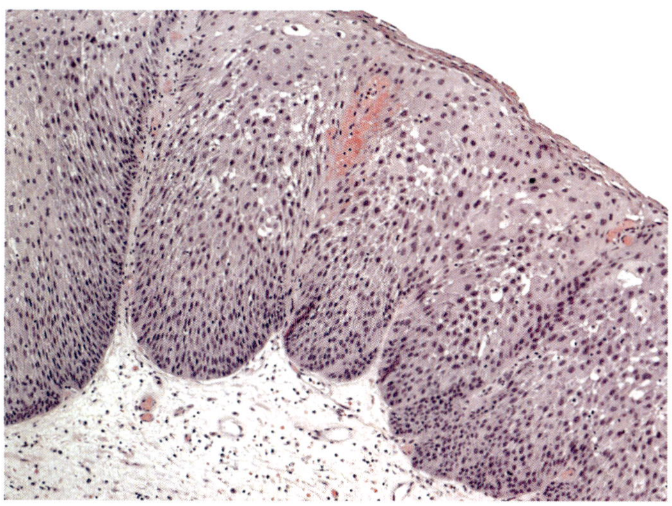

Figure 3.37 — Squamous metaplasia, histologic section. Persistent or repeated injury to the urothelium can cause squamous metaplasia. This type of change is frequently seen in paraplegic patients with indwelling catheters. Squamous metaplasia of the trigone is a normal finding in women, where it happens under the influence of estrogen. This type of metaplasia is composed of glycogenated squamous cells without keratinization and does not predispose to any dysplasia or carcinoma. This image shows keratinizing squamous metaplasia, which can develop dysplasia and eventually squamous cell carcinoma of the bladder. Another predisposing factor to squamous metaplasia is bladder schistosomiasis infection (H&E stain, medium power).

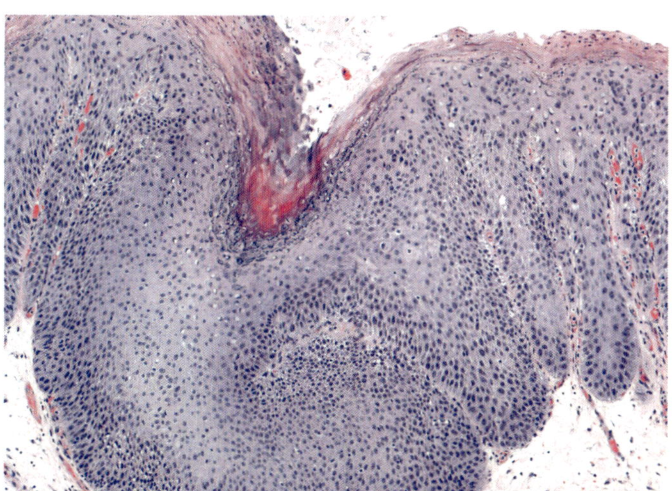

Figure 3.38 — Keratinizing squamous metaplasia, histologic section. Squamous metaplasia can show parakeratosis, hyperkeratosis, and even the formation of a granular cell layer. This type of metaplasia is a risk factor for the development of squamous cell carcinoma of the bladder (H&E stain, medium power).

Figure 3.39 — Granulomatous cystitis, histologic section. Multiple nonnecrotizing granulomas are seen at low magnification in the background of lymphoid follicles. The surface urothelium is benign. The lamina propria is fibrotic, congested, and inflamed. Bacillus Calmette-Guerin (BCG) intravesical therapy for superficial bladder cancer can sometimes result in granuloma formation within the lamina propria. The background is always very inflamed (H&E stain, low power).

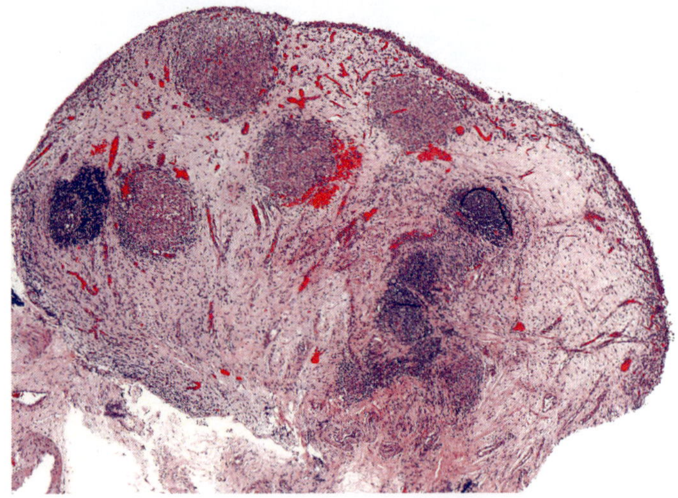

Figure 3.40 — Granulomatous cystitis, histologic section. Nonnecrotizing granuloma comprising of epithelioid histiocytes and some lymphocytic inflammation. The surface urothelium, though intact and benign, shows reactive changes with mild nuclear enlargement and dark opaque cytoplasm. There is lymphoplasmacytic chronic inflammation and congestion within submucosa. Granulomatous inflammation can also occur within adjacent organs such as the prostate after BCG therapy for superficial bladder cancer (H&E stain, medium power).

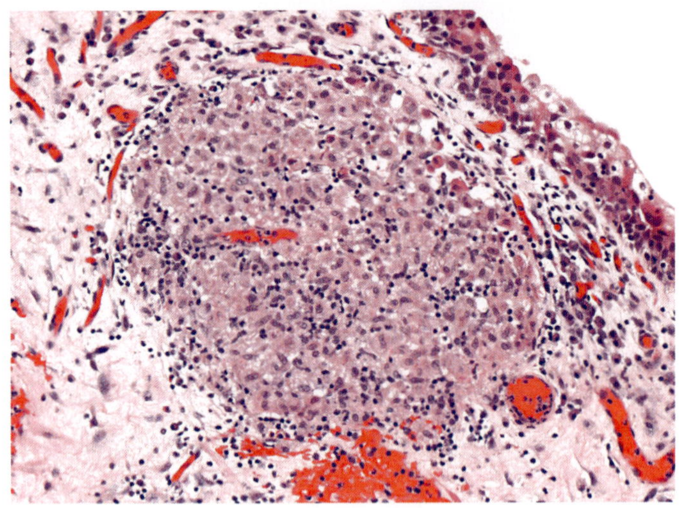

Figure 3.41 — Granulomatous cystitis, voided urine. Intravesical BCG therapy for bladder cancer will provoke a localized or generalized granulomatous response in the submucosa of the bladder. Microscopic granulomas may shed, especially during a bladder washing following therapy. However, the presence of intact granulomas is not unusual in a voided urine specimen (as seen here). Histiocytes, lymphocytes, and fibroblasts compose these classic granulomas. Careful search for persistent tumor is imperative (Papanicolaou stain, high power).

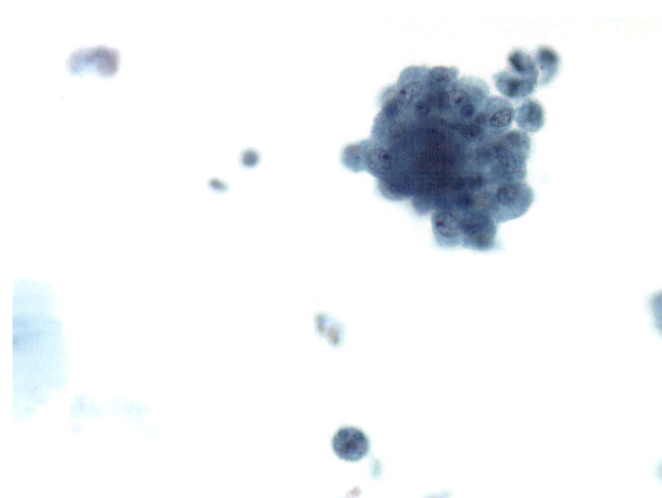

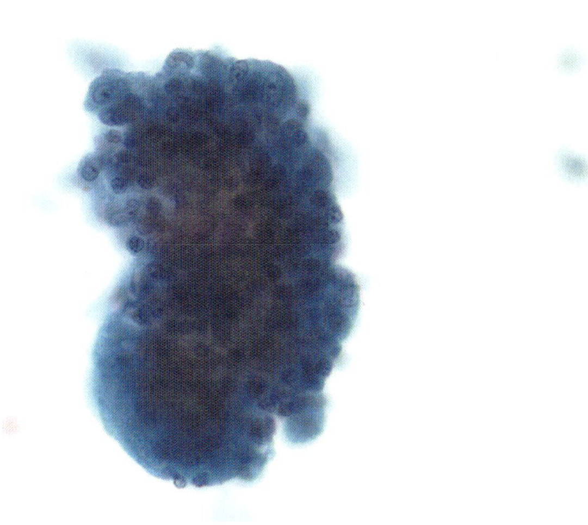

Figure 3.42 — Granulomatous cystitis, instrumented urine. Granulomas caused by BCG therapy appear the same as granulomas elsewhere. Samples following therapy should not be collected unless at least six weeks have passed from the last instillation of BCG to avoid confusing reactive cells with persistent tumor cells (Papanicolaou stain, high power).

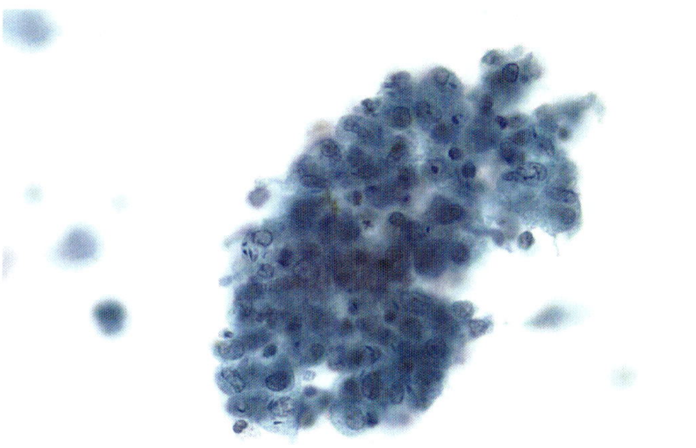

Figure 3.43 — Granulomatous cystitis, instrumented urine. BCG therapy can produce reactive cells that may be confused with residual tumor cells. However, the features of reactive atypia will be present, that is, prominent round nucleoli, bland chromatin and abundant cytoplasm, as well as inflammatory cells within the tissue fragments (Papanicolaou stain, high power).

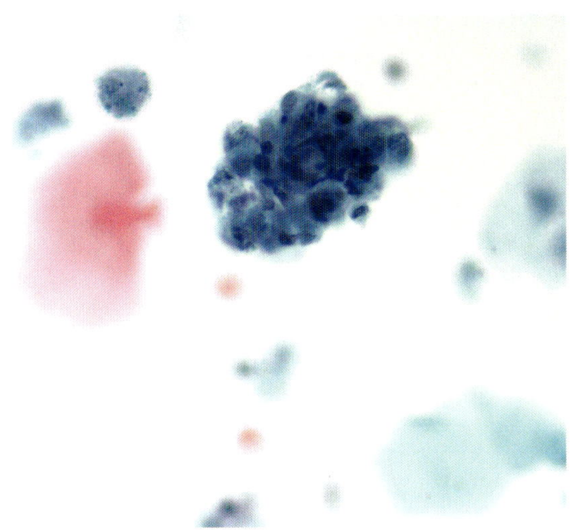

Figure 3.44 — Granulomatous cystitis, voided urine. A large granuloma following BCG therapy comprises histiocytes with reniform nuclei, fibroblasts, lymphocytes, and occasional neutrophils. The aggregate will be loose and should not be confused with an epithelial fragment. Careful consideration to patient's clinical history is imperative to avoid an over call in such scenarios (Papanicolaou stain, high power).

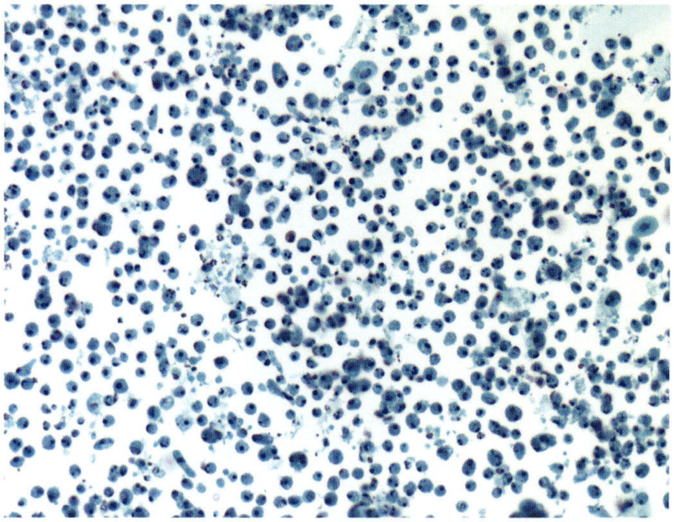

Figure 3.45 — Ileal loop (neobladder), voided urine. Specimens from an ileal loop or neobladder are crowded with small macrophage-like cells, which in reality are degenerated enteric glandular cells. These occasionally cluster, but most frequently are singly occurring. Their distinction from inflammatory cells is sometimes difficult and necessitates a higher power review. Search for neoplastic cells is important, as these patients have a history of urothelial carcinoma and are candidates for new tumors in the upper urinary tract (Papanicolaou stain, low power).

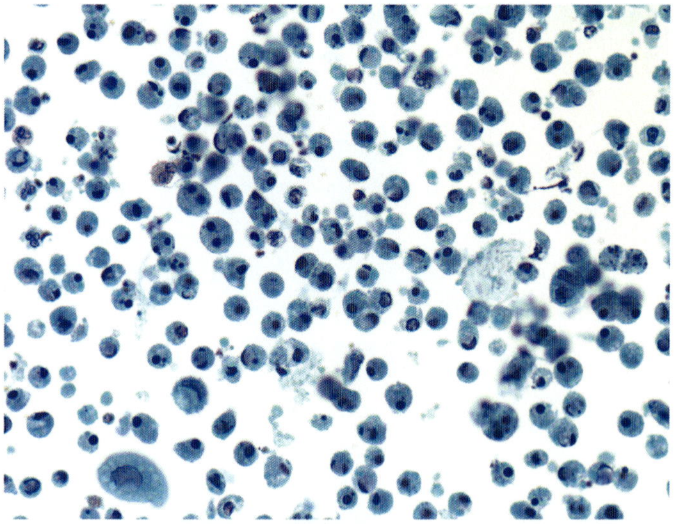

Figure 3.46 — Ileal loop (neobladder), voided urine. Enteric cells from an ileal loop are round with degenerated small, single, or multiple nuclei. Fragments of cytoplasm can also be seen in the background as well as urothelial cells and occasional inflammatory cells (Papanicolaou stain, medium power).

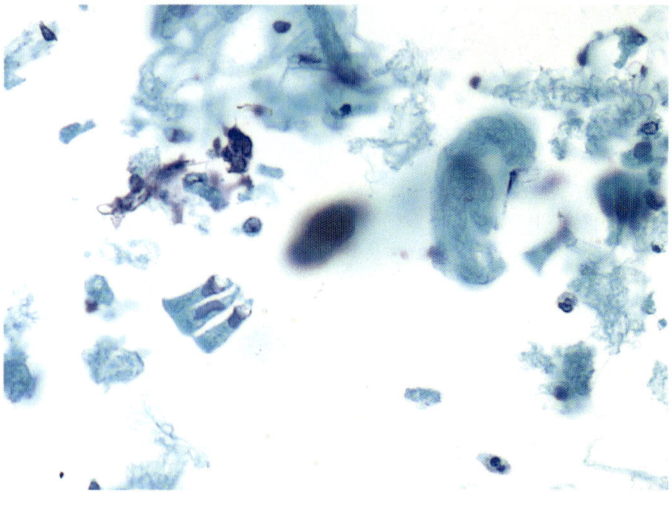

Figure 3.47 — Ileal loop (neobladder), voided urine. Abundant granular and cellular debris contains small strips of intact columnar enteric cells with small basally-placed nuclei and apically cleared cytoplasm. Due to the marked irritant effects of urine on the neobladder lining, the finding of well-preserved columnar cells is unusual (Papanicolaou stain, high power).

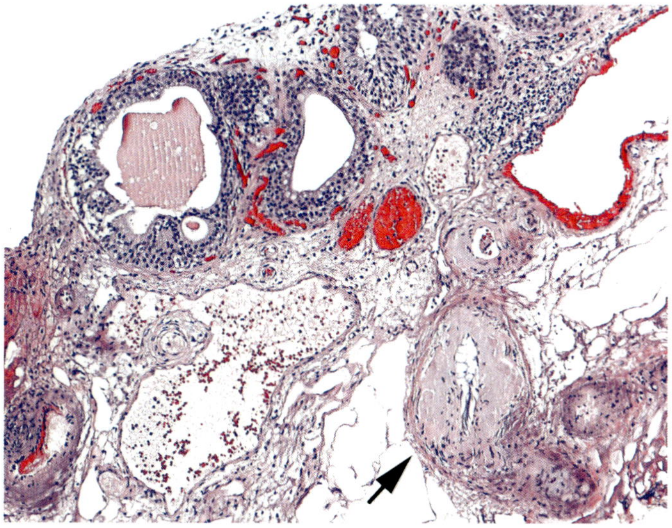

Figure 3.48 — Amyloidosis of the bladder, histologic section. Urinary bladder can be involved in systemic amyloidosis. The presenting symptom is hematuria. Amyloid deposits around the vessels are seen in the lower right side of the image (arrow), with a smooth and eosinophilic appearance. In this image, the surface urothelium is denuded with cystitis cystica.

Primary involvement of the bladder is rare and may occur in the form of a localized mass with amyloid deposition in lamina propria or diffuse involvement that may require radical surgery to control the resulting hemorrhage (H&E stain, medium power).

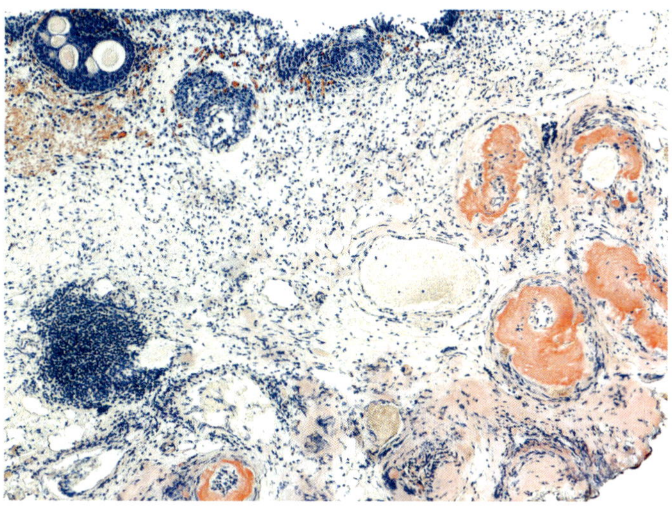

Figure 3.49 — Amyloidosis of the bladder, histologic section. Orange-red staining of the perivascular amyloid deposition by Congo red stain. Other stains that may be utilized include crystal violet (Congo red stain, low power).

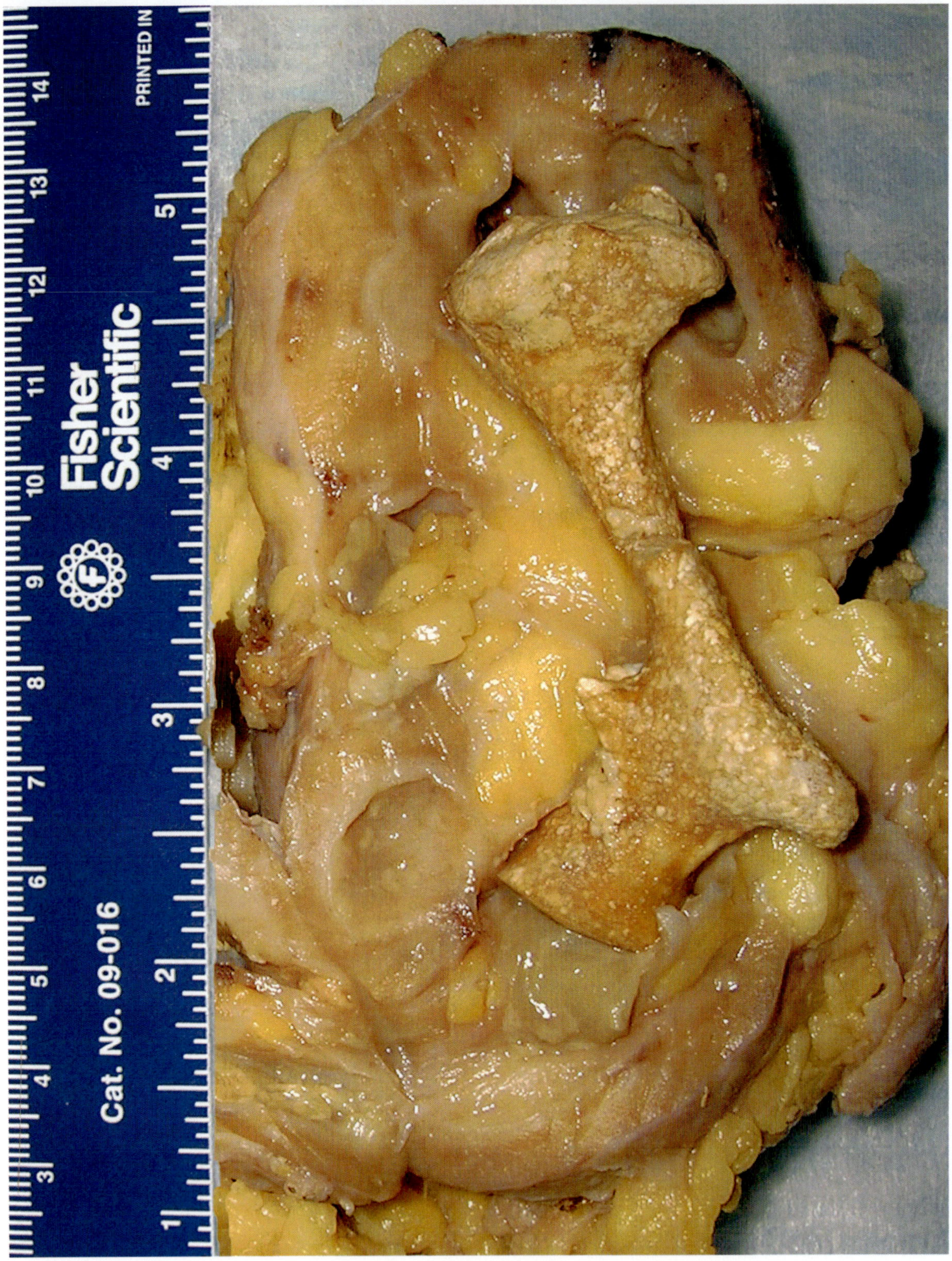

Figure 3.50 — Staghorn calculus associated with xanthogranulomatous pyelonephritis (XGP), gross appearance. Radical nephrectomy specimen. Approximately 70 percent of XGP cases are associated with staghorn calculi within renal pelvis. Also known as the triple phosphate stones (magnesium ammonium phosphate or struvite calculi), they develop secondary to repeated infections by urease-producing proteus, ureaplasma, klebsiella, staphylococcus, and pseudomonas bacterial species, in descending order. E-coli does not produce urease, hence is not associated with struvite calculi.

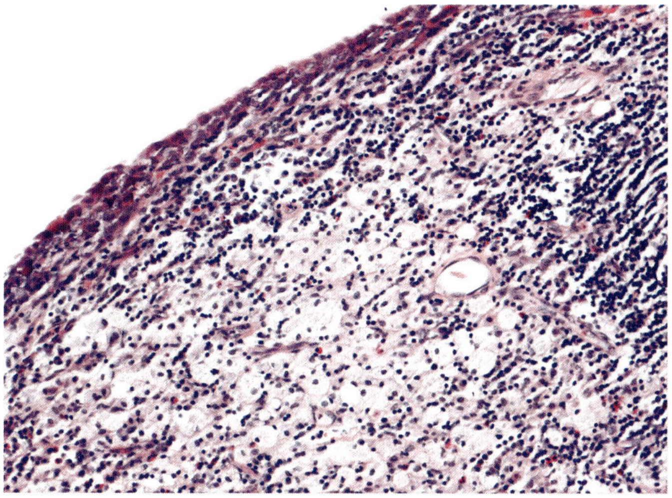

Figure 3.51 — Xanthogranulomatous pyelonephritis, histologic section. A section through the renal pelvic urothelium involved by xanthogranulomatous pyelonephritis (XGP) is shown here. The urothelium is reactive with dark cytoplasm and chronic inflammatory cells infiltrating the mucosa. Within the submucosa foamy histiocytes or xanthoma cells are present, admixed with chronic lymphoplasmacytic inflammation and scattered eosinophils. Occasional giant cells can also be seen (H&E stain, medium power).

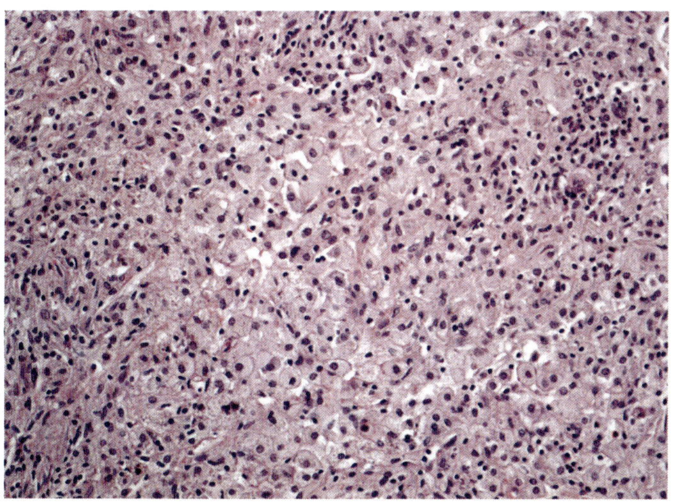

Figure 3.52 — Xanthogranulomatous pyelonephritis, histologic section. Xanthogranulomatous pyelonephritis (XGP) can be mass forming such that on imaging it mimics renal cell carcinoma. This image shows the diagnostic cell—xanthoma cell or foamy histiocyte—which contains debris from the preceding infection. The initial inflammation also has abscess formation or microabscesses with acute inflammation. These abscesses are then replaced by chronic inflammation with occasional giant cells as well. Xanthogranulomatous inflammation can occur anywhere along the urinary tract and can be seen within the bladder itself (H&E stain, medium power).

4

Nonneoplastic Lesions—Infections

- Malakoplakia of Bladder
- Fungal Infections
- Viral Infections
- Parasitic Infections

Figure 4.1 — Malakoplakia of bladder, histologic section. This is a form of chronic cystitis where the bladder mucosa is irregularly thickened and yellow, raised plaques are seen. The lesion comprises inflammatory cells with aggregates of histiocytes or macrophages predominating. These histiocytes have ample eosinophilic granular cytoplasm and are called Von Hansemann cells. Within the cell cytoplasm as well as outside of the cells are characteristic targetoid calcified concretions termed Michaelis-Gutmann bodies. These concretions result from undigested phagocytosed cellular and bacterial materials with deposits of iron and calcium salts. In addition to PAS special stains, these targetoid bodies can be highlighted by iron and calcium stains. This image is a particularly florid example of Michaelis-Gutmann bodies (H&E stain, low power).

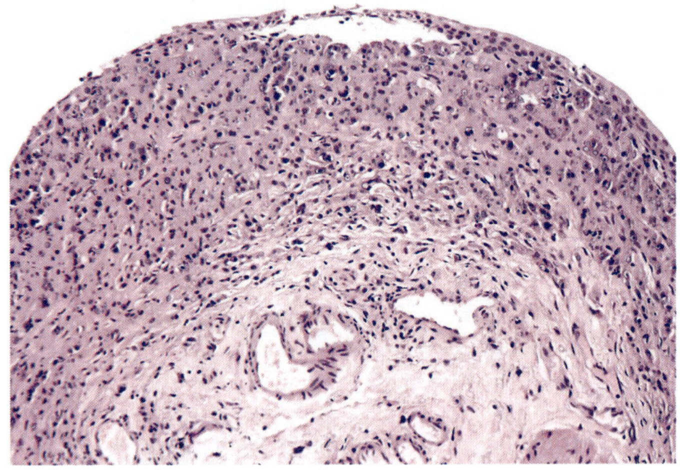

Figure 4.2 — Malakoplakia of bladder, histologic section. High magnification view of the macrophages and Michaelis-Gutmann bodies (arrows). Quite frequently, acute inflammatory cells accompany these lesions in addition to lymphocytes and plasma cells. Pathogenesis is from a defect in the intraphagosomal digestion. Repeated infections, immunocompromised states, and other chronic diseases predispose to malakoplakia. Overlying mucosa may show reactive changes with ulceration or metaplasia. Malakoplakia can occur anywhere in the body; however the urinary bladder is the most common site of involvement (H&E stain, high power).

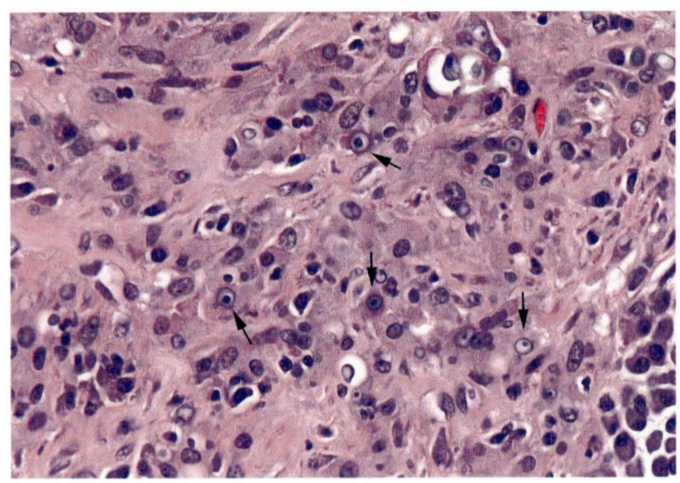

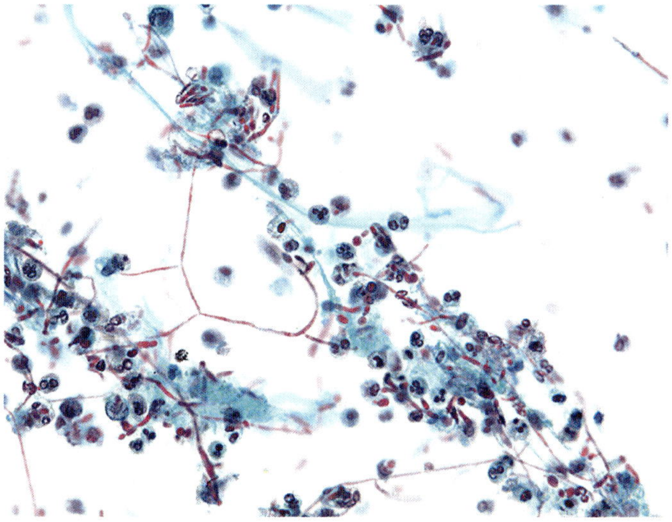

Figure 4.3 — Candidiasis of bladder, voided urine. Candida may be recovered in a urinary specimen, and originate either in the bladder itself, or in the external genitalia, especially in a female. The morphology is the same as any other place in the body. Culture is necessary for speciation (Papanicolaou stain, high power).

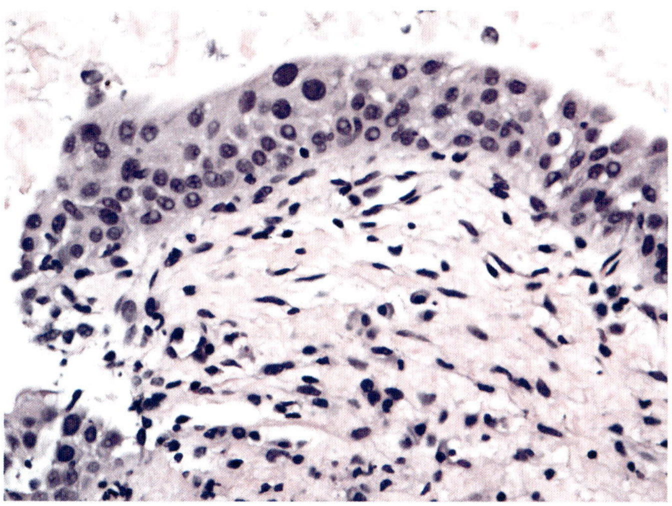

Figure 4.4 — Polyoma (BK) virus infection of the bladder, histologic section. Surface urothelial cells infected by polyoma virus (also known as BK or SV-40 virus) with cytopathic effect (decoy cells) that mimic urothelial carcinoma in situ. This infection is quite commonly observed in urine specimens from immunosuppressed patients. Other viruses involved in bladder infections are herpes and CMV. Adenovirus and herpes simplex virus have been associated with hemorrhagic cystitis (H&E stain, medium power).

Figure 4.5 — Polyoma (BK) virus infection of the bladder, histologic section. The cells infected by the virus are highlighted by nuclear immunolabeling with SV-40 (SV-40 immunostain, medium power).

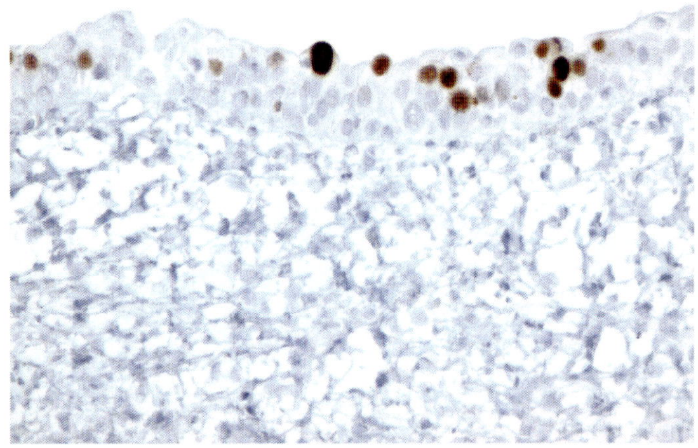

Figure 4.6 — Polyoma (BK) virus infection of the bladder, histologic section. Many urothelial cell nuclei have the typical polyoma virus cytopathic change with enlargement of the nucleus, ground glass inclusion pushing the nucleoli against the nuclear membrane, which is smooth (H&E stain, medium power).

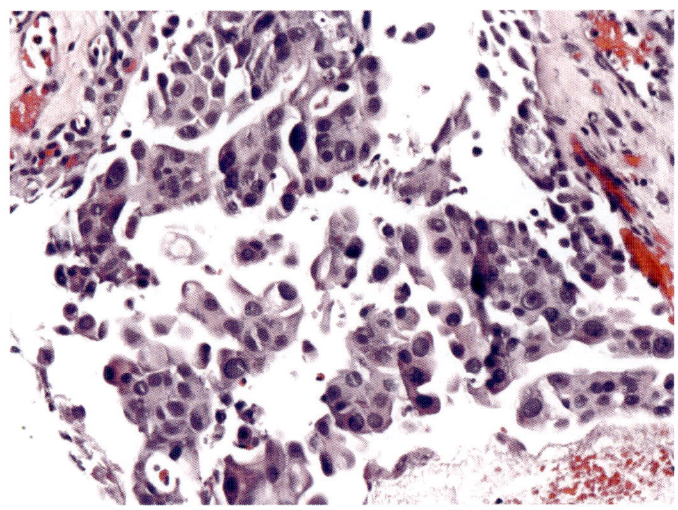

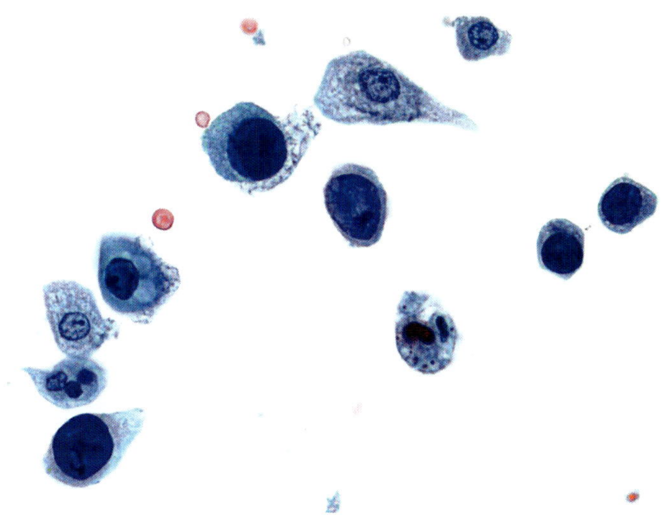

Figure 4.7 — Polyoma (BK) virus infection of the bladder, voided urine. Polyoma (BK) virus produces changes within the cells that are confined to the nucleus. Nuclear enlargement, homogenization of the nuclear chromatin, and a visible margination of the chromatin are features frequently seen. Distinction from high-grade urothelial cancer is sometimes difficult, hence the name "decoy" cells (Papanicolaou stain, high power).

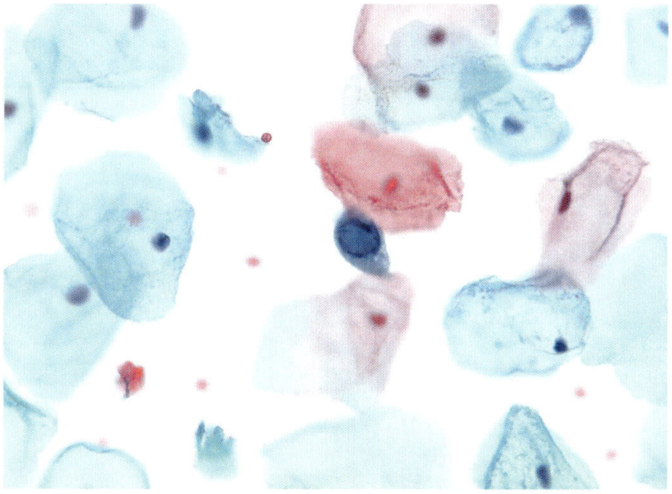

Figure 4.8 — Polyoma (BK) virus infection of the bladder, voided urine. Polyoma virus cells are usually infrequent, and stand out from surrounding urothelial and squamous cells (Papanicolaou stain, high power).

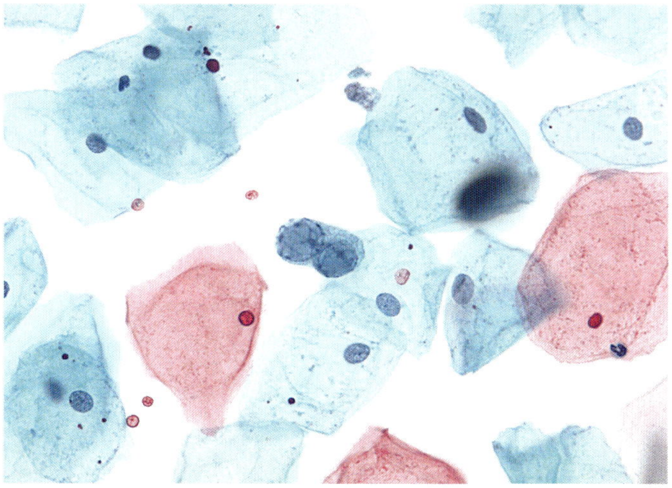

Figure 4.9 — Polyoma (BK) virus infection of the bladder, voided urine. Polyoma virus nuclear changes are not always hyperchromatic, as the stage of degeneration will influence how much chromatin is left in the nuclear sack. This binucleate cell might be confused with herpes change, but the classic molding seen in herpes is not evident here, as each nucleus retains its round shape (Papanicolaou stain, high power).

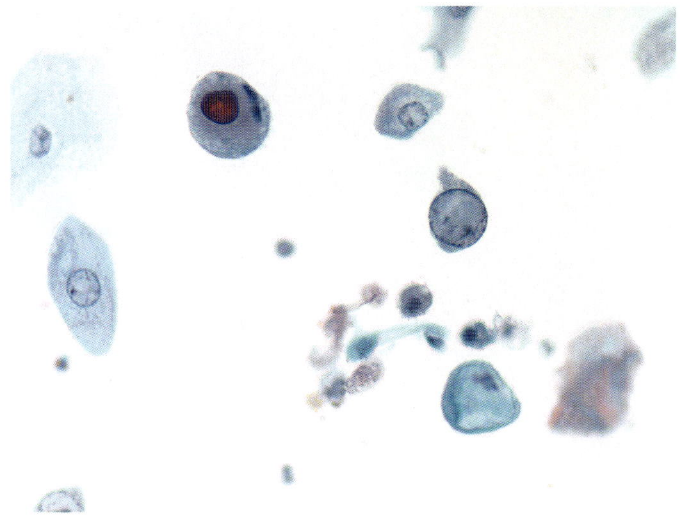

Figure 4.10 — Polyoma (BK) virus infection of the bladder, voided urine. Two different appearances of polyoma viral change are present in this picture. The cell with the very high N/C ratio on the right has a smooth nuclear outline and a round shape. The identification of polyoma virus is comfortable. However, the cell to the left of center (eleven o'clock) has a degenerated, hyperchromatic, and irregularly shaped nucleus, which might indicate origin in a high-grade neoplasm. Careful search of the sample is necessary to eliminate that choice. If in doubt, a notation to the clinician is required (Papanicolaou stain, high power).

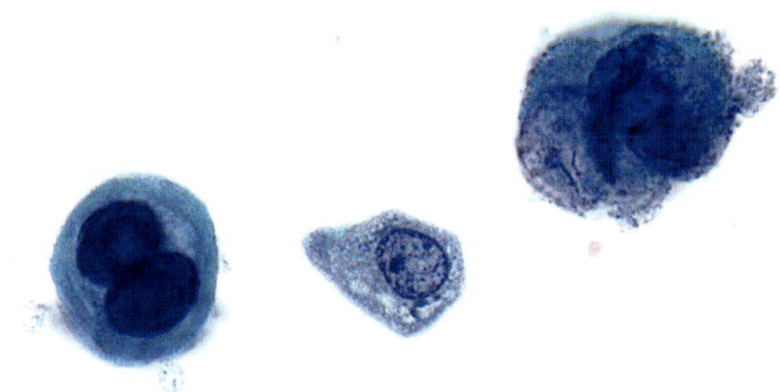

Figure 4.11 — Polyoma (BK) virus infection of the bladder, voided urine. Polyoma virus can infect cancer cells as well as benign cells. If the nucleus is pushing outside of the cytoplasm and the nuclear shape is irregular, neoplasm is a strong consideration. Further confirmation by biopsy is warranted (Papanicolaou stain, high power).

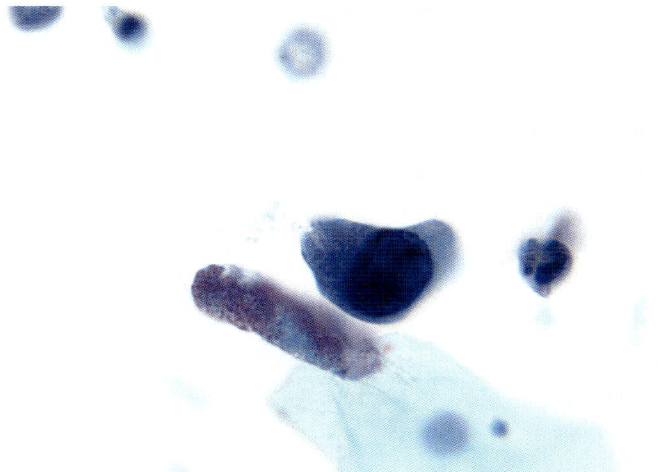

Figure 4.12 — Polyoma (BK) virus infection of the bladder, voided urine. An enlarged urothelial cell is disturbing, and distinction between polyoma virus and high-grade urothelial carcinoma may be difficult if not impossible. Even if only rare abnormal cells are present in the sample, careful search of the patient for a high-grade carcinoma is warranted, as the site of origin may be high in the urinary tract (Papanicolaou stain, high power).

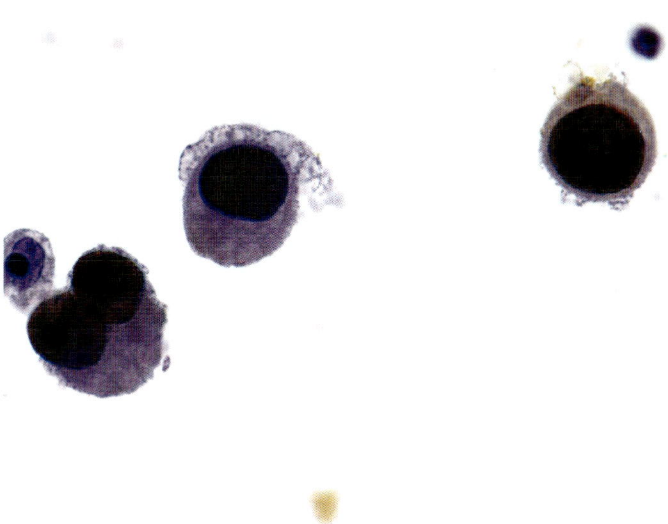

Figure 4.13 — Polyoma (BK) virus infection of the bladder, voided urine. Confirmation of the infection in the sample can be made by immunohistochemistry for SV-40 reacting with the nuclear membrane. However, the polyoma virus can also infect cancer cells, so repeat specimens over time may be necessary to clarify the condition, especially if a lesion is not found immediately. Polyoma virus is usually self limited and the changes will disappear within months (SV-40 immunostain, high power).

Figure 4.14 — HPV infection (condyloma) of the bladder, voided urine. Changes of human papilloma virus may be found in urine specimens. Whether they come from the external genitalia or from inside the bladder cannot be determined unless the specimen is from a catheterized sample. This particular specimen came from a male. (Papanicolaou stain, high power).

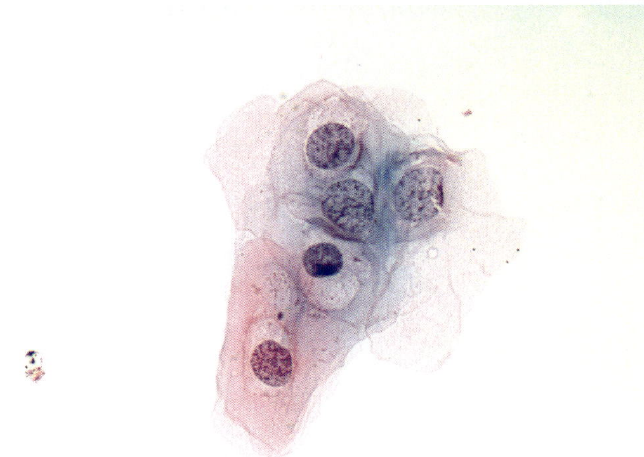

Figure 4.15 — Herpes infection of the urinary tract, voided urine. Herpes simplex infections can affect the urinary bladder, but more commonly seen are the cells captured during voiding from infection of the external genitalia. The cytologic features are the same wherever the cells reside (Papanicolaou stain, high power).

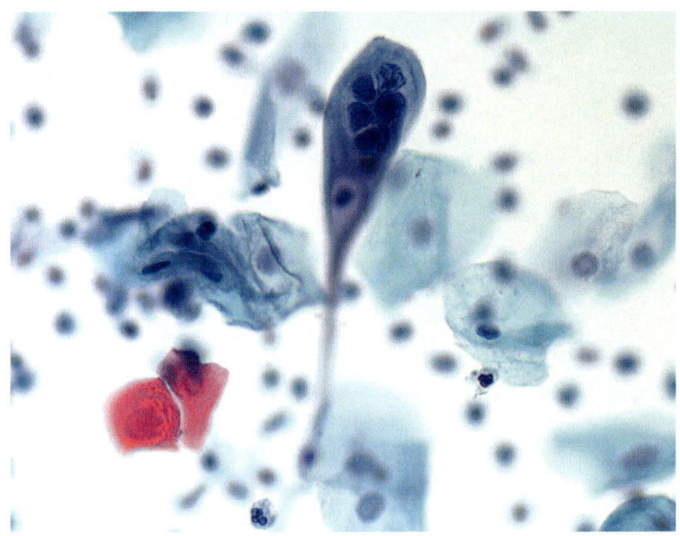

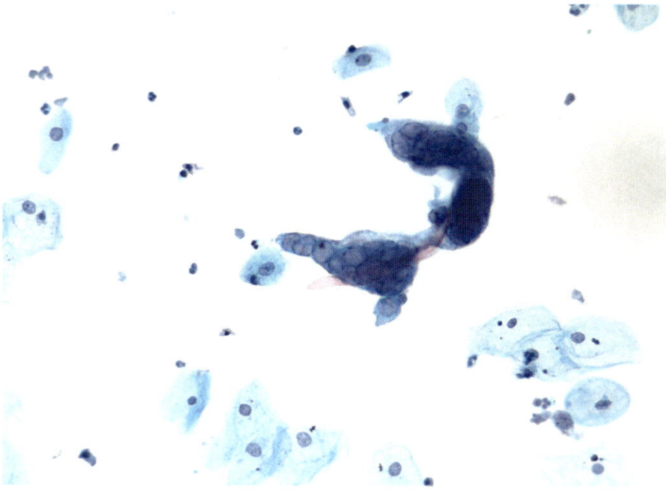

Figure 4.16 — Herpes infection of the urinary tract, voided urine. Infection with herpes virus may be seen in immunocompetent or immunocompromised individuals. If a history of immunosuppression is noted, these herpes changes are indicative of a life-threatening infection. The result should be handled as a panic value (Papanicolaou stain, medium power).

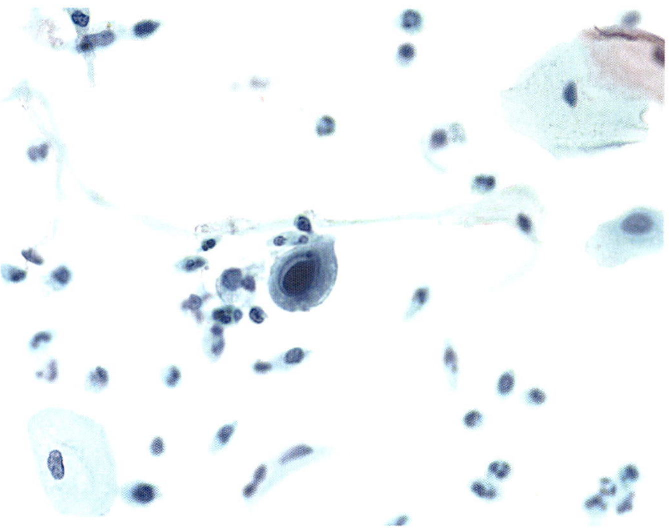

Figure 4.17 — Cytomegalovirus (CMV) infection of the urinary tract, voided urine. Cytomegalovirus is usually an incidental finding, but may indicate a serious infection resulting from immunosuppression, especially in renal transplant patients. The characteristic bull's eye nucleus with the clearing under the nuclear membrane in a greatly enlarged cell is indisputable evidence of CMV infection. Cytoplasmic satellite inclusions may also be seen (Papanicolaou stain, high power).

Figure 4.18 — *Trichomonas* infection of the urinary tract, voided urine. *Trichomonas vaginalis* may infect the bladder, but most commonly is seen in voided urines, having been captured as the urine leaves the bladder, especially in women. Characteristic features are oval shape, flagellum and multiple small inclusions, and are the same anywhere these organisms reside (Papanicolaou stain, high power).

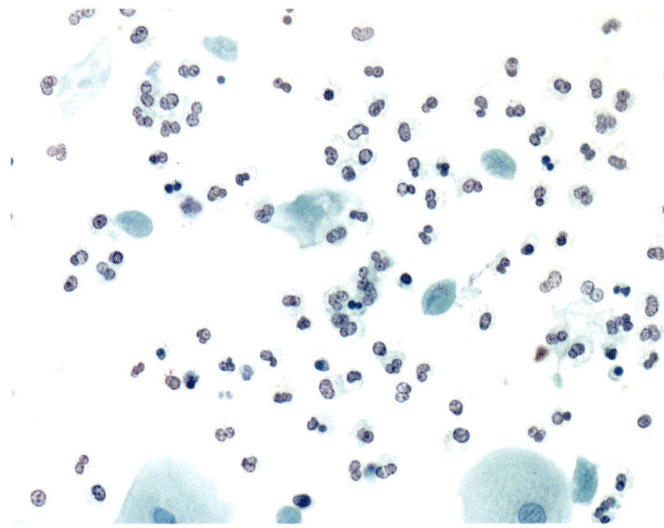

Figure 4.19 — *Schistosoma hematobium* infection of the bladder, histologic section. Low power view of bladder with schistosomiasis. Male and female worms migrate to the pelvic and bladder veins, where the female worms lay eggs. The eggs are seen within the submucosa but with intense infestation, eggs may be seen at all levels of the bladder wall. There is intense accompanying eosinophilic infiltrate surrounding the granulomatous reaction around the recently laid parasite eggs. This can give rise to polypoid hyperemic mucosal masses. Bladder infection is caused by larvae of *Schistosoma hematobium* species. This chronic disease involving the bladder most commonly occurs in the Middle East and the African continent. Patients most often suffer frequency, dysuria, pyuria, and hematuria (H&E stain, low power).

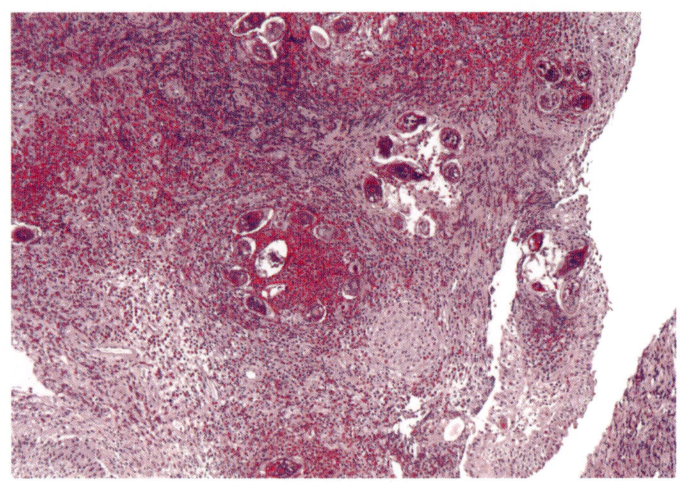

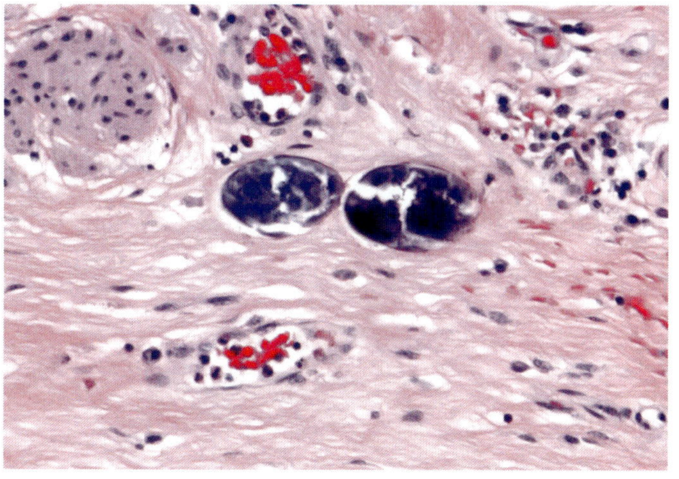

Figure 4.20 — *Schistosoma hematobium* infection of the bladder, histologic section. In later stages, the eggs are destroyed and become calcified, inflammation subsides, and fibrosis occurs. Some of the complications of bladder schistosomiasis include ureteral strictures, bladder neck obstruction, and development of bladder carcinoma. Up to 90 percent of the carcinomas associated with this infection are squamous cell carcinomas (H&E stain, medium power).

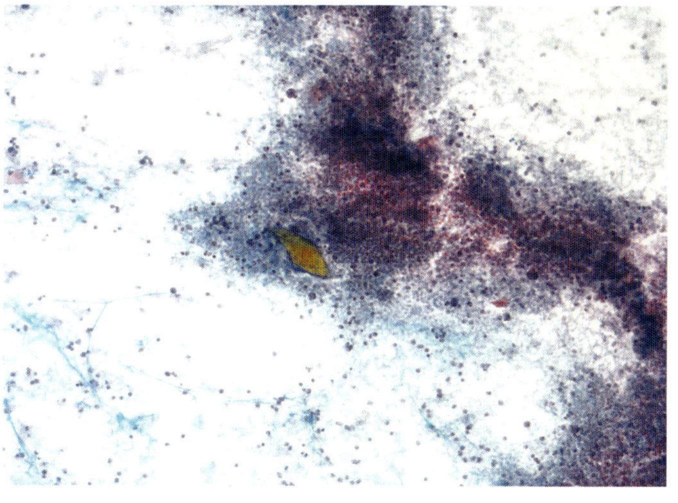

Figure 4.21 — *Schistosoma hematobium* infection of the bladder, voided urine. *Schistosoma hematobium,* also called the bladder fluke, is a common parasite in urinary samples, and is often associated with squamous carcinoma of the bladder in endemic areas. Not only is the organism seen, but also an exuberant inflammatory reaction frequently accompanies the characteristic egg (Papanicolaou stain, low power).

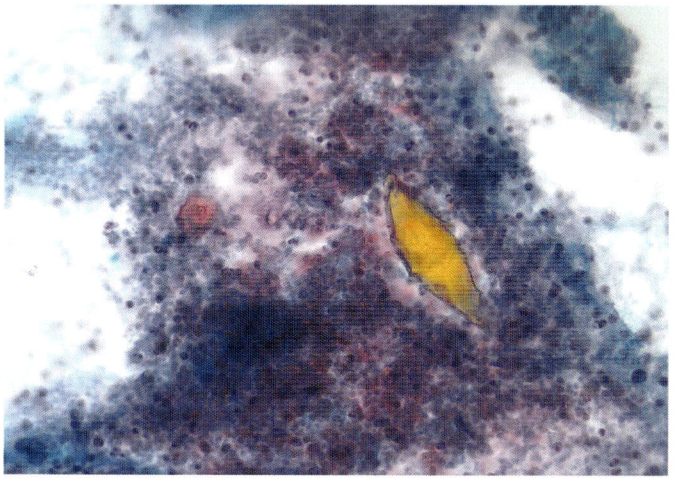

Figure 4.22 — *Schistosoma hematobium* infection of the bladder, voided urine. The organism has a characteristic spine, which should be identified because the location of the spine will distinguish between *japonicum* species (subterminal spine) and *hematobium* (terminal spine) (Papanicolaou stain, high power).

Figure 4.23 — *Schistosoma hematobium* infection of the bladder, voided urine. Two eggs of the parasite displaying the characteristic terminal spine are embedded in dense, acute, inflammatory exudate (Papanicolaou stain, high power).

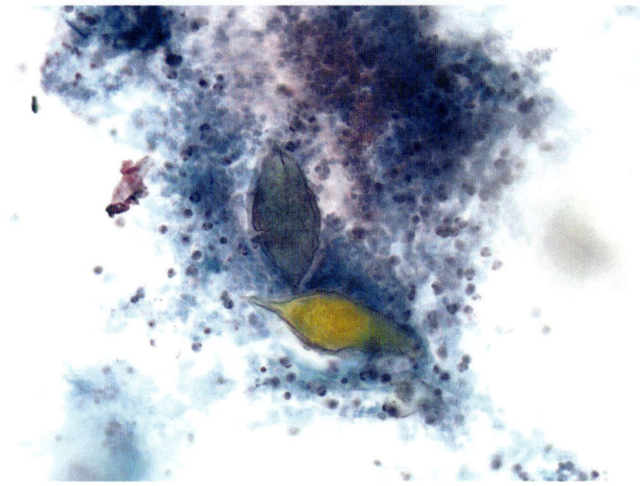

5

Hyperplasia, Benign, and Borderline Urothelial Neoplasms

- Denuded Papillae
- Urothelial Dysplasia
- Papillary Urothelial Hyperplasia
- Villous Adenoma
- Intestinal Metaplasia with Low-Grade Dysplasia
- Urothelial Papilloma
- Inverted Papilloma
- Condyloma Acuminatum of Bladder
- Papillary Urothelial Neoplasm of Low Malignant Potential (PUNLMP)

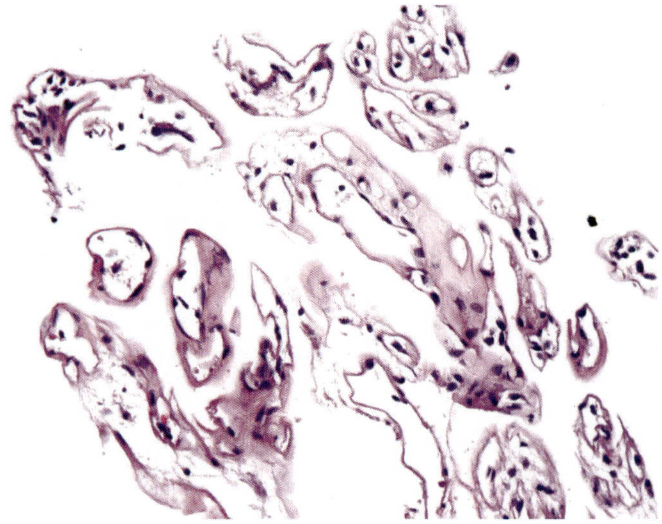

Figure 5.1 — Denuded papillae, histologic section. Prior instrumentation or shedding of cells from a high-grade urothelial carcinoma may cause a papillary neoplasm to lose the epithelial cells, and what remains are naked or denuded fibrovascular cores. Unless these are recognized as the residual fibrovascular cores of a papillary neoplasm, the biopsy or sometimes resection may be falsely called "negative." More often, high-grade lesions have dyscohesive cells, which slough off readily, but low-grade lesions may lose their epithelium particularly after instrumentation (H&E stain, medium power).

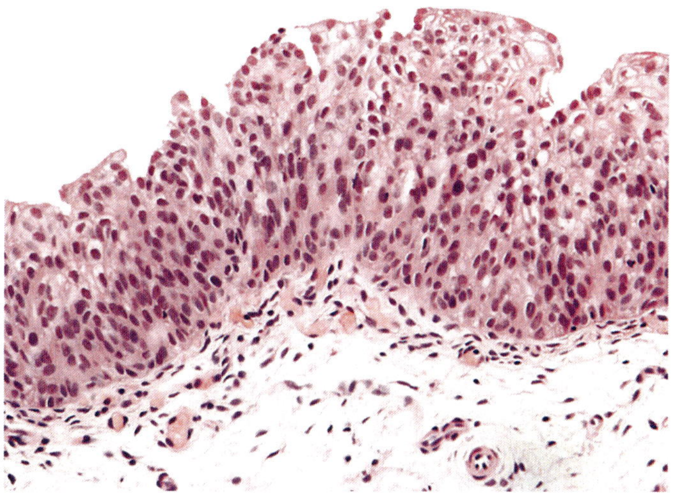

Figure 5.2 — Urothelial dysplasia, histologic section. This is a low-grade lesion and is most often seen in patients with a history of cancer on a follow-up biopsy or in resection specimens for carcinoma. Urothelium is usually intact and is of normal thickness with maintained polarity. There are occasional hyperchromatic enlarged nuclei seen among normal-appearing cells. Scattered mitotic figures may be seen at all levels of the urothelium (H&E stain, medium power).

Figure 5.3 — Papillary urothelial hyperplasia, histologic section. This lesion is most often seen adjacent to a papillary tumor. This may represent a precursor to low-grade papillary tumors. The urothelium is thrown into folds with a tented appearance. At the base of some folds capillaries are seen reaching upwards. The urothelium may be of normal thickness as seen in this image, or could be thicker than usual (H&E stain, low power).

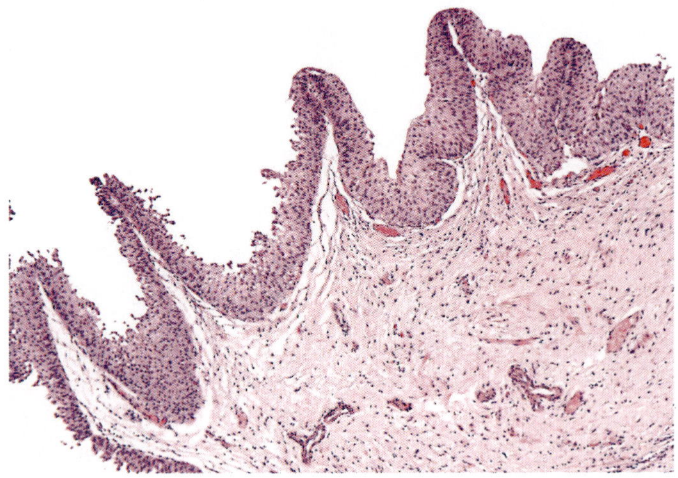

Figure 5.4 — Papillary urothelial hyperplasia with dysplasia, histologic section. This low-power image shows the undulations of papillary urothelial hyperplasia. Capillaries are seen at the base of the tented urothelium, making early fibrovascular cores. As mentioned earlier, these lesions are commonly seen adjacent to papillary tumors. A well-formed papillary frond is seen at the bottom of the image (H&E stain, low power).

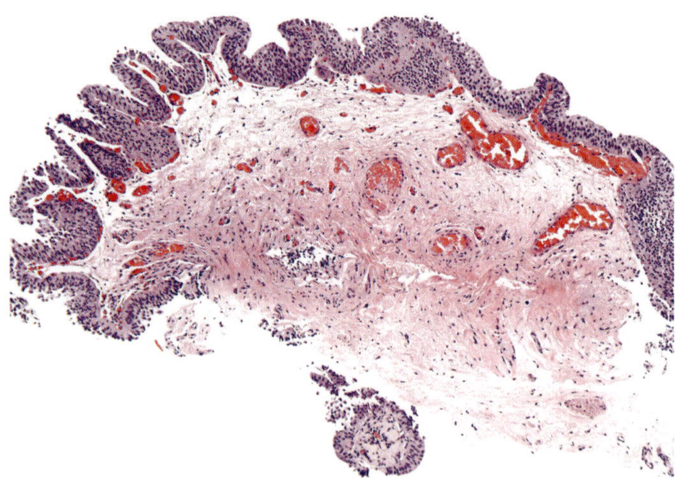

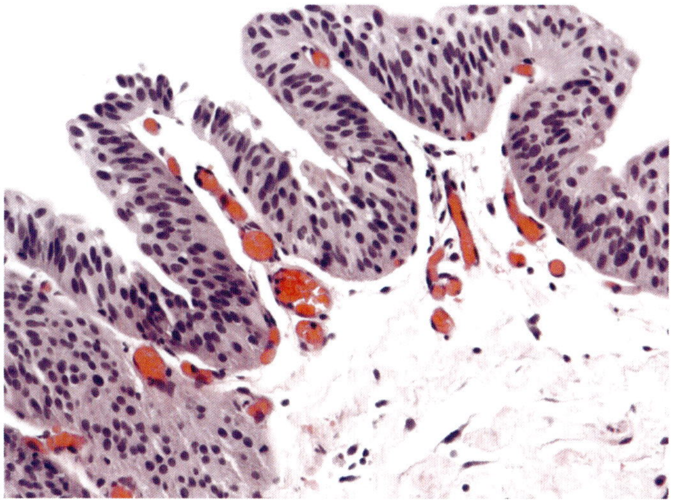

Figure 5.5 — Papillary urothelial hyperplasia with dysplasia, histologic section. Scattered enlarged, hyperchromatic cells are visible. The rest of the urothelium has retained polarity and cohesiveness. These are features of dysplasia, similar to what is seen in low-grade papillary carcinoma (H&E stain, medium power).

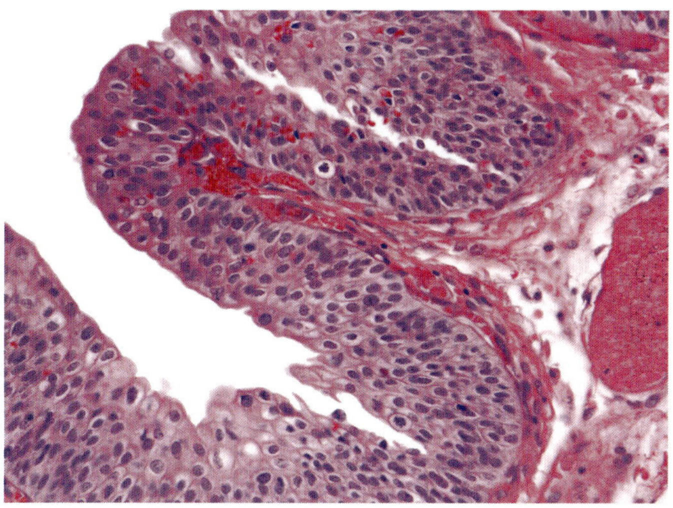

Figure 5.6 — Papillary urothelial hyperplasia with dysplasia, histologic section. Another example with scattered normal appearing mitotic figures seen at all levels of the urothelium. This lesion represents the precursor to low-grade papillary urothelial carcinoma (H&E stain, high power).

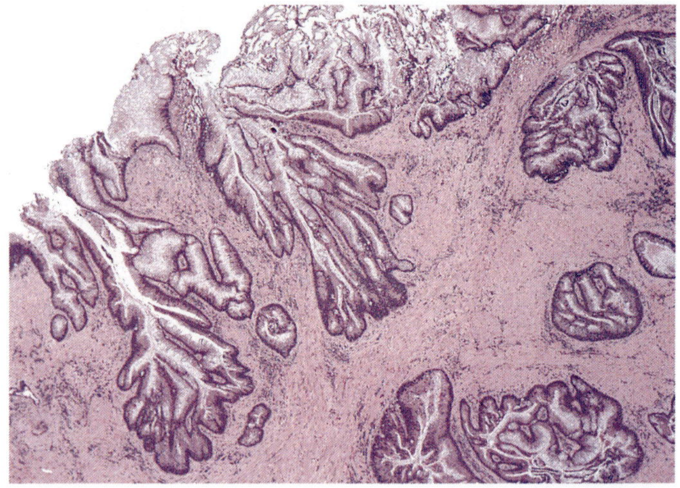

Figure 5.7 — Villous adenoma, histologic section. Villous adenomas have inherent low-grade dysplasia similar to that seen in its counterpart in the bowel. Villous adenomas have been reported to arise within the bladder, prostatic urethra, or the urachus. Patients present with hematuria and irritative symptoms. This image is of a villous adenoma of the urachus. The adenomatous glands are seen within the muscle layers of the bladder wall (pseudoinvasion). There are fingerlike villi and glandular spaces lined by pseudostratified columnar epithelium (H&E stain, low power).

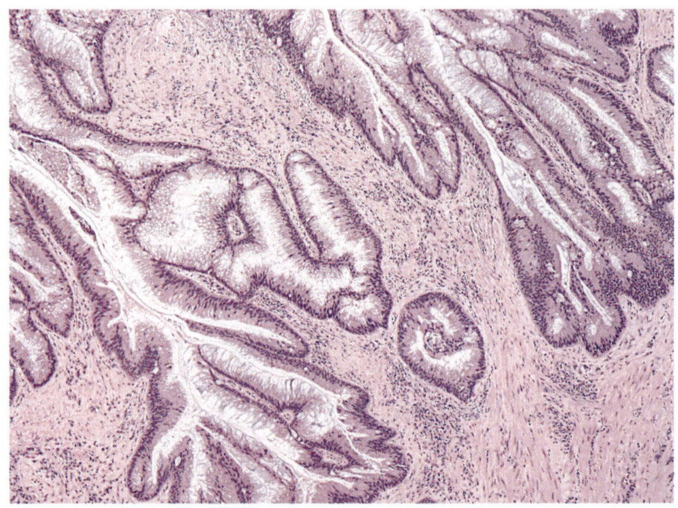

Figure 5.8 — Villous adenoma, histologic section. Higher magnification with epithelial cell nuclear stratification, nuclear crowding, and hyperchromasia. These lesions may show occasional prominent nucleoli and mitotic figures. Mucin is seen within the lumina. Thorough sampling of the tissue received is imperative to look for associated high-grade dysplasia or in-situ or infiltrating adenocarcinoma. Complete resection of villous adenoma is recommended. These have an excellent prognosis as long as no associated infiltrating carcinoma is present (H&E stain, medium power).

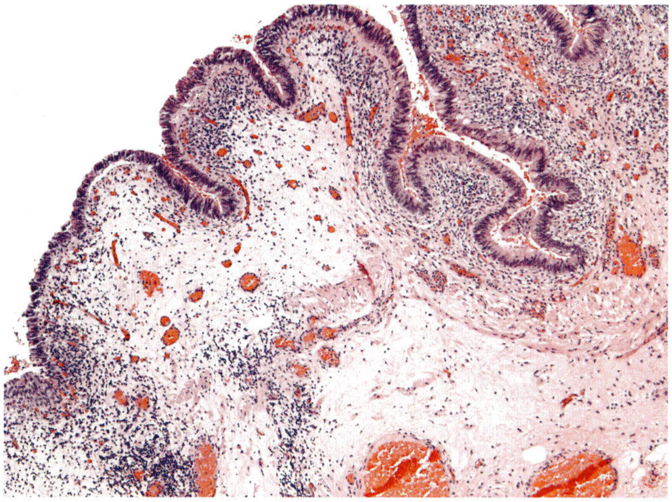

Figure 5.9 — Intestinal metaplasia with low-grade dysplasia, histologic section. Surface urothelium is replaced by intestinal metaplasia with low-grade dysplasia. The nuclei are elongated, pseudostratified, and hyperchromatic (H&E stain, low power).

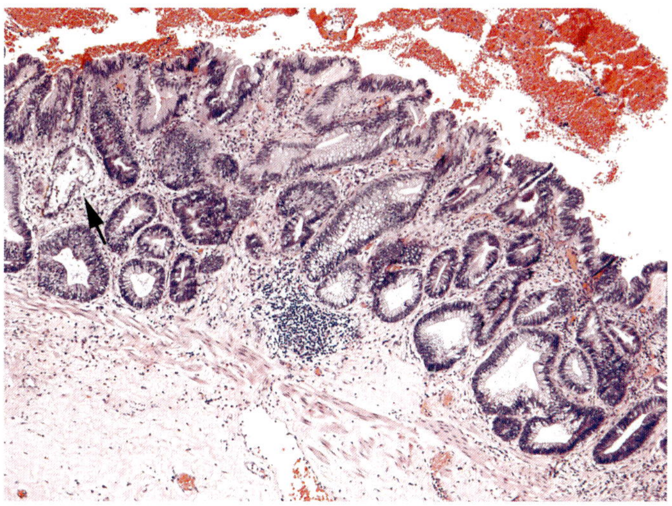

Figure 5.10 — Intestinal metaplasia with low-grade dysplasia, histologic section. Low grade dysplasia is evident in this lesion similar to that seen in gastrointestinal tract adenomas. The glandular spaces are lined by pseudostratified columnar epithelium. The architecture is also becoming complex. A residual nondysplastic gland is seen (arrow). Low-grade dysplasia can progress into high-grade dysplasia or adenocarcinoma in-situ and eventually infiltrating adenocarcinoma (H&E stain, low power).

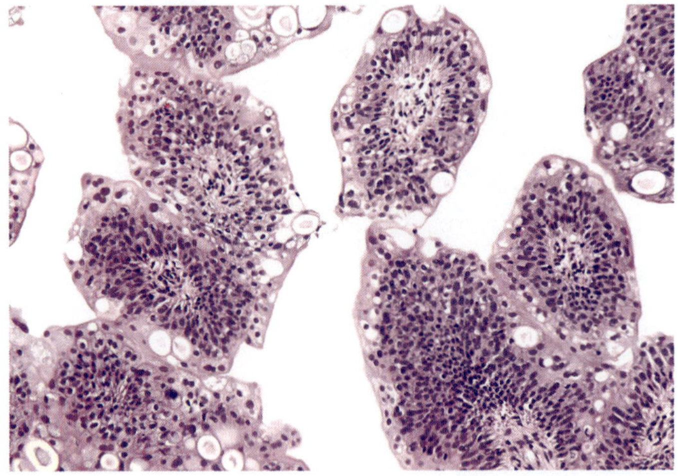

Figure 5.11 — Urothelial papilloma, histologic section. These are considered benign papillary urothelial neoplasms. According to the WHO (2003) ISUP system, the diagnosis of papilloma requires the fibrovascular cores lined by urothelium that resembles normal urothelium. These are usually small unifocal lesions. There is minimal branching, and the cells lining the papillary fronds are cohesive. In this case, the umbrella cells have prominent cytoplasmic vacuolization (H&E stain, low power).

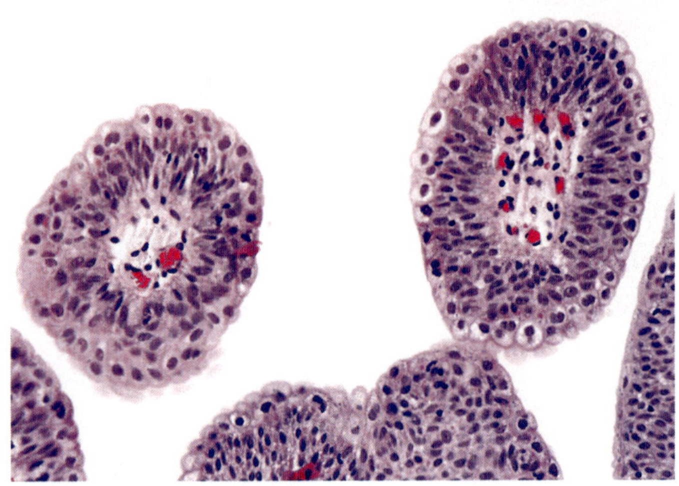

Figure 5.12 — Urothelial papilloma, histologic section. This papilloma has a prominent cuboidal umbrella cell layer. The urothelium is of normal thickness and the cells are bland with maintained polarity; nuclear grooves are also present. Cellular atypia excludes the diagnosis of urothelial papilloma (H&E stain, medium power).

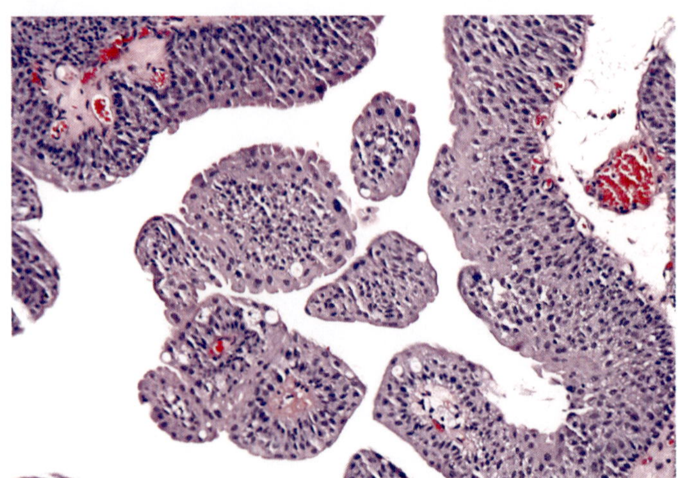

Figure 5.13 — Urothelial papilloma, histologic section. This papilloma has a prominent umbrella cell layer. The rest of the cells lining the fibrovascular cores are uniform and bland (H&E stain, low power).

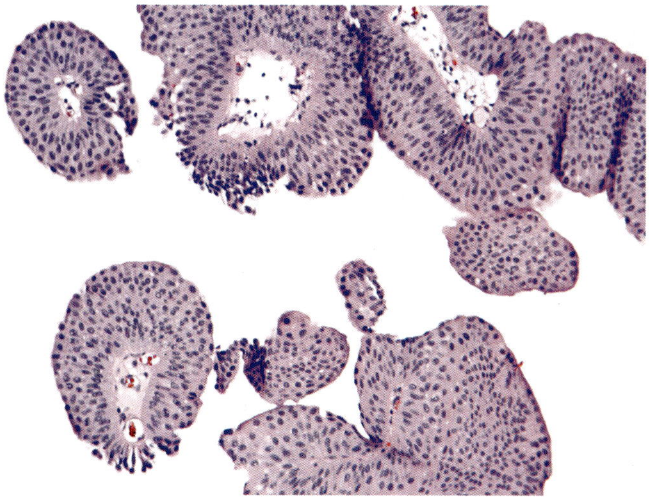

Figure 5.14 — Urothelial papilloma, histologic section. These are rare lesions, and most of them do not recur following excision (H&E stain, low power).

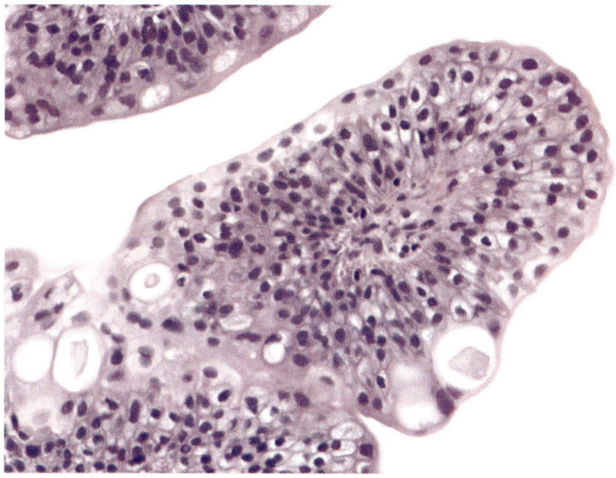

Figure 5.15 — Urothelial papilloma, histologic section. Well-formed fibrovascular cores are lined by normal-appearing urothelium (H&E stain, medium power).

Figure 5.16 — Inverted papilloma, histologic section. Inverted papillomas are considered benign lesions. The surface is smooth with minimal if any exophytic growth; urothelium grows inwards with interconnected cords, trabeculae, and sometimes nests. The stroma is delicate without any inflammation. The cords are made up of uniform cells that stream towards the center and are palisaded at the edges (H&E stain, low power).

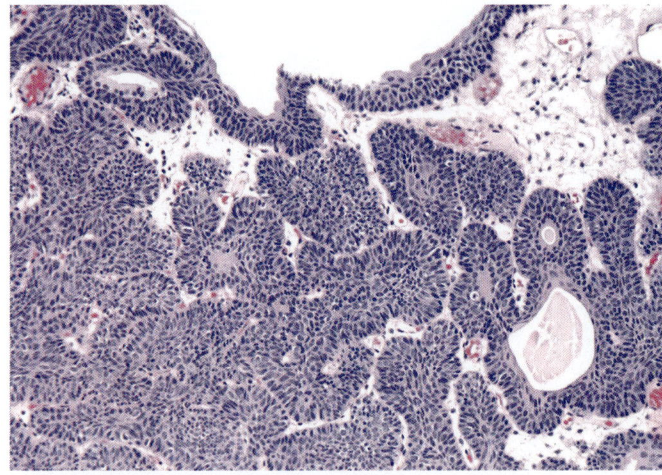

Figure 5.17 — Inverted papilloma, histologic section. Interanastomosing cords of inverted papilloma with streaming uniform nuclei. The stroma is delicate and edematous. These rare lesions comprise about one percent of the neoplasms involving the bladder. The presenting symptom is hematuria, with a male predilection (H&E stain, medium power).

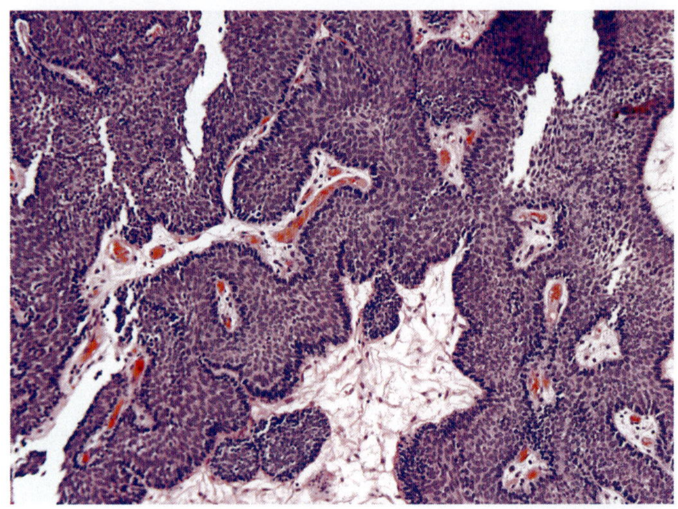

Figure 5.18 — Inverted papilloma, histologic section. Close-up view shows the grooved, uniform nuclei and the typical peripheral palisading. These outer cells represent the basal cells (H&E stain, high power).

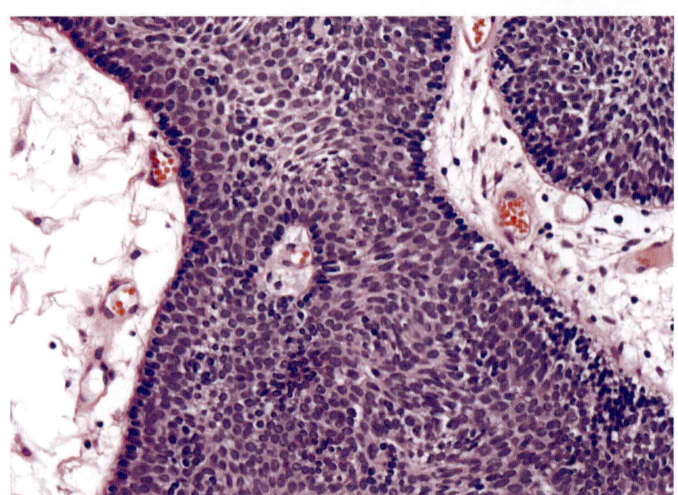

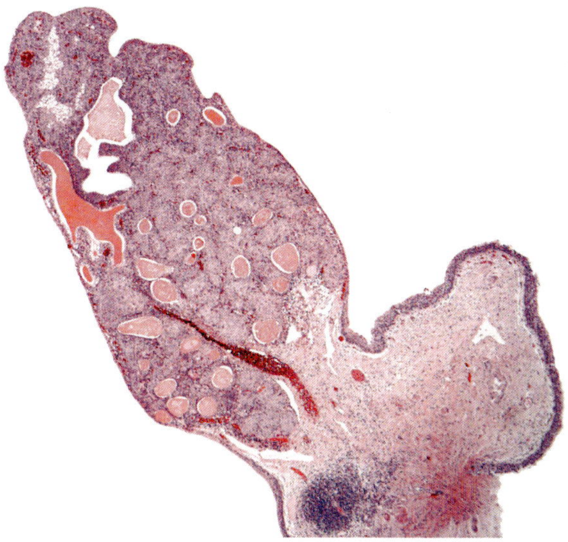

Figure 5.19 — Inverted papilloma, histologic section. These are usually solitary lesions with a pedunculated, smooth-surfaced, gross appearance. This low power image shows an entire small inverted papilloma. Typical features of an inverted papilloma helpful in establishing a diagnosis include: smooth surface, circumscribed lesion without infiltrative growth, minimal to absent cytological atypia (H&E stain, low power).

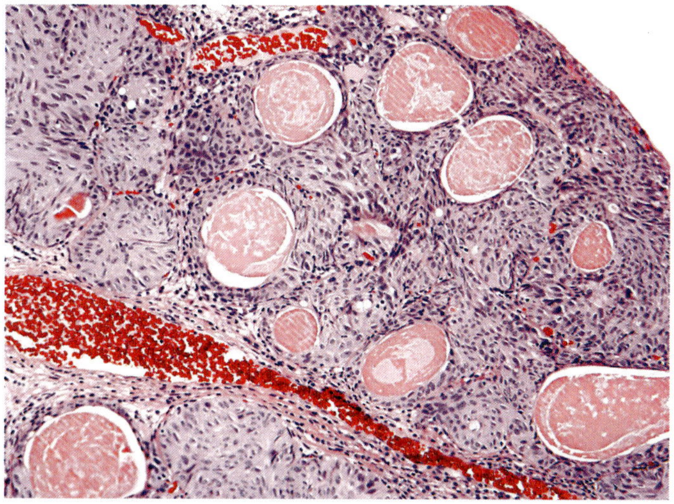

Figure 5.20 — Inverted papilloma, histologic section. This higher power image shows colloid cyst formation in addition to nests of streaming cells with bland ovoid nuclei (H&E stain, medium power).

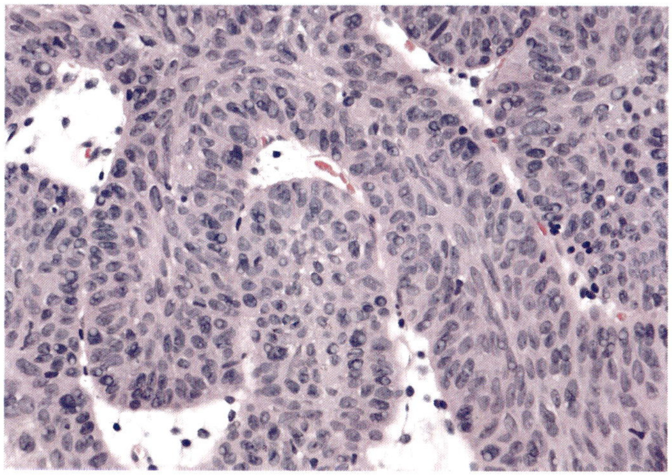

Figure 5.21 — Inverted papilloma, histologic section. There may be squamoid features within the trabeculae or nests of inverted papilloma; however, these are without keratinization. In contrast, papillary urothelial carcinoma may have squamous differentiation with keratinization (H&E stain, high power).

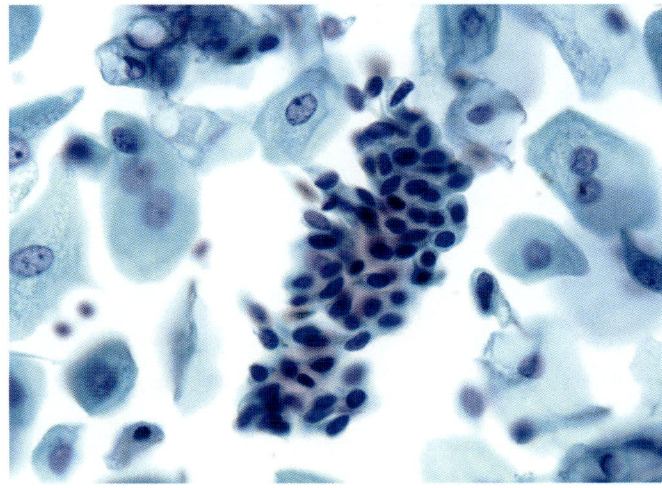

Figure 5.22 — Inverted papilloma, voided urine. This haphazardly arranged cluster of urothelial cells has characteristics of a low-grade urothelial lesion, characterized by opaque and distinct cytoplasm, high N/C ratios, and oval nuclei with darkened chromatin. The actual diagnosis of inverted papilloma cannot be made on cytology and relies on tissue correlation (Papanicolaou stain, high power).

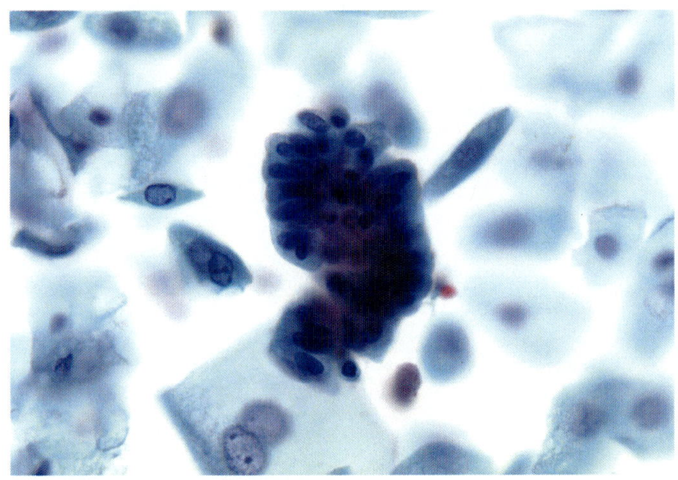

Figure 5.23 — Inverted papilloma, voided urine. This compact fragment of urothelial cells has well-defined cytoplasmic boundaries and oval nuclei with high N/C ratios. Although the tissue follow-up is inverted papilloma, the cytologic diagnosis should be strictly limited and interpreted as "suspicious for a low-grade urothelial lesion." Additionally, the presence of a tissue fragment in this voided urine sample is an abnormal finding and should raise a red flag for a urothelial lesion (Papanicolaou stain, high power).

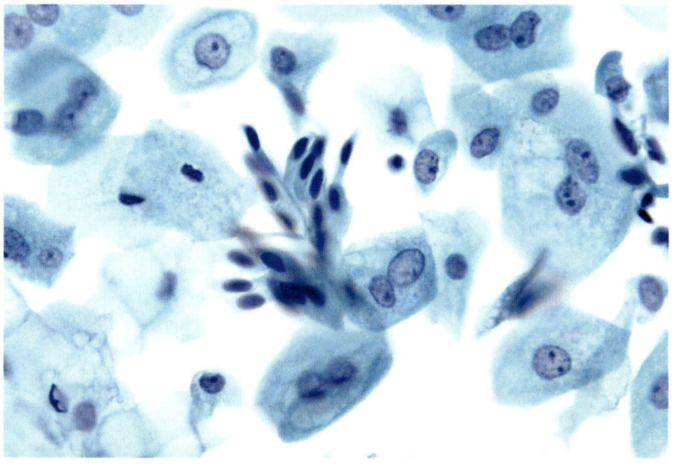

Figure 5.24 — Inverted papilloma, voided urine. Columnar-appearing cells are dissociated but in close contact with each other by filamented cytoplasmic processes. This characteristic is frequently seen in low-grade urothelial lesions, including inverted papilloma. However, that diagnosis is made only on tissue; the cytologic interpretation of this particular sample should be "atypical urothelial cells consistent with low-grade urothelial lesion" (Papanicolaou stain, high power).

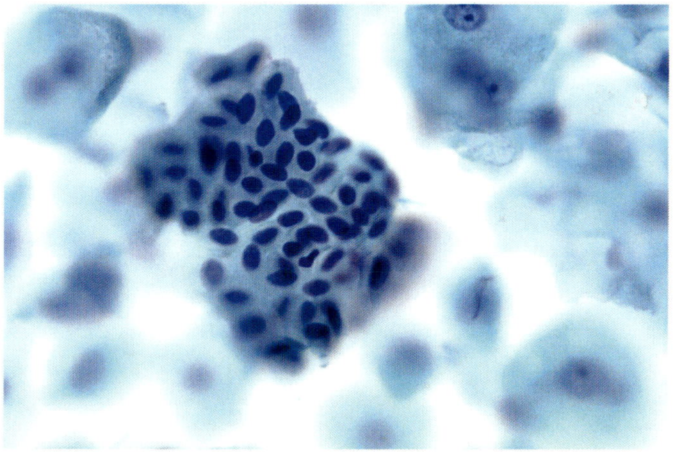

Figure 5.25 — Inverted papilloma, voided urine. This group of urothelial cells has characteristics of a low-grade lesion, complete with uniform oval nuclei, high N/C ratios, haphazard arrangement, and even moderately dark chromatin. Cytoplasmic borders are well defined (Papanicolaou stain, high power).

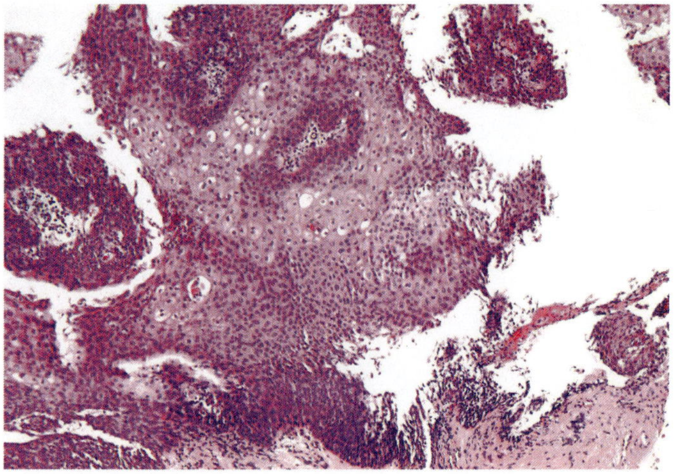

Figure 5.26 — Condyloma acuminatum of bladder, histologic section. Condyloma acuminatum, a human papilloma virus (HPV) associated sexually transmitted disease of the urinary bladder is a rare lesion. Involvement of the bladder as extension of condylomata of the external genitalia and urethra is the common pathway. As seen in this image, fibrovascular cores are lined by squamous epithelium with clear cytoplasm. These can be focal or diffusely involve the bladder urothelium, causing hematuria or irritative symptoms for the patient (H&E stain, low power).

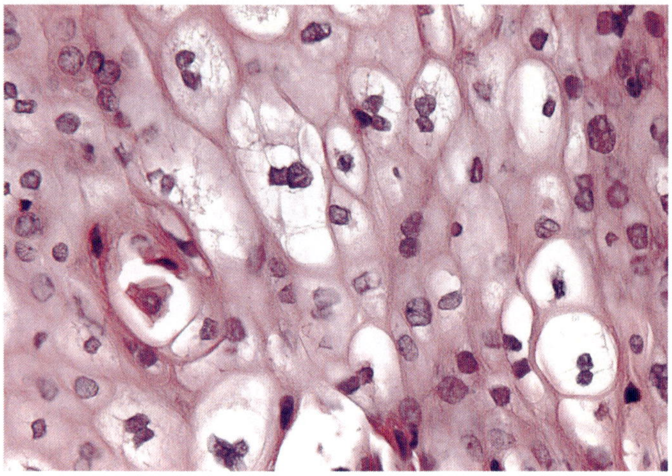

Figure 5.27 — Condyloma acuminatum of bladder, histologic section. Higher magnification shows wrinkled nuclei with surrounding halo in some of the virus-affected cells (koilocytes). Condyloma of the bladder can give rise to squamous cell carcinoma. Focal lesions can be managed by transurethral resection; for diffuse involvement of the bladder, a more radical procedure may be required (H&E stain, high power).

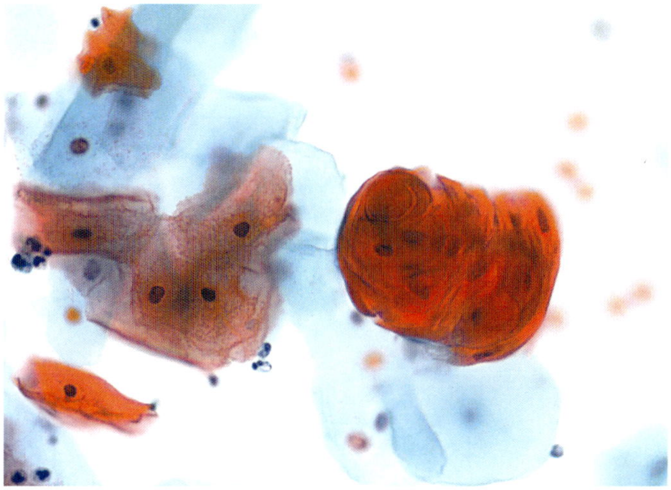

Figure 5.28 — Condyloma acuminatum of bladder, voided urine. Bladder condylomata are uncommonly encountered in urinary cytology. These lesions release cells singly or in clusters and may display overt characteristics of HPV infection, including hyperkeratosis and parakeratosis. Most classic for this group of cells is the hyperchromasia and irregular nuclear shapes in addition to the keratinized and very opaque cytoplasm of each cell (Papanicolaou stain, high power).

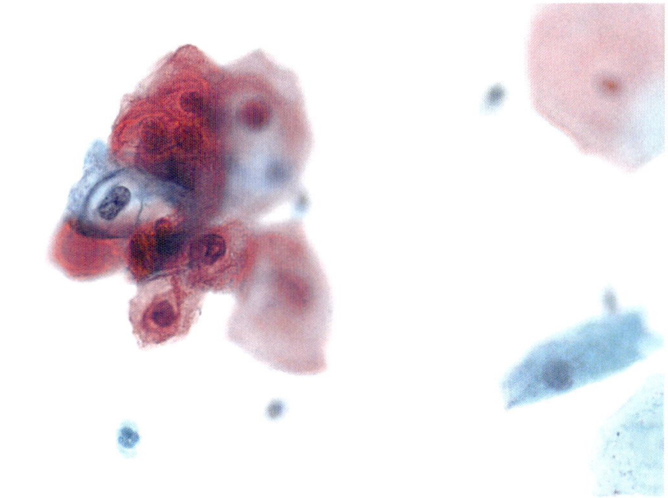

Figure 5.29 — Condyloma acuminatum of bladder, voided urine. HPV-related koilocytic changes can be quite apparent in urine samples of bladder condylomata. Note enlarged nuclei with smudgy chromatin and well-formed large perinuclear cytoplasmic halo (Papanicolaou stain, high power).

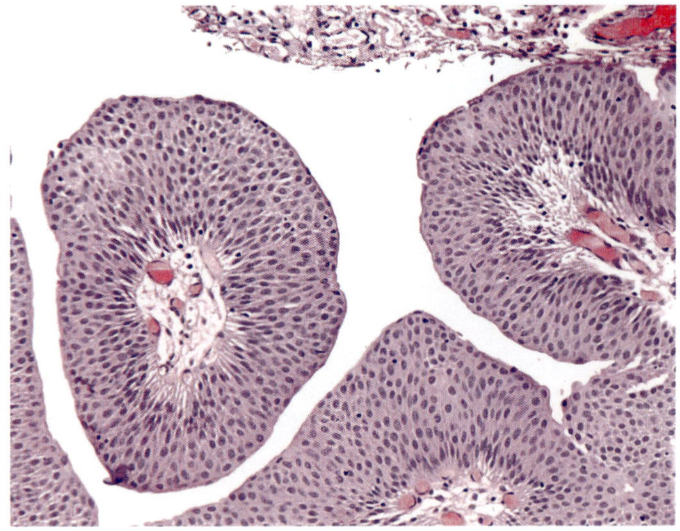

Figure 5.30 — Papillary urothelial neoplasm of low malignant potential (PUNLMP), histologic section. PUNLMP category was introduced in the WHO (2003) ISUP system. This papillary neoplasm has fibrovascular cores that are lined by bland-appearing urothelium, which is thicker than is seen in papilloma. The nuclei may be only slightly enlarged but maintain polarity (H&E stain, medium power).

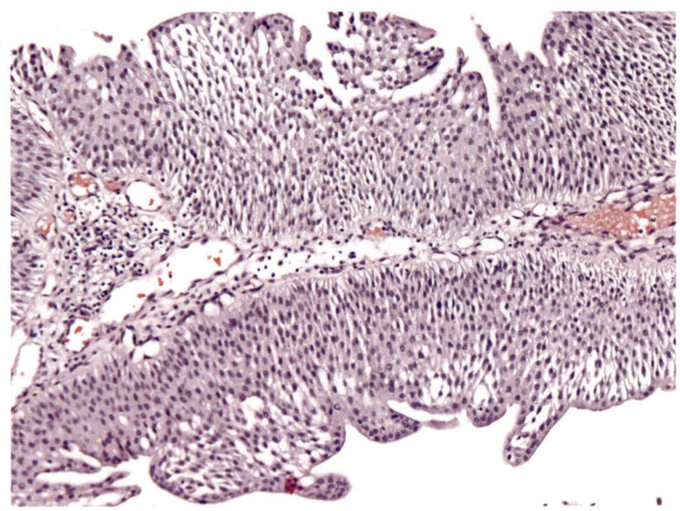

Figure 5.31 — PUNLMP, histologic section. There is orderly arrangement of the nuclei, with only rare basal mitosis; nuclear grooves may be present, as seen in benign urothelium (H&E stain, low power).

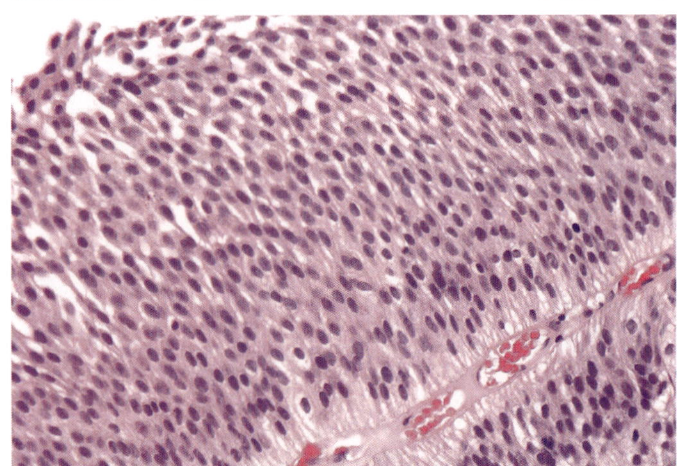

Figure 5.32 — PUNLMP, histologic section. High-power image of PUNLMP, the chromatin of the nuclei is uniform (H&E stain, high power).

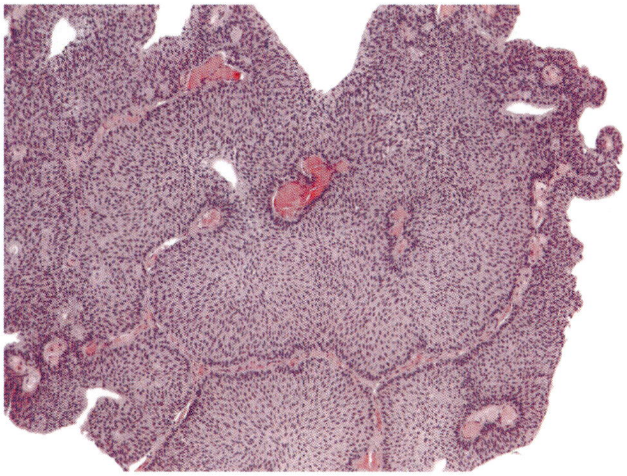

Figure 5.33 — PUNLMP, histologic section. Occasionally in PUNLMP the cells appear to stream (H&E stain, low power).

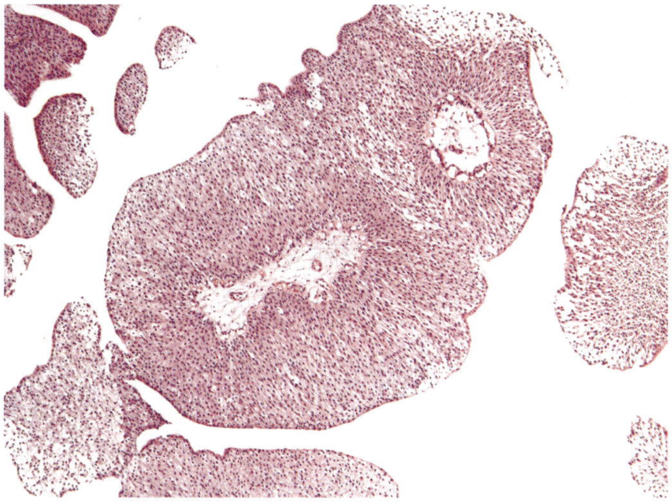

Figure 5.34 — PUNLMP, histologic section. The cells are uniform with maintained polarity and identical appearance. There is much thicker urothelial lining than in urothelial papilloma (H&E stain, low power).

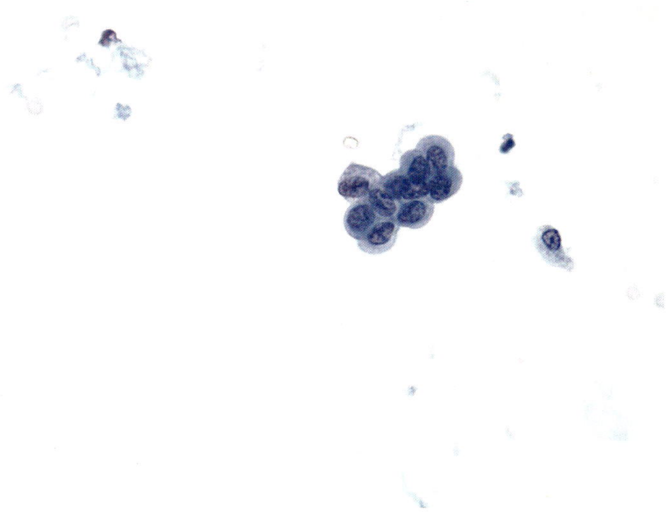

Figure 5.35 — PUNLMP, voided urine. This is usually a retrospective diagnosis, correlated with the subsequent tissue biopsy. The most telling characteristics of this particular cell group include high N/C ratios, irregular nuclear outlines, and loss of polarity. The cell size is small, indicating a low-grade urothelial lesion (Papanicolaou stain, medium power).

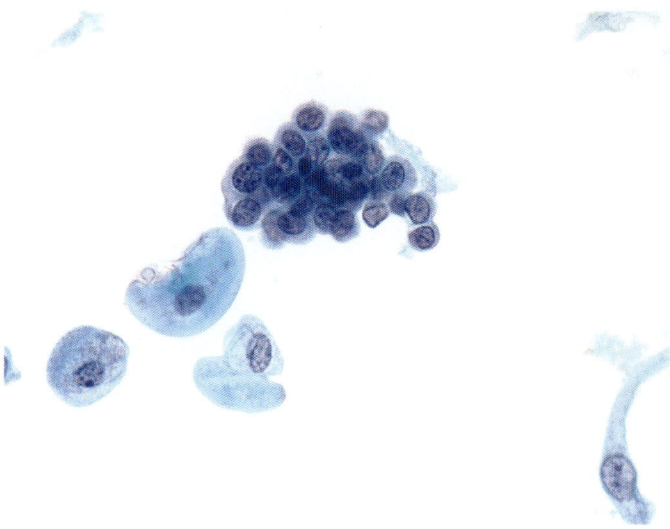

Figure 5.36 — PUNLMP, voided urine. PUNLMP is usually *not* a prospective diagnosis in urinary cytology. The cells in this photograph suggest a low-grade urothelial neoplasm characterized by haphazard orientation, oval nuclei, and opaque cytoplasm (Papanicolaou stain, medium power).

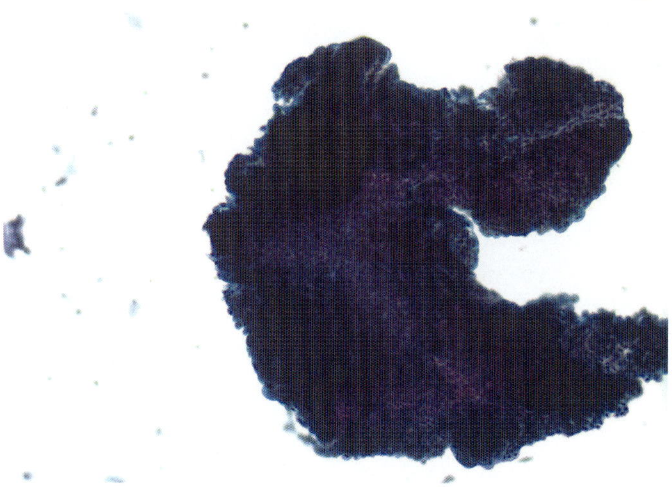

Figure 5.37 — PUNLMP, instrumented urine. A very large fragment of a papillary lesion is thick enough to make light transmission very difficult. The central fibrovascular core can be appreciated, however, and small nuclear size is suggested at the periphery of the large fragment (Papanicolaou stain, low power).

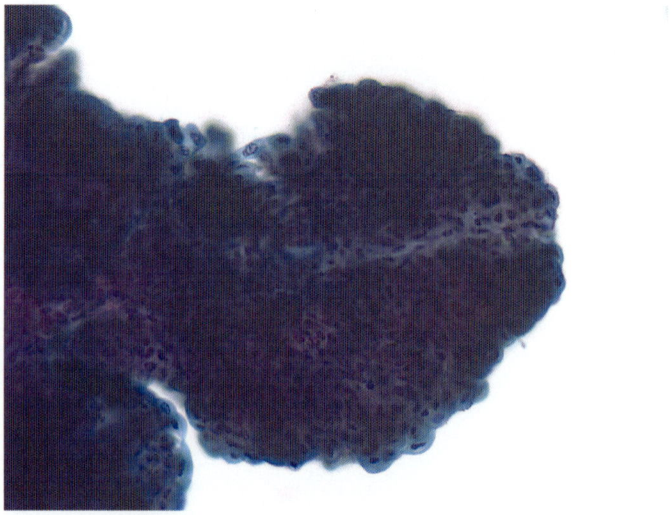

Figure 5.38 — PUNLMP, instrumented urine. A higher-power photograph of the previous case confirms the very low grade of this papillary lesion (Papanicolaou stain, medium power).

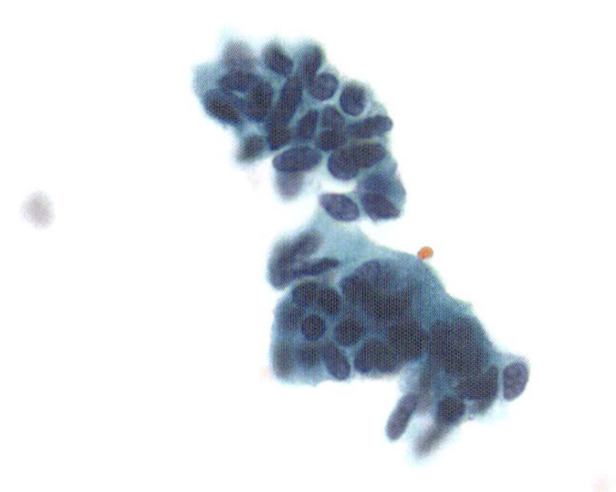

Figure 5.39 — PUNLMP, voided urine. The two tissue fragments in this voided urine depict fairly uniform small cells with round to oval nuclei suggesting a low-grade urothelial lesion. However, tissue verification is essential in all such cases (Papanicolaou stain, medium power).

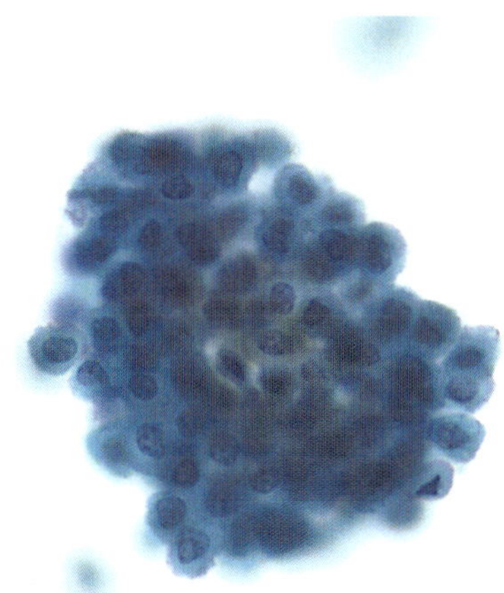

Figure 5.40 — PUNLMP, voided urine. An aggregate of urothelial cells displays neoplastic characteristics of irregular nuclear chromatin. However their round nuclear shapes and small size suggest a very low-grade lesion (Papanicolaou stain, high power).

Urothelial Atypia

6

- Atypical Urothelial Cells/Fragments, NOS
- Atypical Urothelial Cells, Cannot Exclude a High-grade Urothelial Carcinoma

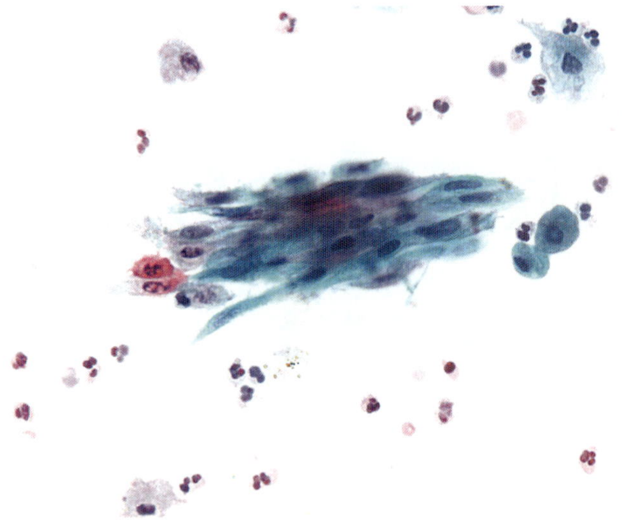

Figure 6.1 — Atypical urothelial cells, voided urine. (Follow-up: benign) Reactive changes are the same in the bladder as in any place else in the body, assuming a squamoid appearance. N/C ratio should be low and polarity preserved, or else a neoplasm should be considered. Usually, the reactive cells are accompanied by inflammation, as in this photograph (Papanicolaou stain, medium power).

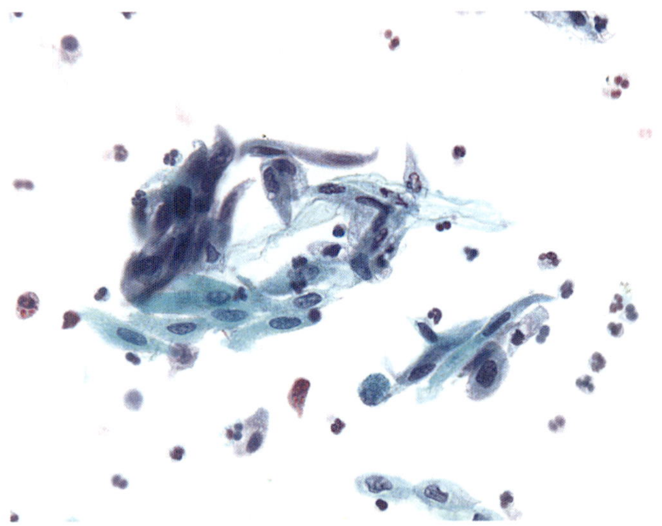

Figure 6.2 — Atypical urothelial cells, voided urine. (Follow-up: benign) Bipolar cells with low N/C ratios are the classic reparative changes seen in the bladder as elsewhere. Nuclear chromatin is slightly granular, but the low N/C ratios and preserved polarity confirm the benign process. Acute inflammation accompanies these changes (Papanicolaou stain, medium power).

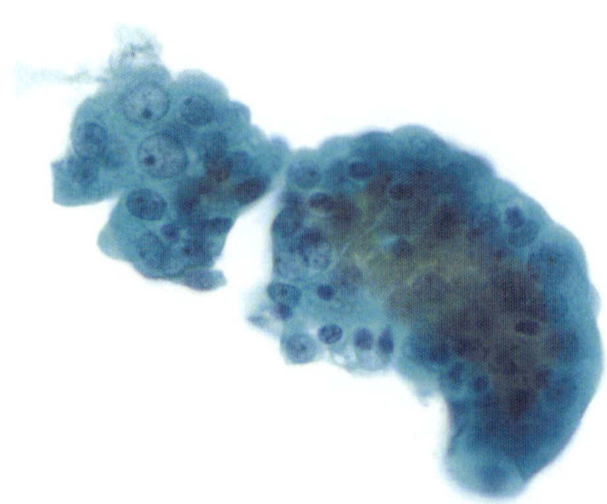

Figure 6.3 — Atypical urothelial cells, voided urine. (Follow-up: benign with bladder calculi). The usual reactive changes in the bladder subsequent to stone formation vary. Usually, benign urothelial cells, often in fragments (as in this case of voided urine), will contain a prominent central nucleolus in a round nucleus. Occasional cells will have hyperchromatic and degenerated nuclei, suggesting neoplasia. Calculi frequently accompany neoplastic lesions, a conundrum of urologic cytopathology (Papanicolaou stain, high power).

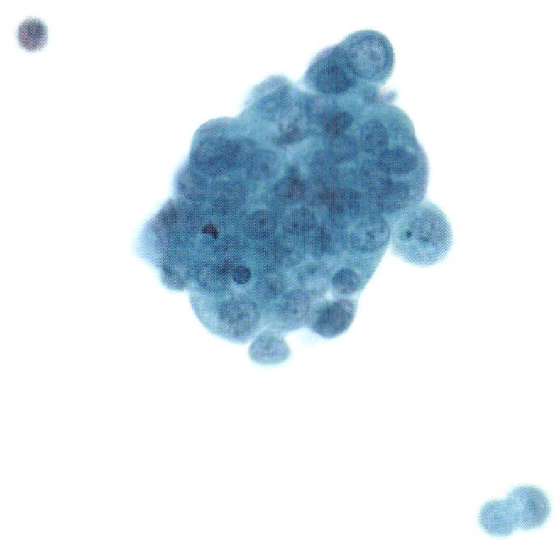

Figure 6.4 — Atypical urothelial cells, voided urine. (Follow-up: benign with bladder calculi). Another group of urothelial cells from a patient who had passed a stone. The prominent nucleoli and inflammatory cells within the fragment are typical reactive changes. Also, groups of urothelial cells in a voided urine without instrumentation may indicate neoplasia. Sometimes clusters of renal tubular epithelial cells can be mistaken for clusters of small urothelial cells. A true tissue fragment will have shared cell borders. Approximately 20 percent of all voided urines with benign follow-up will have small fragments of spontaneously exfoliated urothelium (Papanicolaou stain, high power).

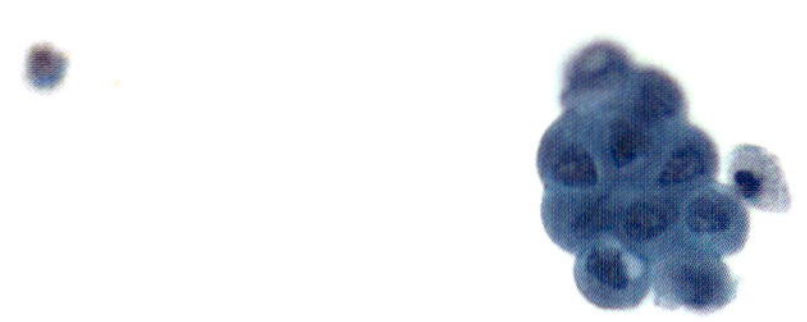

Figure 6.5 — Atypical urothelial fragments, voided urine. (Follow-up: low-grade urothelial carcinoma). Groups of small urothelial cells may be perfectly benign but also may be seen in patients with low-grade urothelial lesions. Frequent surveillance of a patient with spontaneously exfoliated fragments is prudent to rule out a neoplasm from the urinary tract. The low-grade lesions are not life threatening, so time may be allowed to pass before intervention is considered (Papanicolaou stain, high power).

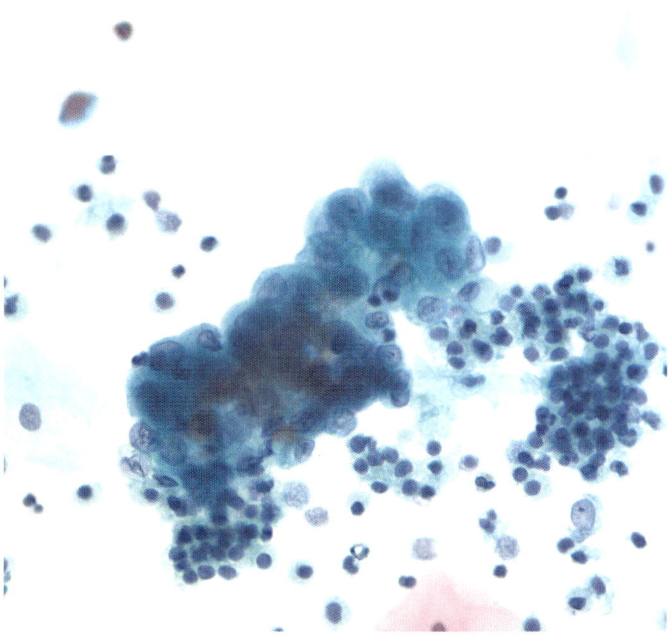

Figure 6.6 — Atypical urothelial fragments, voided urine. (Follow-up: low-grade urothelial carcinoma). Fragments of umbrella cells with underlying basal cells attached are rarely seen spontaneously exfoliated. They almost always are a result of instrumentation. Assessment of the basal cells for atypia is crucial to an accurate diagnosis (Papanicolaou stain, high power).

Figure 6.7 — Atypical urothelial fragments, voided urine. (Follow-up: low-grade urothelial carcinoma). Careful inspection of nuclear morphology in tissue fragments may suggest a neoplasm rather than a benign process. This group of cells has oval shaped nuclei, irregular nuclear outlines and granular chromatin. A low-grade carcinoma should be suspected (Papanicolaou stain, high power).

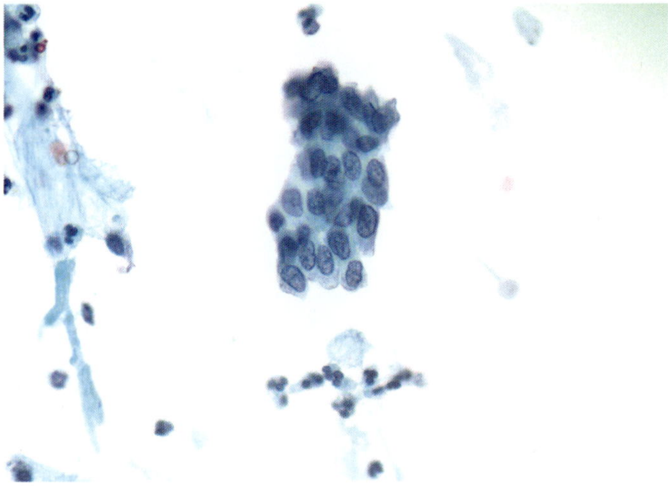

Figure 6.8 — Atypical urothelial fragments, voided urine. (Follow-up: low-grade urothelial carcinoma). When inspecting a tissue fragment in a voided urine, carefully focusing through the group will reveal the true N/C ratios, critical to deciding whether or not the fragment is significant. In this group, nuclear membrane irregularity and granular nuclear chromatin makes a low-grade lesion suspect (Papanicolaou stain, high power).

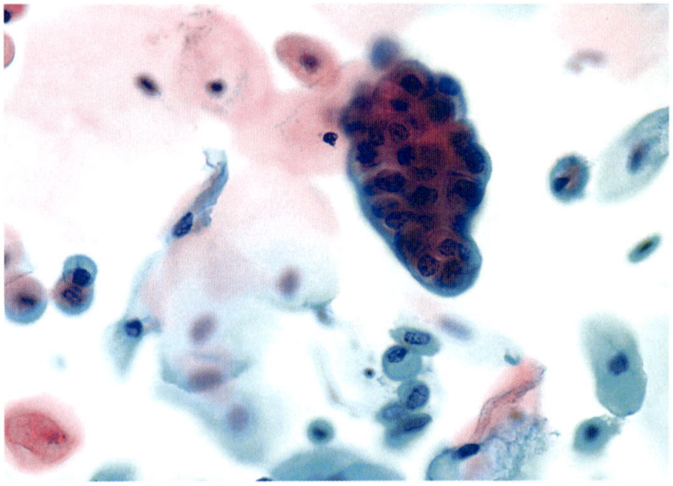

Figure 6.9 — Atypical urothelial fragments, voided urine. (Follow-up: low-grade urothelial carcinoma). Although this tissue fragment is covered by umbrella cells, the variation in nuclear size of the basal cells and the disorganization within the fragment are suggestive of a neoplasm (Papanicolaou stain, medium power).

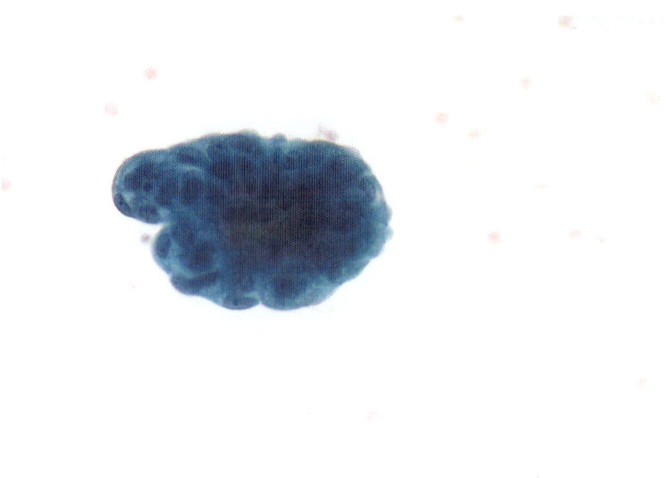

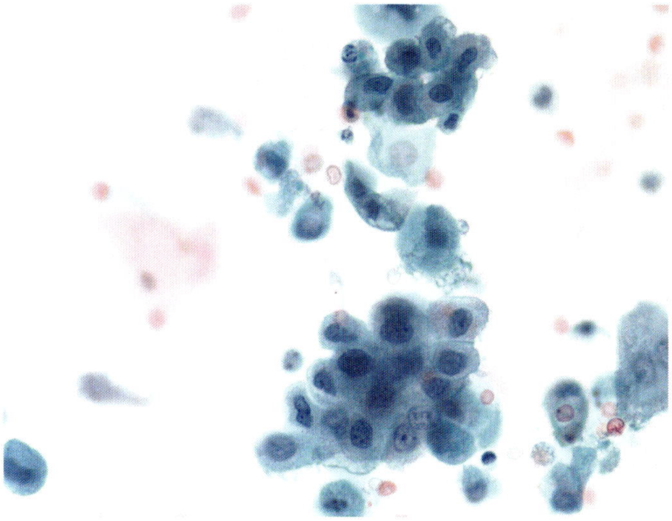

Figure 6.10 — Atypical urothelial cells, voided urine. (Follow-up: low-grade urothelial carcinoma). These two groups of urothelial cells are distinctly abnormal, although the nuclei themselves are relatively small and N/C ratios are only moderately increased. The irregular nuclear outlines and hyperchromasia of the nuclei are ominous features (Papanicolaou stain, high power).

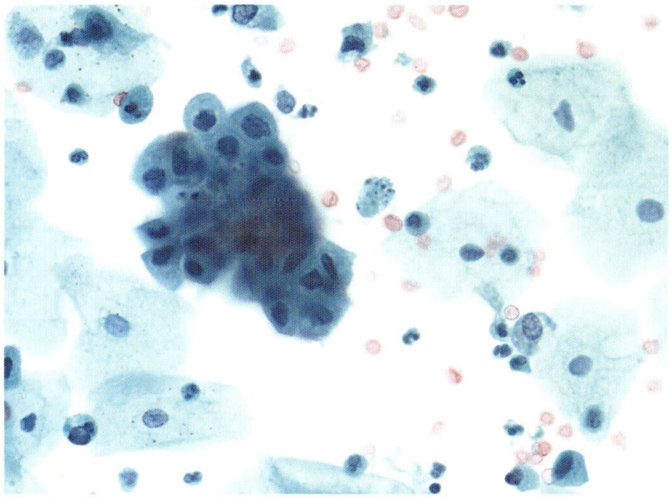

Figure 6.11 — Atypical urothelial cells, voided urine. (Follow-up: low-grade urothelial carcinoma). Although degeneration can produce hyperchromatic nuclei with irregular shapes, the cells in question should be compared with the well-preserved urothelial or squamous cells in the same sample. This group of cells has distinctly abnormal nuclei, but only moderately increased nuclear cytoplasmic ratios. They are strongly suspicious for a neoplastic process (Papanicolaou stain, high power).

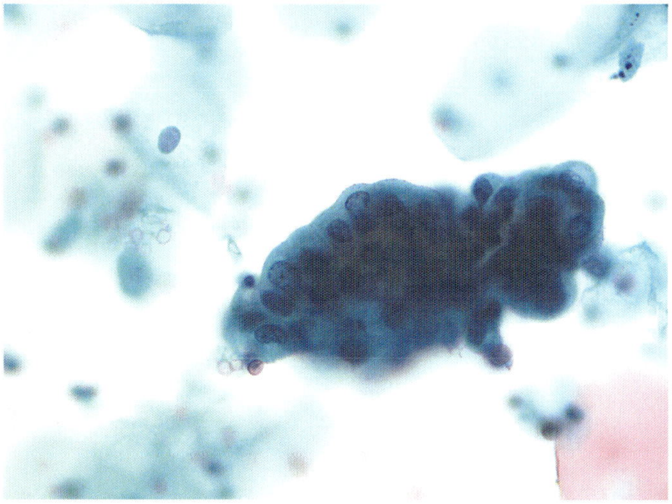

Figure 6.12 — Atypical urothelial fragments, voided urine. (Follow-up: low-grade urothelial carcinoma). Despite the presence of umbrella cells on the surface of the fragment, a neoplasm cannot be excluded based on the atypical nuclear shapes and dark chromatin of the basal cells (Papanicolaou stain, high power).

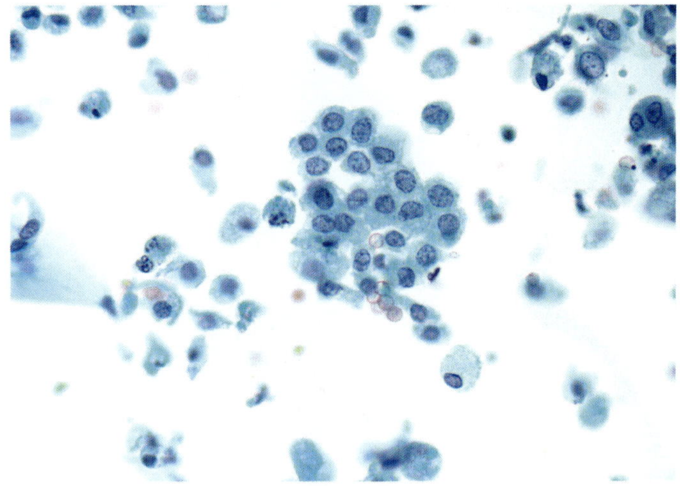

Figure 6.13 — Atypical urothelial cells, voided urine. (Follow-up: low-grade urothelial carcinoma). Only mild atypia is present in this case. Some low-grade lesions are so cytologically bland that careful search of the urine does not reveal any discernable abnormalities, as in this case. Such samples account for the poor sensitivity of urine cytology for detecting low-grade lesions (Papanicolaou stain, medium power).

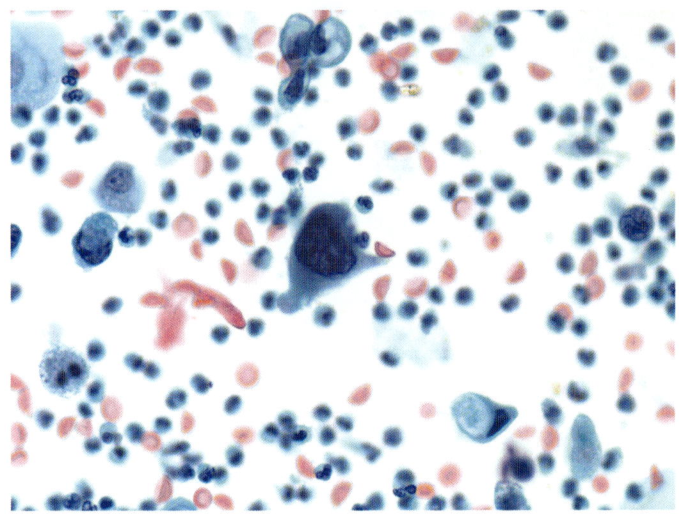

Figure 6.14 — Atypical urothelial cells cannot exclude a high-grade carcinoma, voided urine. (Follow-up: high-grade urothelial carcinoma). Within a severely inflamed sample, rare markedly atypical cells may be disregarded as reactive; however, the cell in the center of the photograph should not be ignored, and an interpretation of at least suspicious for high-grade carcinoma is indicated. Other cells in the field are also suspect based on their hyperchromatic nuclei and abnormal shapes (Papanicolaou stain, high power).

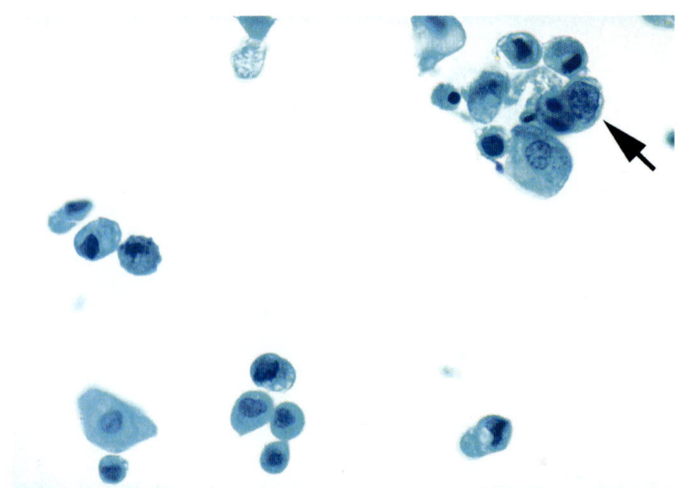

Figure 6.15 — Atypical urothelial cells cannot exclude a high-grade carcinoma, voided urine. (Follow-up: high-grade urothelial carcinoma). Contrary to expectation, some high-grade lesions shed small cells with highly atypical nuclei, as in this case. Only one cell has an enlarged nucleus with malignant characteristics (arrow). An interpretation of "suspicious for high-grade urothelial lesion" should be considered when small cells with very atypical hyperchromatic nuclei are present in the sample (Papanicolaou stain, high power).

7

Urothelial Carcinoma

- Low-grade Papillary Carcinoma
- High-grade Papillary Carcinoma
- Flat Urothelial Carcinoma In-situ
- Invasive Urothelial Carcinoma
- Urothelial Carcinoma in Ileal Loop (Neobladder)

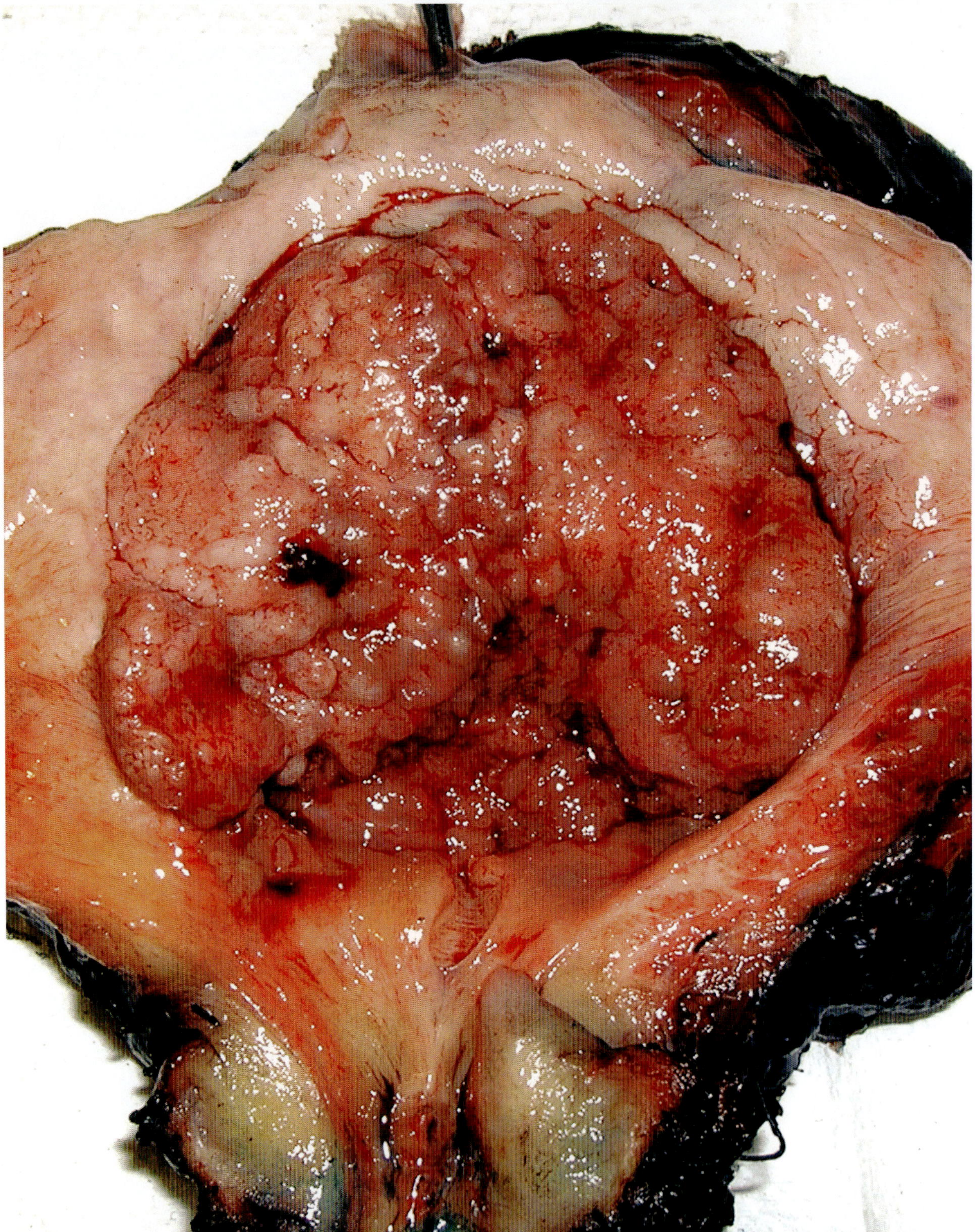

Figure 7.1 — Papillary urothelial carcinoma, Gross specimen. Cystoprostatectomy specimen opened anteriorly via a Y incision has a large cauliflower-like polypoid mass arising from the posterior wall and filling the bladder lumen. This was a case of invasive low-grade papillary urothelial carcinoma from a man in his thirties. After an initial diagnosis of noninvasive low-grade papillary urothelial carcinoma, he did not follow up for the next five years, until he had severe obstructive symptoms. The tumor was still low grade, and it invaded the muscle layer with a broad front to the extent of near extravesicular extension. No metastases were present.

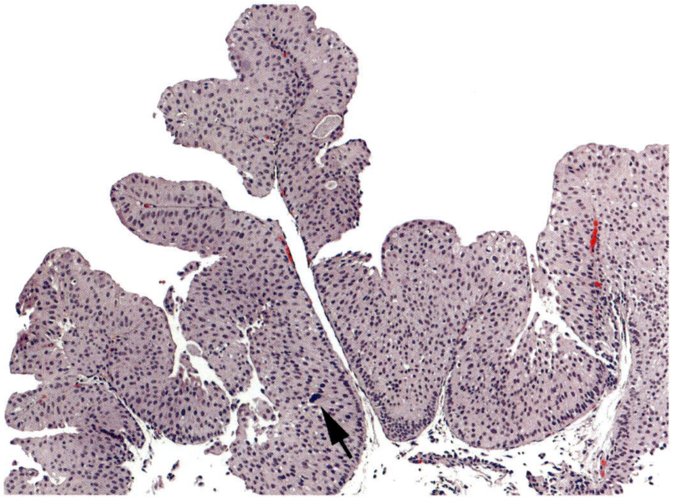

Figure 7.2 — Low-grade urothelial carcinoma, histologic section. These papillary tumors have an overall orderly appearance. There are well formed fibrovascular cores that can be lined by urothelium of any thickness. The papillae are arborizing with minimal fusion. These lesions can be small to fairly large. The cellular polarity is maintained for the most part with mild enlargement of the nuclei. Occasional hyperchromatic nuclei are seen. Mitoses may be scattered and present at any level. This image shows a small lesion with orderly cells and scattered hyperchromatic cells (arrow; H&E stain, low power).

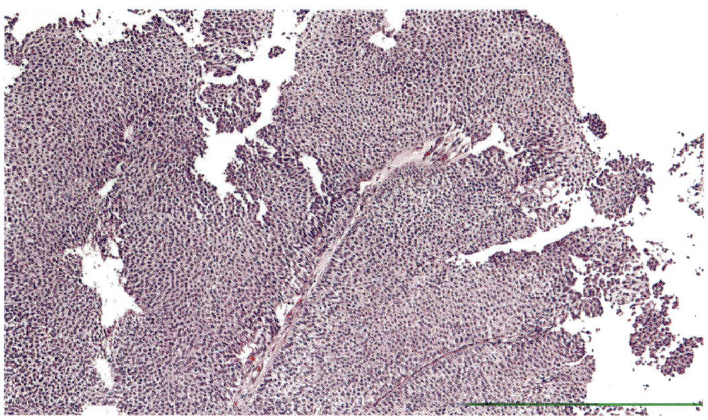

Figure 7.3 — Low-grade papillary urothelial carcinoma, histologic section. Fibrovascular cores are lined by thickened urothelium with cells maintaining their polarity to each other. There is no invasion seen. Compared with papillary urothelial neoplasm of uncertain malignant potential (PUNLMP), low-grade papillary urothelial carcinoma recurs twice as often (H&E stain, low power).

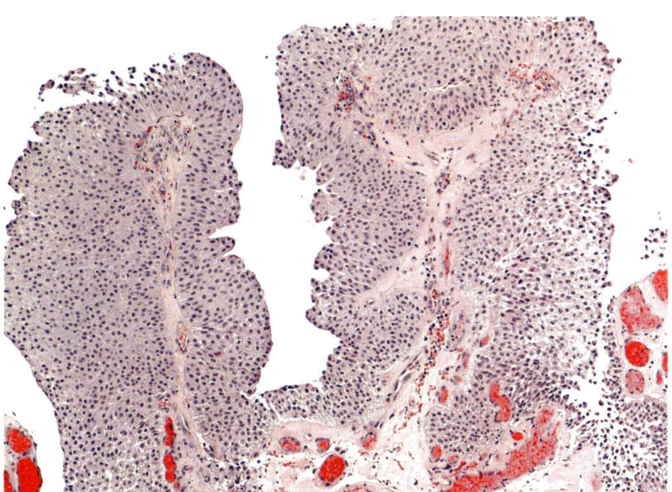

Figure 7.4 — Low-grade papillary urothelial carcinoma, histologic section. Minimal atypia is noted and neoplastic cells have low N/C ratios (H&E stain, low power).

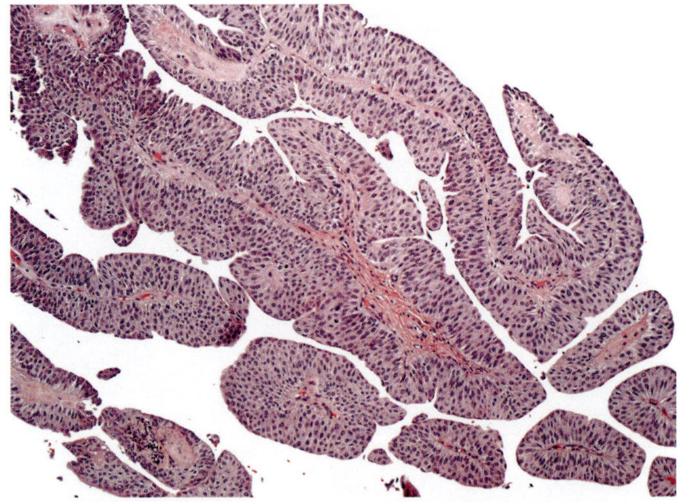

Figure 7.5 — Low-grade papillary urothelial carcinoma, histologic section. Arborizing papillae with low-grade morphology are seen. Scattered mitoses were present (H&E stain, low power).

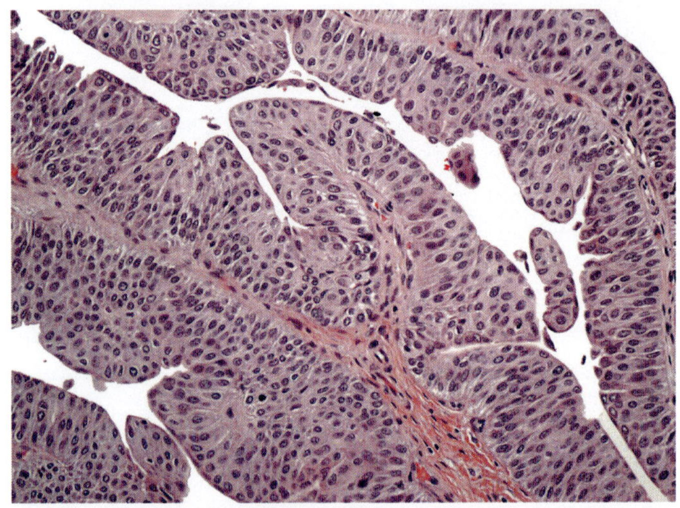

Figure 7.6 — Low-grade papillary urothelial carcinoma, histologic section. Orderly arrangement of minimally variable cells. The urothelium is intact without dyscohesiveness (H&E stain, medium power).

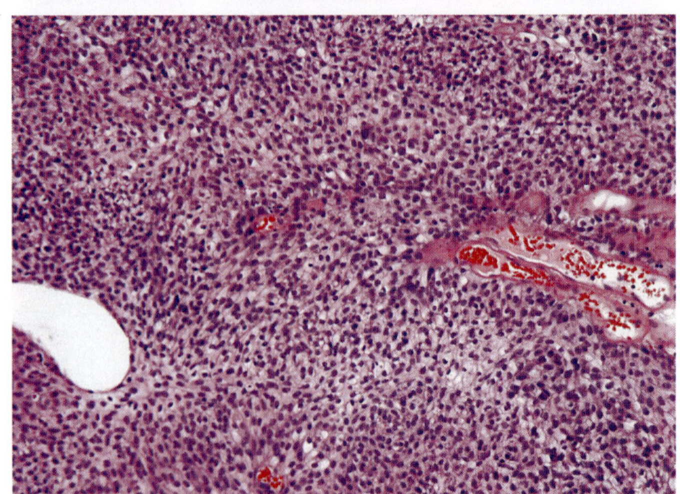

Figure 7.7 — Low-grade papillary urothelial carcinoma, histologic section. Neoplastic urothelial cells have low N/C ratios with scattered mildly enlarged hyperchromatic nuclei. Fibrovascular cores are evident (H&E stain, medium power).

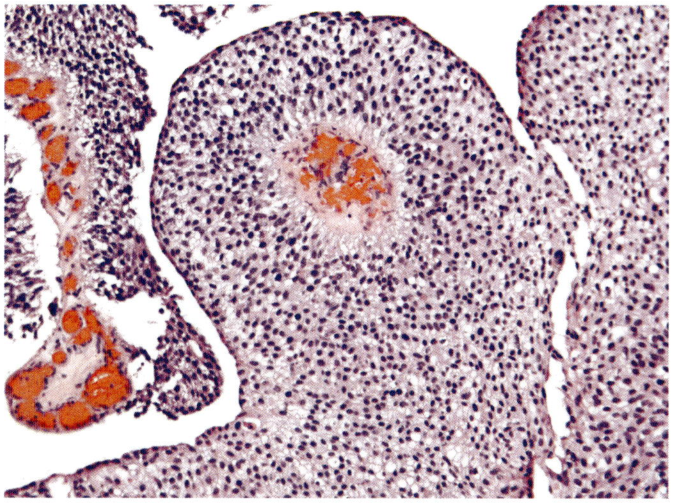

Figure 7.8 — Low-grade papillary urothelial carcinoma, histologic section. A papilla displaying cells with minimal architectural disarray and low N/C ratios. Scattered mildly enlarged and hyperchromatic nuclei are present (H&E stain, medium power).

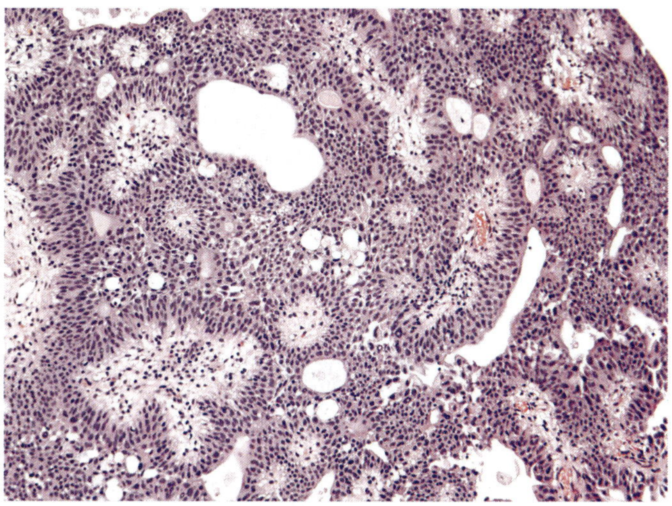

Figure 7.9 — Low-grade papillary urothelial carcinoma, histologic section. Bland-appearing cells with maintained polarity and fused papillae. Additionally, microcystic spaces are seen known as "gland-like lumina." This feature of urothelium may be seen with carcinoma in-situ (CIS) and invasive high-grade tumors as well. These are not true glandular spaces (H&E stain, medium power).

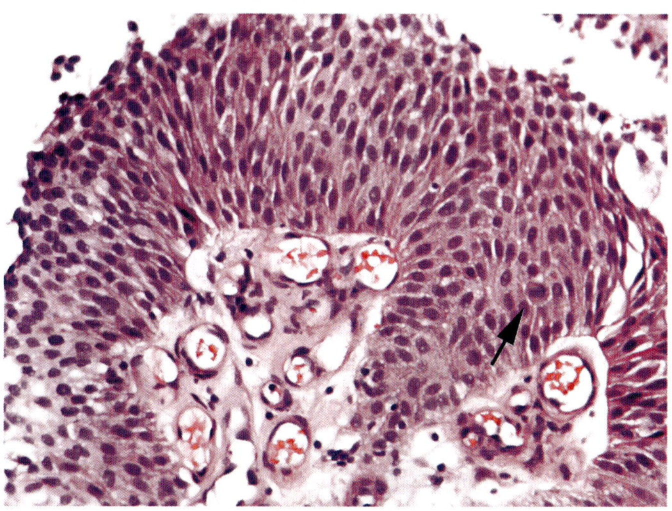

Figure 7.10 — Low-grade papillary urothelial carcinoma, histologic section. Cells lining the core are mildly enlarged with orderly arrangement. Mildly enlarged hyperchromatic nuclei are scattered throughout in addition to a mid-level mitosis (arrow; H&E stain, high power).

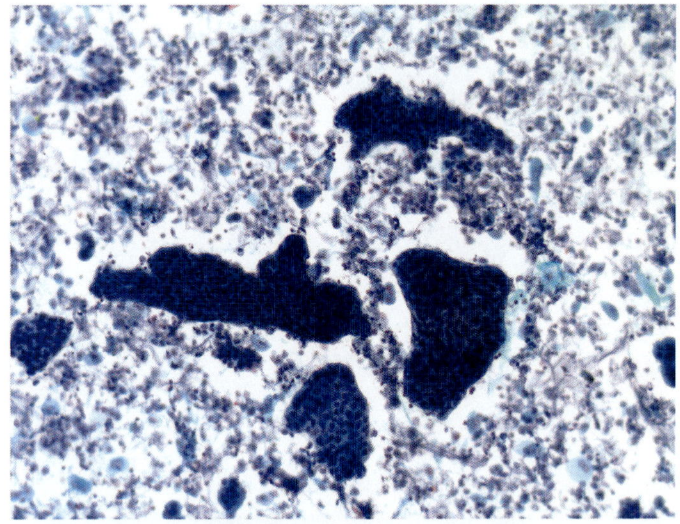

Figure 7.11 — Low-grade urothelial carcinoma, instrumented urine. This low power view of a low-grade papillary urothelial lesion is dramatic in its cellularity and large fragments. Depending upon the method of sample collection, voided versus bladder washing, the cellularity will vary. This bladder washing contains fragments of benign urothelium, suggested by the abundant cytoplasm and therefore less hyperchromatic appearance of the fragment, in contrast with the very dense, hyperchromatic and crowded fragments suggesting origin in the papillary urothelial lesion. Higher power is needed for confirmation (Papanicolaou stain, low power).

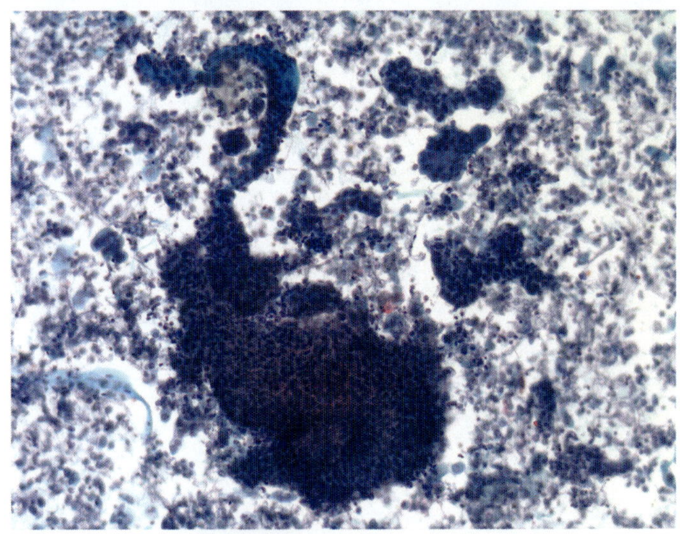

Figure 7.12 — Low-grade urothelial carcinoma, instrumented urine. A dense fragment of urothelium contains a branching fibrovascular stalk supporting the dense and haphazardly arranged urothelial cells. These are small cells with uniform nuclear size, very characteristic of a low-grade urothelial lesion. Other benign fragments can be identified by their abundant cytoplasm surrounding small nuclei (Papanicolaou stain, low power).

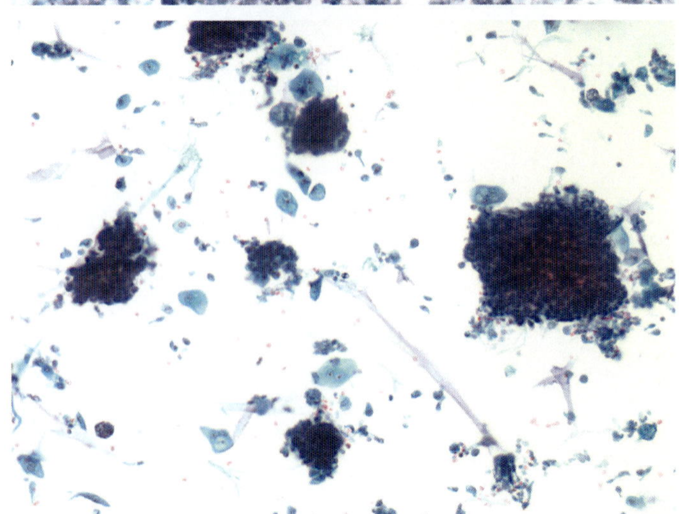

Figure 7.13 — Low-grade urothelial carcinoma, instrumented urine. Even though most low-grade lesions are papillary, the papillary nature of cellular fragments is not always apparent. More important is the grading of the individual cells within the group, that is, are they small and uniform, as from a low-grade lesion, or are they large, characteristic of a high-grade urothelial lesion? (Papanicolaou stain, low power).

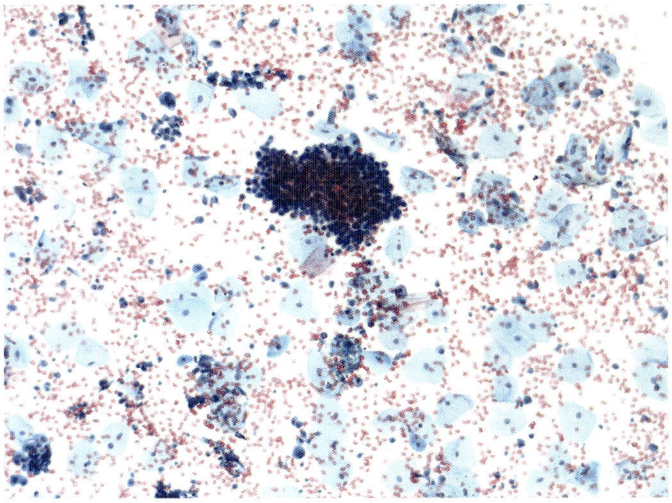

Figure 7.14 — Low-grade urothelial carcinoma, voided urine. The presenting symptom of most low-grade urothelial lesions is hematuria, as is expressed in the background of this sample. The hyperchromatic fragment of urothelium is the diagnostic proof of a urothelial lesion, and the grading can be made on the small size and uniform nature of these cells within the fragment (Papanicolaou stain, low power).

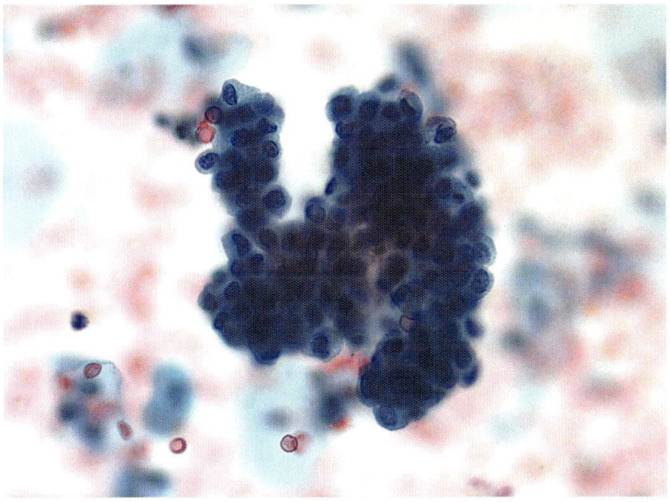

Figure 7.15 — Low-grade urothelial carcinoma, voided urine. Examination of the fragments on high power indicates the uniformity and high N/C ratios. Many of the nuclei are oval, and most have irregular outlines as well as dark chromatin. These characteristics separate this lesion from that of a PUNLMP, which has a more uniform appearance of the nuclei. Nuclear enlargement is not appreciated, and that separates this lesion from a high-grade urothelial lesion (Papanicolaou stain, high power).

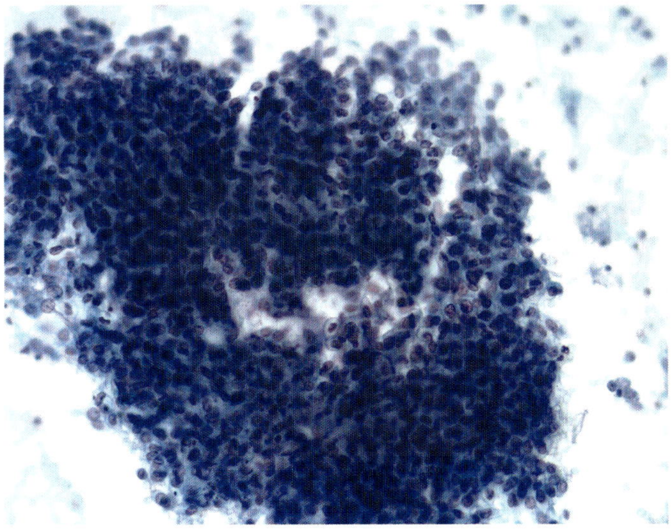

Figure 7.16 — Low-grade urothelial carcinoma, instrumented urine. Instrumentation of a low-grade urothelial lesion will dislodge large fragments, essentially equivalent to a biopsy. Uniform nuclear size and chromasia of the nuclei is characteristic of a low-grade urothelial carcinoma, separating it from a high-grade lesion with its variable chromatin, enlarged overall cell size and very high N/C ratios (Papanicolaou stain, medium power).

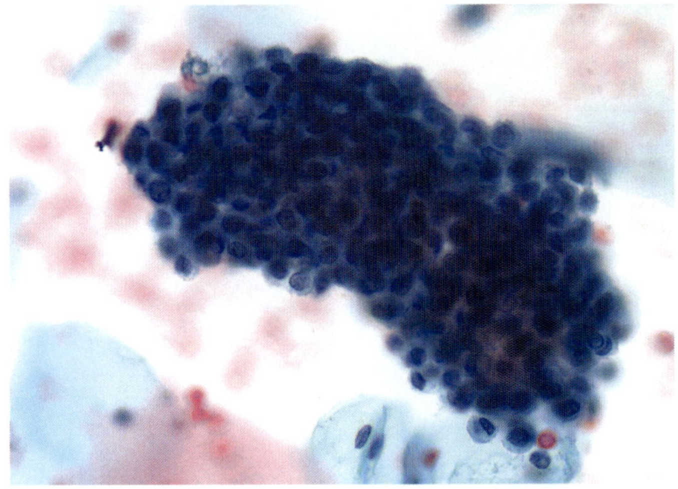

Figure 7.17 — Low-grade urothelial carcinoma, instrumented urine. Close-up view of a low-grade urothelial lesion displays opaque cytoplasm, high N/C ratios, and round to oval nuclei without nucleoli. Depending upon the size of the fragments, fibrovascular stalks are variably seen (Papanicolaou stain, high power).

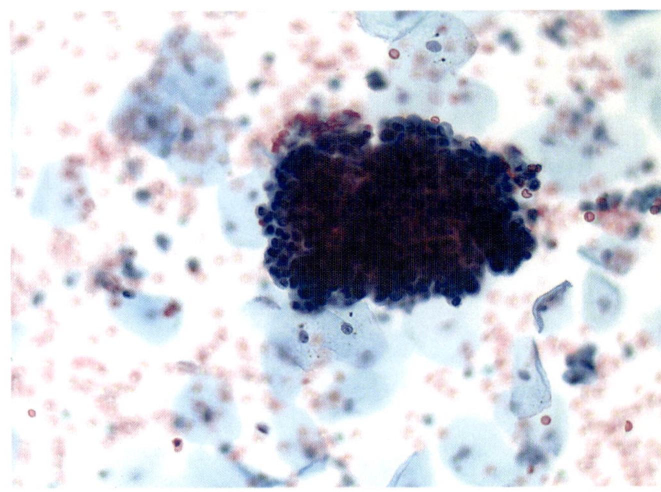

Figure 7.18 — Low-grade urothelial carcinoma, instrumented urine. This fragment of a low-grade urothelial carcinoma has evident fibrovascular support that enables the observer to definitely identify it as a papillary lesion. However, this is not essential for the diagnosis, which can be made strictly on the cytomorphology of the individual cells (Papanicolaou stain, medium power).

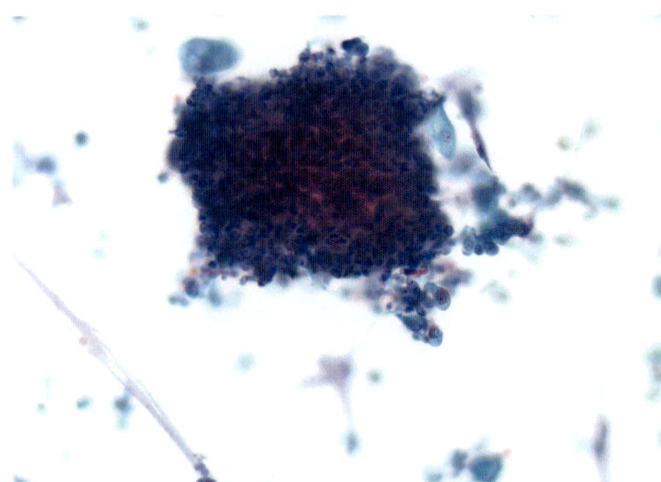

Figure 7.19 — Low-grade urothelial carcinoma, instrumented urine. A large fragment of tissue from a low-grade urothelial carcinoma demonstrates a haphazard arrangement of uniform but clearly neoplastic cells (Papanicolaou stain, medium power).

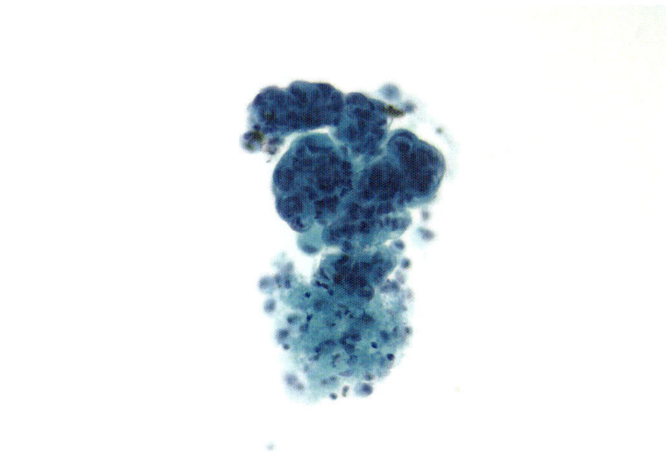

Figure 7.20 — Low-grade urothelial carcinoma, instrumented urine. The presence of umbrella cells covering these basal cells is frequently seen in a low-grade urothelial carcinoma and should not persuade against that diagnosis. As long as the characteristics of neoplasia are present in the basal cells, the diagnosis may be at least suggested (Papanicolaou stain, medium power).

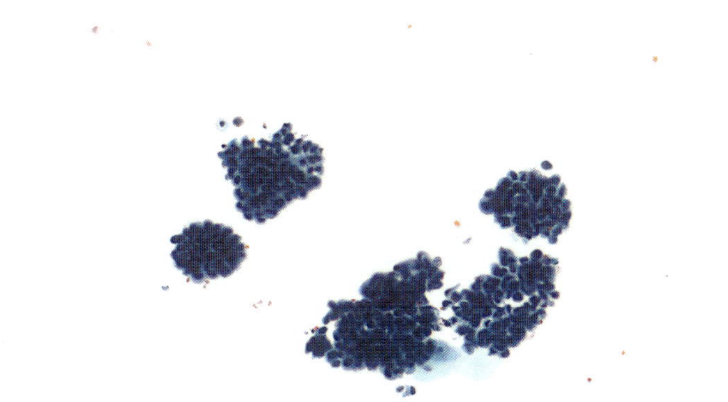

Figure 7.21 — Low-grade urothelial carcinoma, instrumented urine. Even on low power, the diagnosis of a low-grade urothelial lesion is evident by the hyperchromatic crowded groups comprising small uniform urothelial cells. The background is relatively clean, implying absence of invasion (Papanicolaou stain, low power).

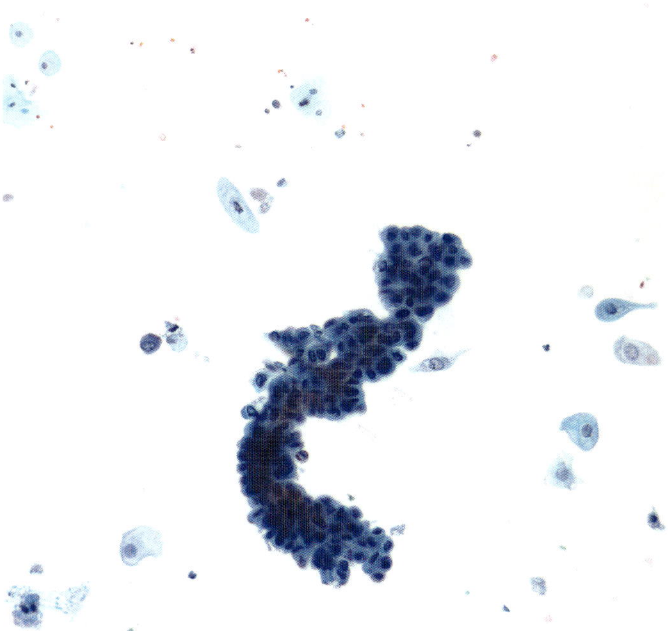

Figure 7.22 — Low-grade urothelial carcinoma, instrumented urine. When a sample is obtained by catheterization, the strip of epithelium dislodged by the catheter may contain both normal and abnormal cells. The most abnormal cells will determine the grading of this particular lesion (Papanicolaou stain, medium power).

Figure 7.23 — Low-grade urothelial carcinoma, instrumented urine. This large fragment of urothelial cells has highly irregularly shaped nuclei, which might change the grade from low to high. However, the size of the nuclei is approximately the same as the intermediate cell nucleus and only two to three times the size of red cells, eliminating a high-grade urothelial carcinoma from the diagnosis. Also, the uniformity from nucleus to nucleus speaks more in favor of a low-grade lesion than a high-grade lesion (Papanicolaou stain, medium power).

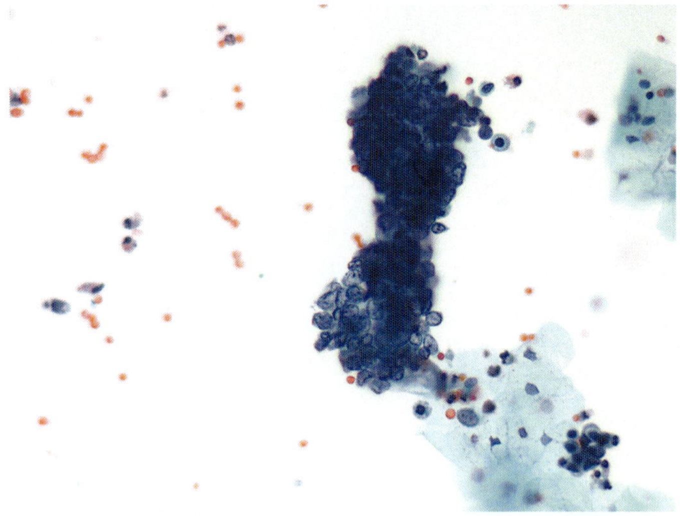

Figure 7.24 — Low-grade urothelial carcinoma, instrumented urine. Large fragments of obviously papillary tissue immediately suggest a diagnosis of papillary carcinoma. Higher power is necessary for grading the lesion (Papanicolaou stain, low power).

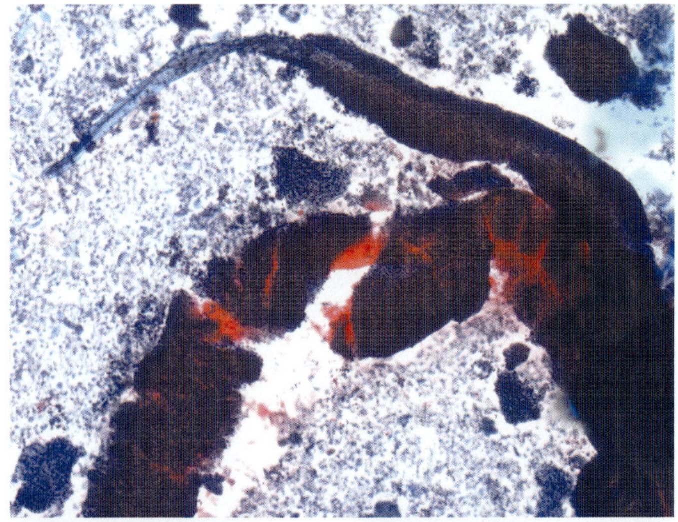

Figure 7.25 — Low-grade urothelial carcinoma, instrumented urine. Higher power investigation of the fragments seen in the previous photograph indicates small uniform nuclei surrounded by a moderate amount of cytoplasm, adherent to a fibrovascular stalk. The diagnosis of low-grade papillary carcinoma is appropriate (Papanicolaou stain, medium power).

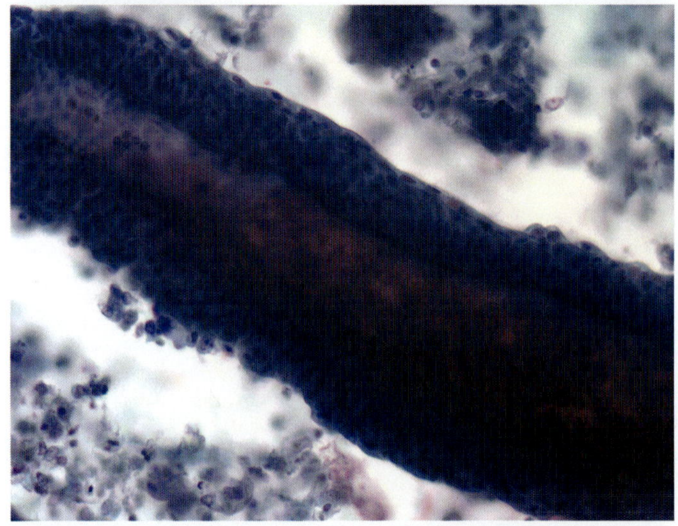

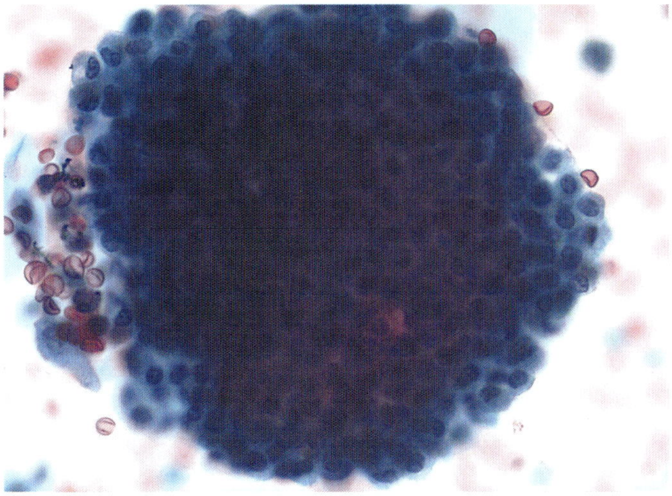

Figure 7.26 — Low-grade urothelial carcinoma, instrumented urine. A higher power view of the previous epithelium confirms the small size of the cells and moderate nuclear cytoplasmic ratios, all conclusive for a low-grade lesion (Papanicolaou stain, high power).

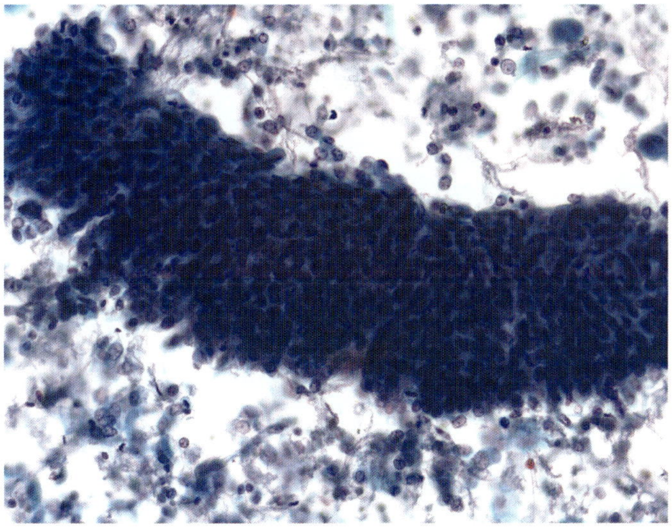

Figure 7.27 — Low-grade urothelial carcinoma, instrumented urine. While the diagnosis of "papillary" cannot be established on this dislodged fragment of urothelium, the impression of low-grade urothelial carcinoma is suggested by the crowding of the nuclei and the hyperchromasia as well as the disorganization of the fragment (Papanicolaou stain, medium power).

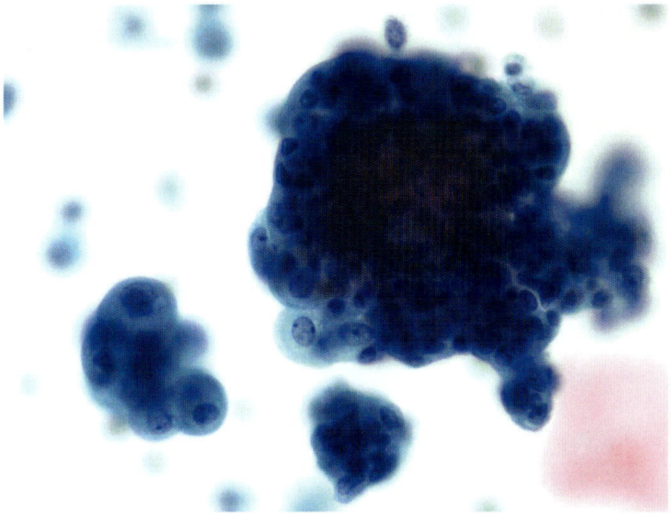

Figure 7.28 — Low-grade urothelial carcinoma, voided urine. The group in the lower left hand corner consists of umbrella cells. The larger fragment that predominates in the photograph is covered by umbrella cells, but also contains crowded and haphazardly arranged basal type cells with increased N/C ratios and hyperchromasia. The presence of umbrella cells should not dissuade the observer from entertaining the diagnosis of a low-grade lesion. That impression is established by the morphology of the basal-type cells (Papanicolaou stain, high power).

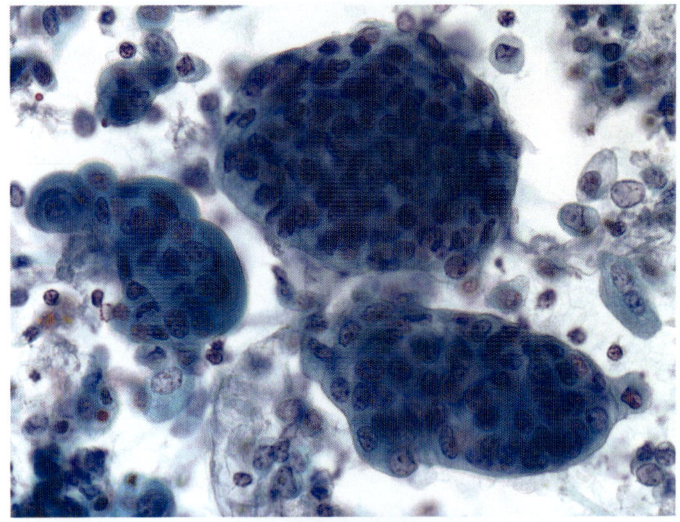

Figure 7.29 — Low-grade urothelial carcinoma, instrumented urine. These three fragments of urothelium display changes of reactive (lower portion) low-grade urothelial carcinoma (upper portion) and benign umbrella cells (left group). Variations in the N/C ratios, chromatin pattern and presence or absence of nucleoli are helpful clues to the nature of each of the cell groups. Careful search of the sample is important to establish presence or absence of a higher grade lesion in which single cells are the rule rather than the exception (Papanicolaou stain, medium power).

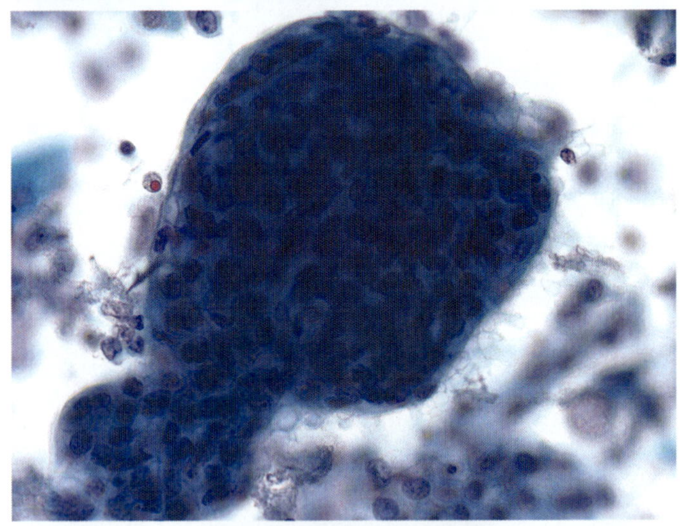

Figure 7.30 — Low-grade urothelial carcinoma, instrumented urine. A compact group of urothelial cells, even without a fibrovascular stalk, suggests a papillary lesion by its smooth outline on all sides. The uniformly small cells indicate a low-grade lesion (Papanicolaou stain, medium power).

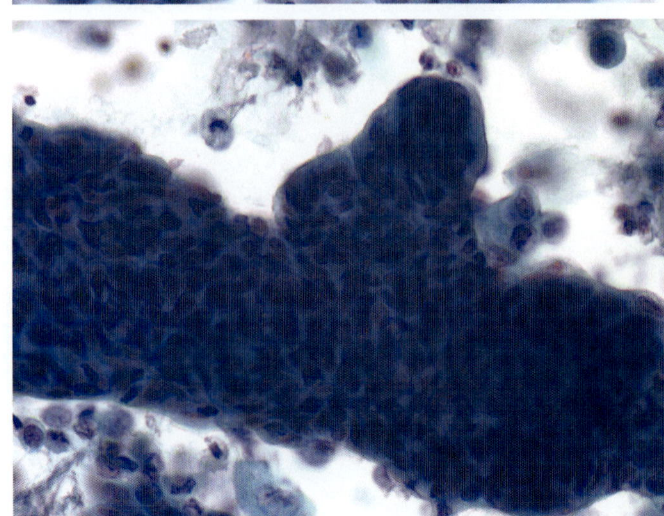

Figure 7.31 — Low-grade urothelial carcinoma, instrumented urine. The haphazard arrangement of nuclei within this tissue fragment suggests a neoplastic lesion, although the abundant cytoplasm indicates numerous umbrella cells. No fibrovascular stalk is observed, but the smooth outer covering on all sides suggests a papillary lesion (Papanicolaou stain, medium power).

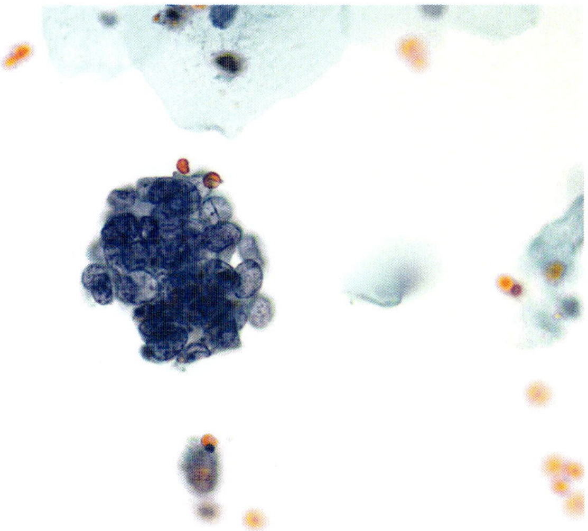

Figure 7.32 — Low-grade urothelial carcinoma, voided urine. A small cluster of uniform cells that have very high N/C ratios is worrisome for a high-grade lesion. However, the size of the nuclei is small, the chromatin is pale and fine, so a low-grade lesion is the better choice (Papanicolaou stain, high power).

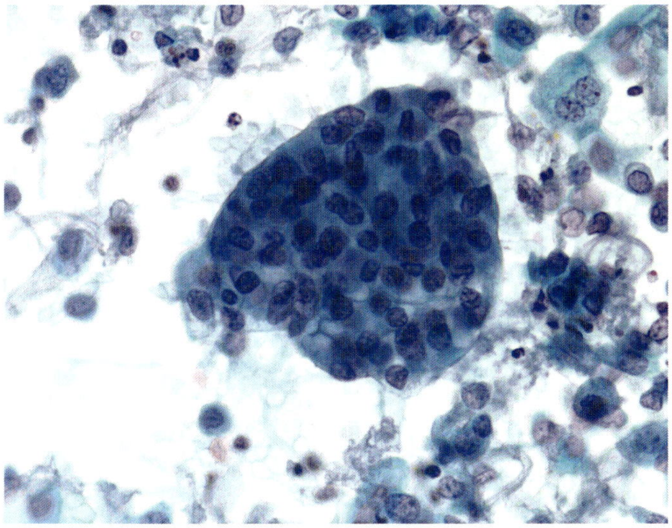

Figure 7.33 — Low-grade urothelial carcinoma, instrumented urine. Uniform round to oval nuclei within this tissue fragment are haphazardly arranged, some of the nuclei overlap, others are separated by variable distances from each other, indicating architectural disorganization. These characteristics of a low-grade lesion are all that is necessary for the diagnosis (Papanicolaou stain, medium power).

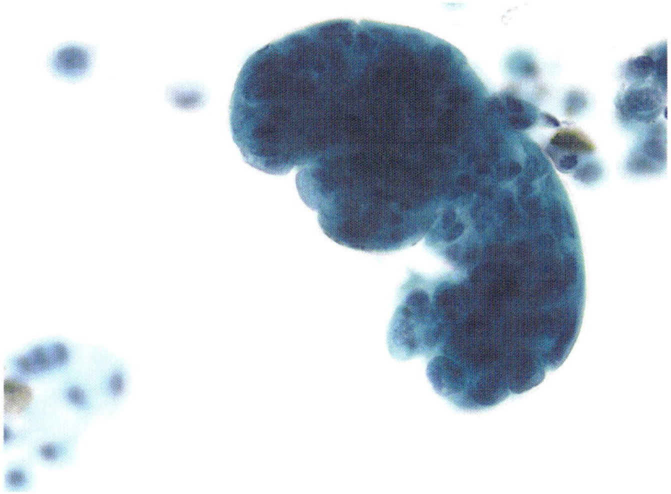

Figure 7.34 — Low-grade urothelial carcinoma, instrumented urine. Although umbrella cells are covering the surface of this fragment, the central cells are small with high N/C ratios and are tightly packed. This characteristic suggests a low-grade papillary lesion. Umbrella cells are frequently seen in such instances (Papanicolaou stain, high power).

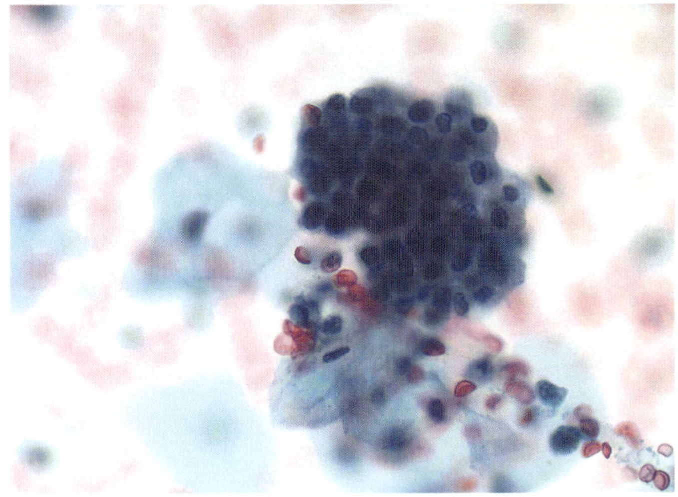

Figure 7.35 — Low-grade urothelial carcinoma, voided urine. In contrast to the preceding photograph this fragment has a shaggy boundary, so that the diagnosis of a papillary lesion cannot be made with certainty. However, the morphology of the individual cells within the fragment is suitable for the diagnosis of a low-grade lesion. Abundant red blood cells are present in the background (Papanicolaou stain, high power).

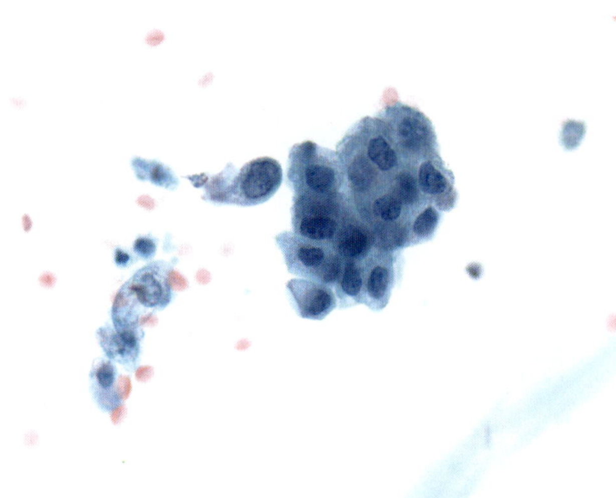

Figure 7.36 — Low-grade urothelial carcinoma, voided urine. Although this fragment is neither papillary nor crowded, the individual cells within it are sufficiently variable and hyperchromatic to place a suspicion of a low-grade lesion in the mind of the observer (Papanicolaou stain, medium power).

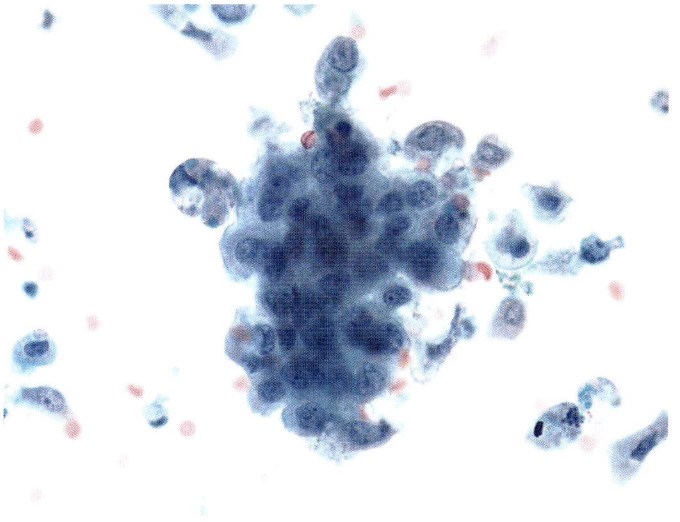

Figure 7.37 — Low-grade urothelial carcinoma, voided urine. Variation in size and shape of the nuclei is worrisome for a higher grade lesion. However the N/C ratios are low and substantial degeneration has occurred in the sample. "Suspicious for a urothelial lesion" is probably the best interpretation, without grading (Papanicolaou stain, medium power).

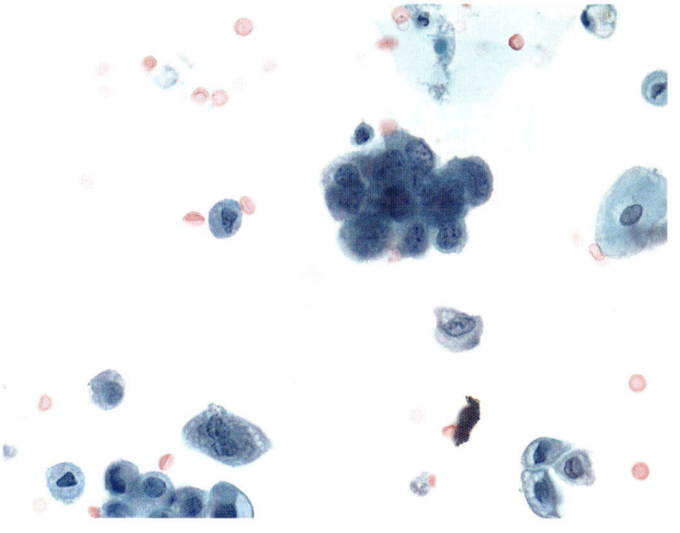

Figure 7.38 — Low-grade urothelial carcinoma, voided urine. Within this tissue fragment are tightly packed cells with overlapping nuclei and granular nuclear chromatin. N/C ratios are high, but the cell size is relatively small, making the interpretation of a low-grade urothelial carcinoma appropriate (Papanicolaou stain, medium power).

Figure 7.39 — High-grade papillary urothelial carcinoma, histologic section. The image highlights the marked cytologic atypia associated with high-grade lesions. There is extreme cellular crowding, pleomorphism, increased apoptosis, and small areas of necrosis. The cytologic and architectural abnormalities are visible at low magnification (H&E stain, low power).

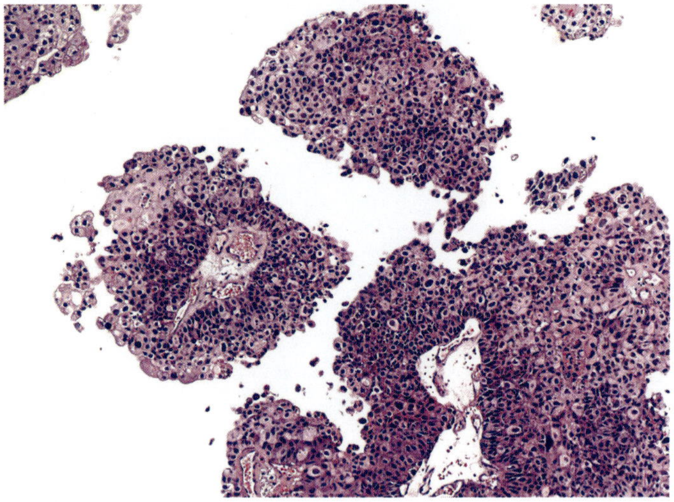

Figure 7.40 — High-grade papillary urothelial carcinoma, histologic section. This neoplasm shows increased dyscohesiveness and cellular disarray. Nuclei are hyperchromatic (H&E stain, medium power).

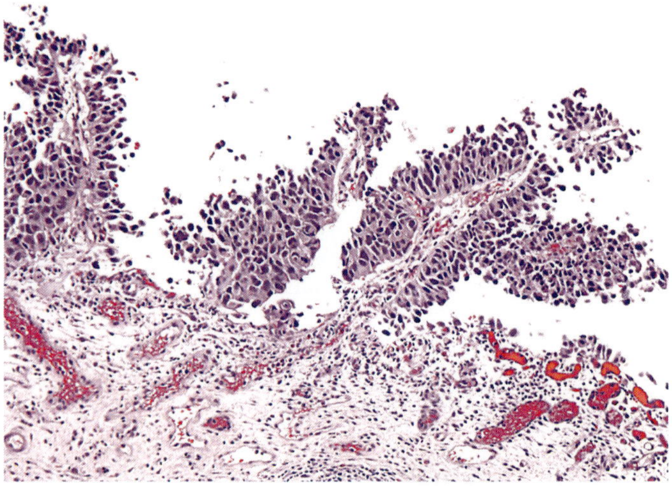

Figure 7.41 — High-grade papillary urothelial carcinoma, histologic section. The carcinoma shows obvious high-grade features with loss of polarity, increased N/C ratios, hyperchromatic nuclei, increased apoptosis, and mitoses (H&E stain, high power).

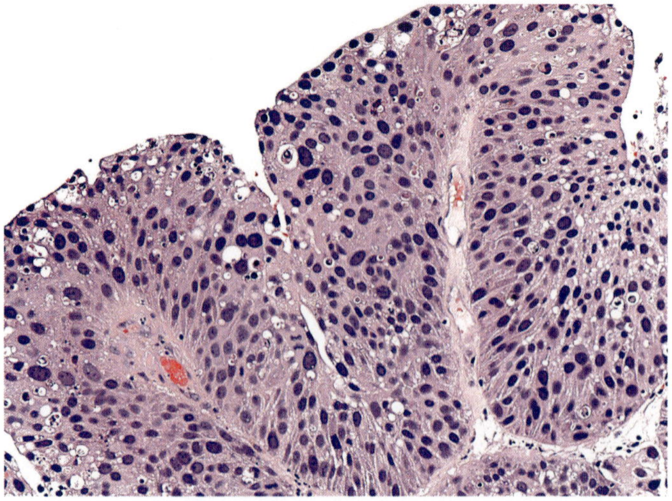

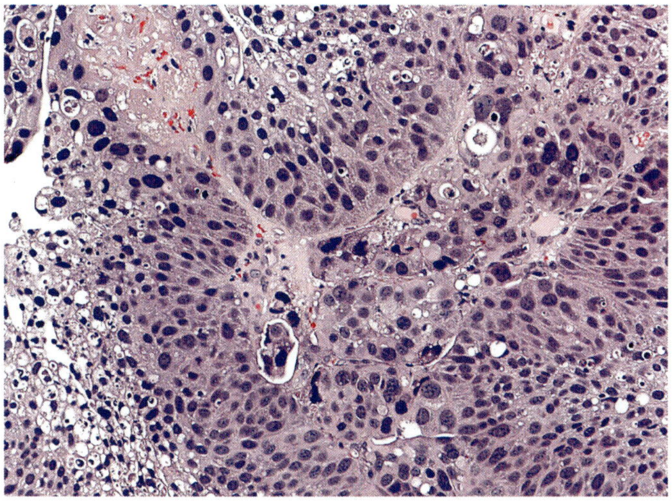

Figure 7.42 — High-grade papillary urothelial carcinoma with lamina propria invasion, histologic section. Within the fibrovascular cores, there is invasion of the lamina propria. Note the early invasion in the form of infiltrating nests surrounded by "clefting" artifact (H&E stain, high power).

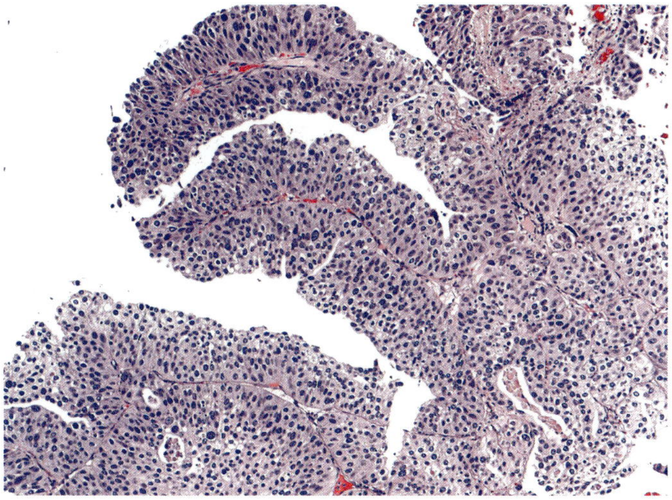

Figure 7.43 — High-grade papillary urothelial carcinoma, histologic section. High-grade carcinomas have at ninety months a 51 percent risk of progression, while low-grade carcinomas have a 13 percent risk of progression. Fibrovascular cores lined by cells of high-grade morphology are depicted here. Small areas of necrosis are noted. Necrosis is usually associated with high-grade lesions (H&E stain, low power).

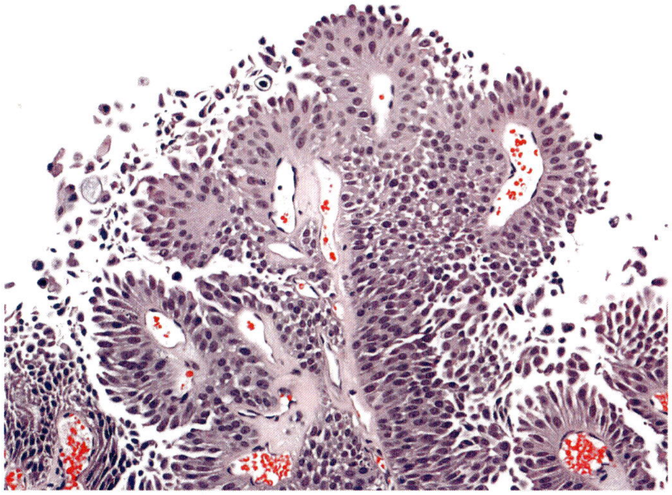

Figure 7.44 — High-grade papillary urothelial carcinoma, histologic section. This noninvasive, high-grade papillary carcinoma shows dyscohesiveness and increased apoptosis. The nuclei are hyperchromatic, and prominent nucleoli are seen. The cellular pleomorphism is less pronounced than the carcinomas shown earlier (H&E stain, medium power).

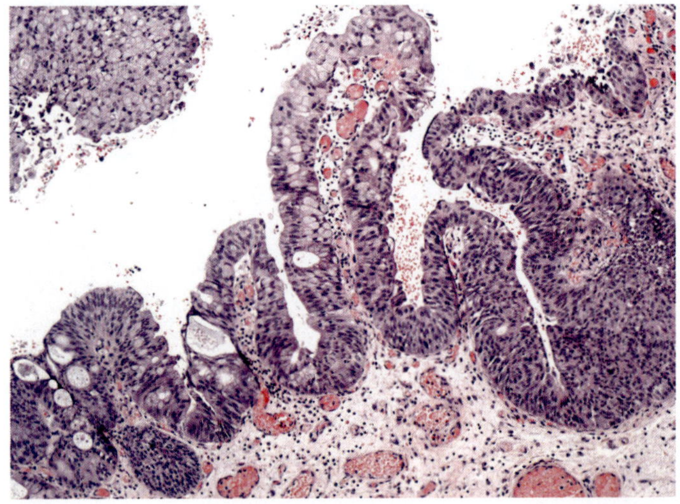

Figure 7.45 — High-grade papillary urothelial carcinoma with signet-ring cell features, histologic section. High-grade urothelial tumors can show divergent differentiation, as seen in this image. In addition to high-grade papillary and flat urothelial CIS, there are mucin containing signet-ring cells and glandlike lumina associated with the carcinoma (H&E stain, medium power).

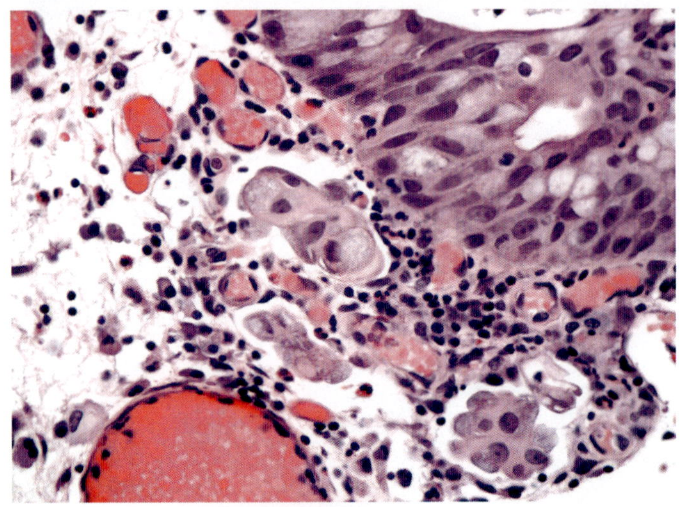

Figure 7.46 — High-grade papillary urothelial carcinoma, histologic section. Same neoplasm as seen in the previous image shows involvement of a von Brunn's nest by CIS and from there a small area of microinvasion into the lamina propria is present. The invading nests have the peculiar "clefting" artifact commonly seen in early invasive urothelial carcinomas. Additionally, the phenomenon of paradoxical differentiation is also noted, where the invasive carcinoma develops more eosinophilic cytoplasm (H&E stain, high power).

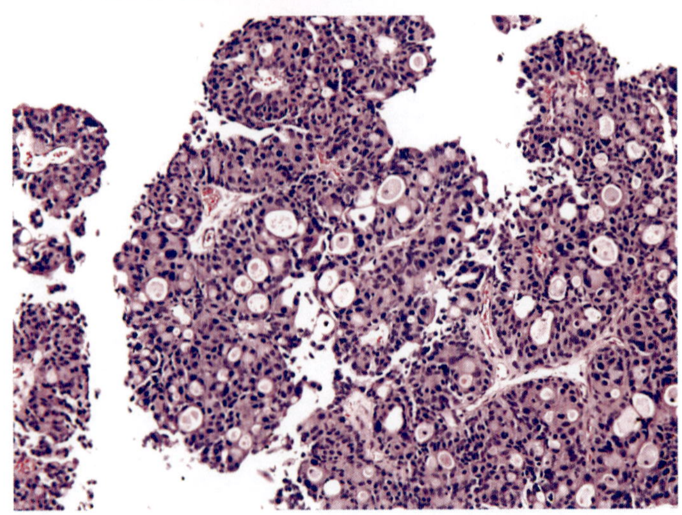

Figure 7.47 — High-grade papillary urothelial carcinoma, histologic section. This high-grade carcinoma has prominent glandlike lumina. The latter are not true glands (H&E stain, medium power).

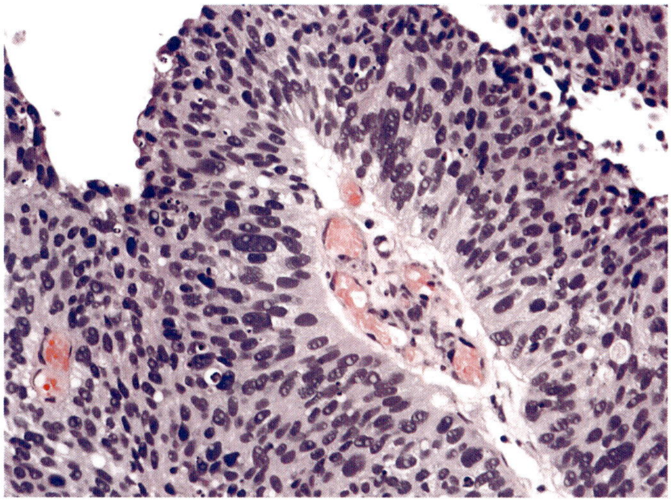

Figure 7.48 — High-grade papillary urothelial carcinoma, histologic section. Variation in nuclear size, crowding, hyperchromasia, increased mitoses, and apoptoses are seen in this high-grade lesion (H&E stain, high power).

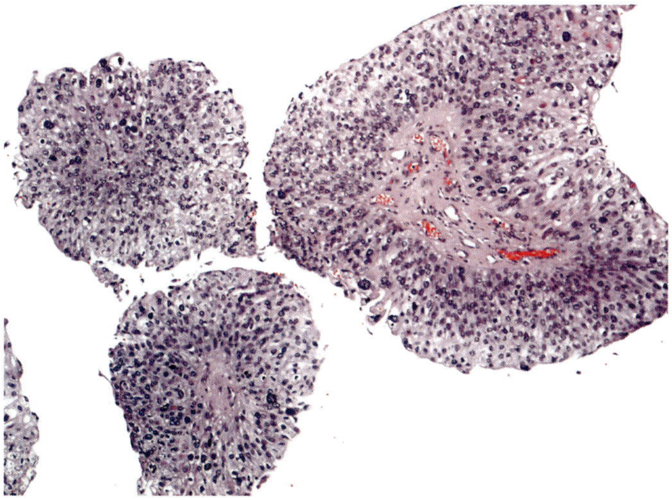

Figure 7.49 — High-grade papillary urothelial carcinoma, histologic section. Focal anisonucleosis is depicted here with occasional large hyperchromatic cells associated with this high-grade papillary carcinoma (H&E stain, medium power).

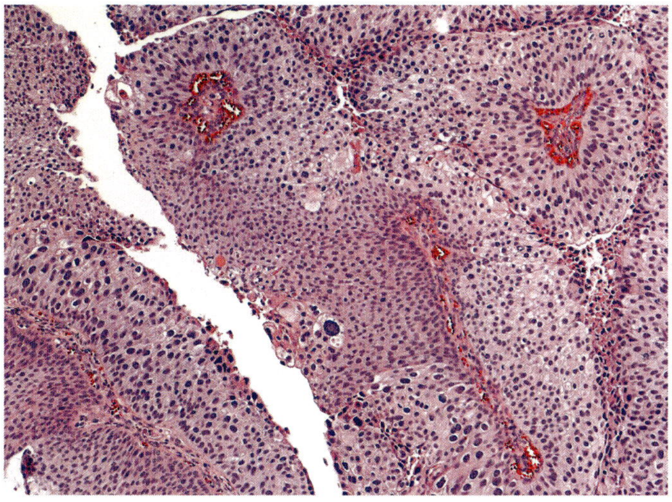

Figure 7.50 — High-grade papillary urothelial carcinoma, histologic section. An example of mixed, high- and low-grade tumor morphology is shown in this image. The papillae are fused. When high-grade morphology occupies at least 5 percent of the tumor, the entire tumor should be graded as a high-grade carcinoma (H&E stain, medium power).

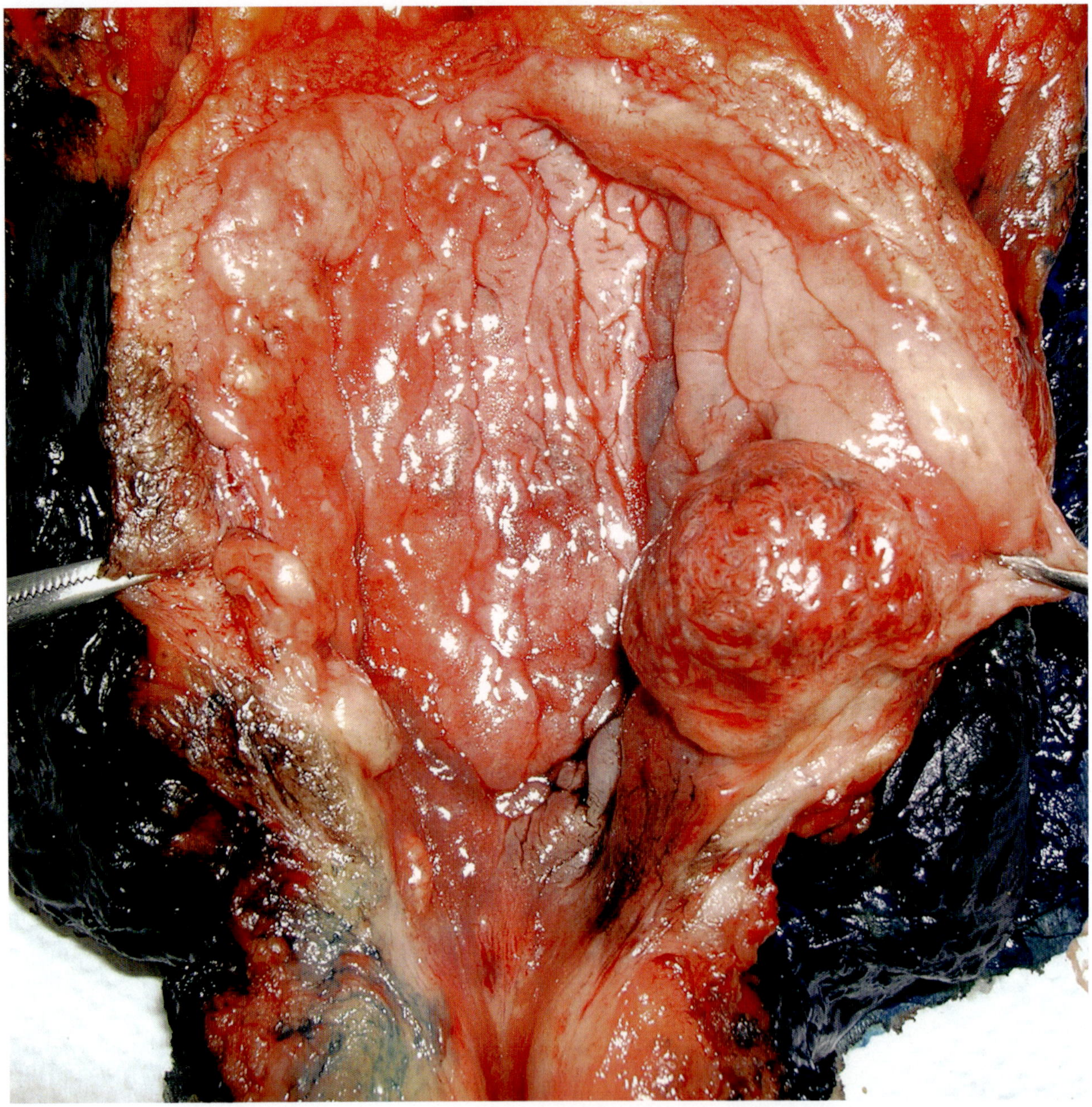

Figure 7.51 — Invasive high-grade urothelial carcinoma, gross appearance. Anteriorly opened cystoprostatectomy specimen shows a polypoid mass on the left anterior wall of the bladder. This was an invasive high-grade papillary urothelial carcinoma that invaded the muscularis propria.

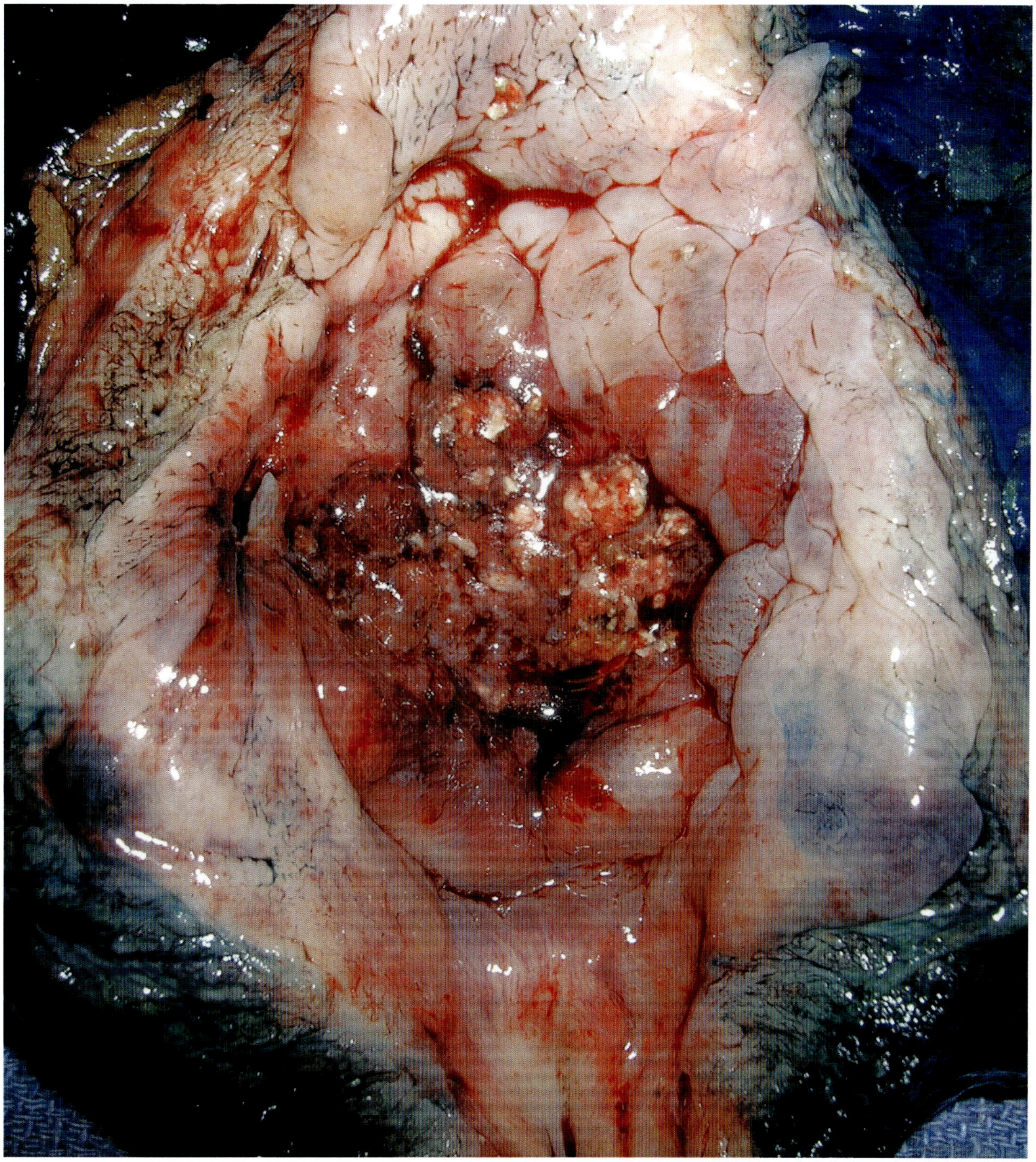

Figure 7.52 — Invasive high-grade urothelial carcinoma, gross appearance. Cystoprostatectomy specimen opened anteriorly via a Y-incision shows a large ulcerated mass in the posterior wall. The invasive high-grade urothelial carcinoma showed extravesicular extension. The uninvolved mucosa is markedly edematous.

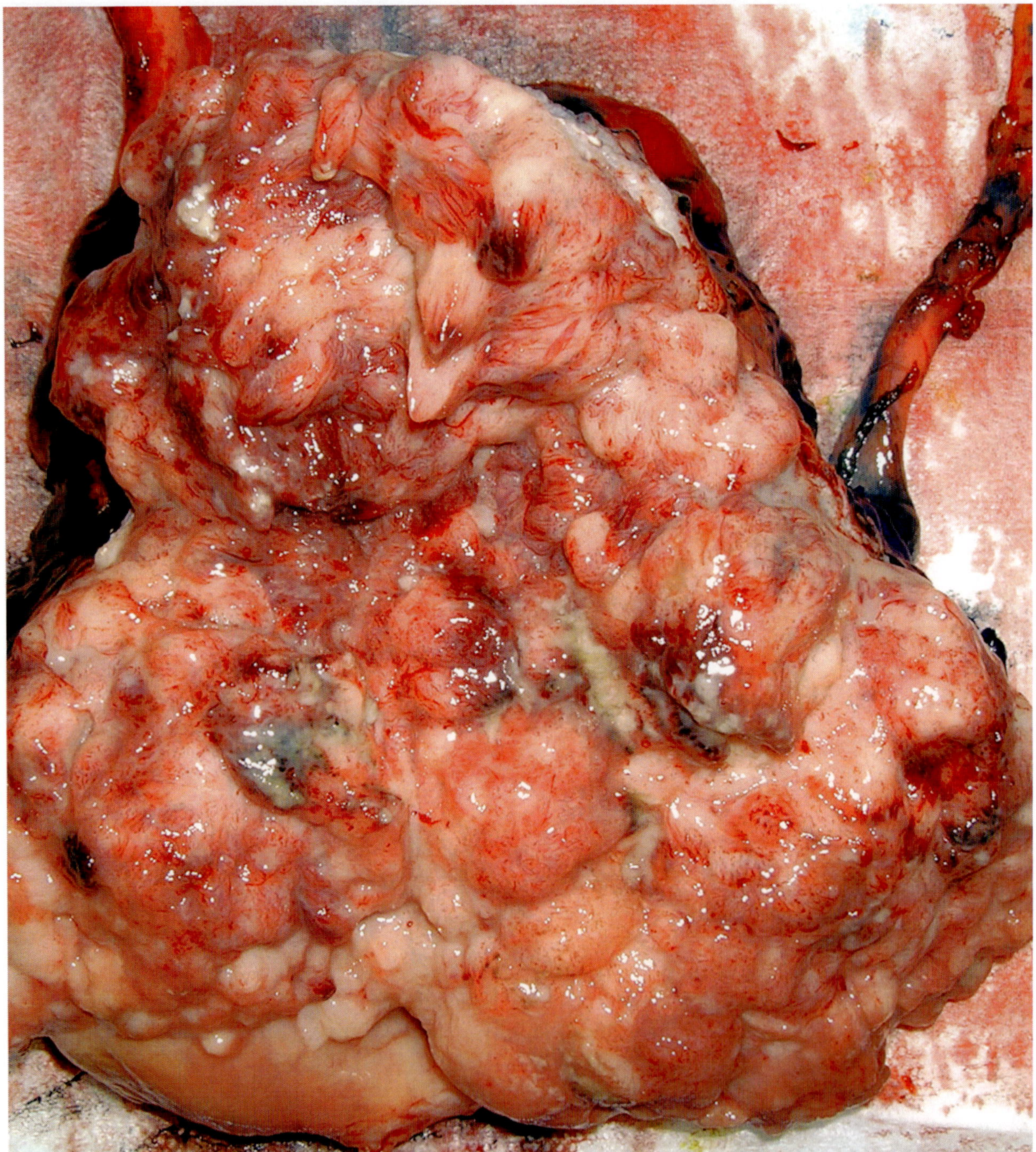

Figure 7.53 — Invasive high-grade urothelial carcinoma, gross appearance. The bladder is part of an en bloc bilateral nephrectomy and cystectomy specimen from a woman. The patient suffered recurrent multifocal disease. The entire bladder surface is involved by carcinoma, with areas of necrosis and ulceration. This multifocal high-grade urothelial carcinoma was myoinvasive but organ confined.

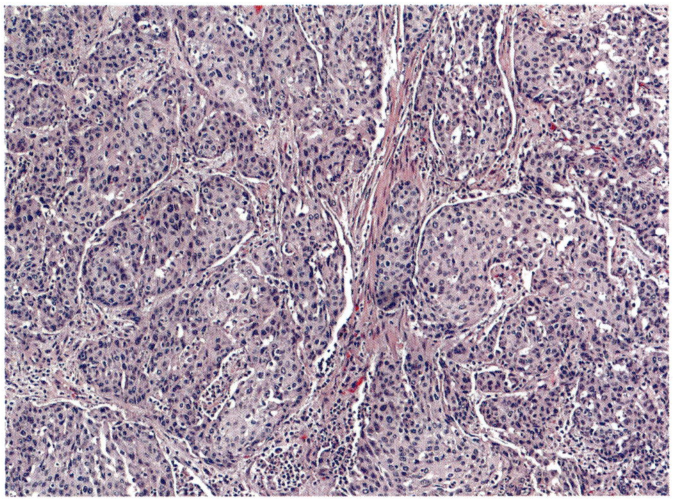

Figure 7.54 — Invasive high-grade urothelial carcinoma, histologic section. This urothelial carcinoma is growing in large nests and sheets as it invades the bladder wall. Urothelial carcinoma often makes nests and cords as it invades with surrounding desmoplastic and inflamed stroma. In the center of the image, thin strips of muscle layer remain. The nuclei have coarse, clumped chromatin and are pleomorphic. There is ample eosinophilic cytoplasm (H&E stain, low power).

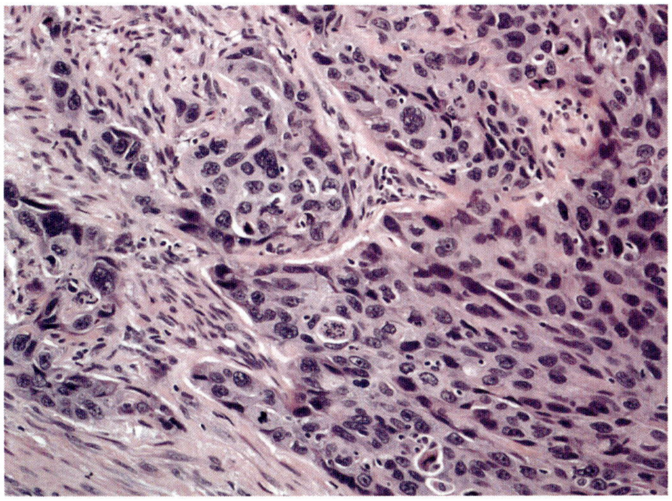

Figure 7.55 — Invasive high-grade urothelial carcinoma, histologic section. Nuclear pleomorphism and scattered atypical mitoses are seen in this invasive carcinoma (H&E stain, high power).

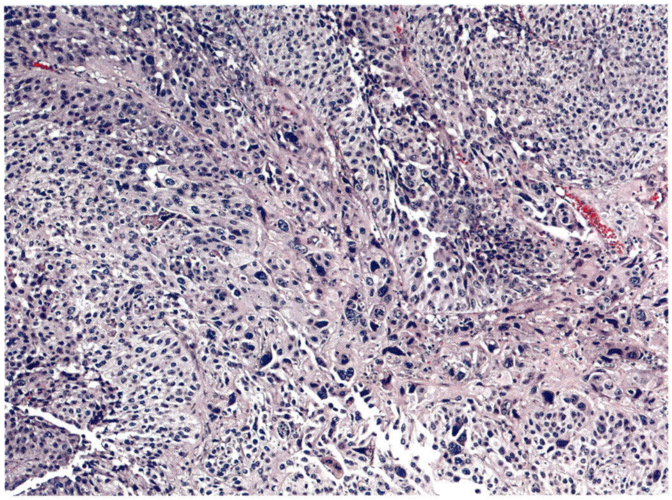

Figure 7.56 — Invasive high-grade urothelial carcinoma, histologic section. The carcinoma is seen invading with irregular nests that show intense nuclear pleomorphism, features inherent in most high-grade urothelial carcinomas. Necrosis is a common feature of these neoplasms (H&E stain, medium power).

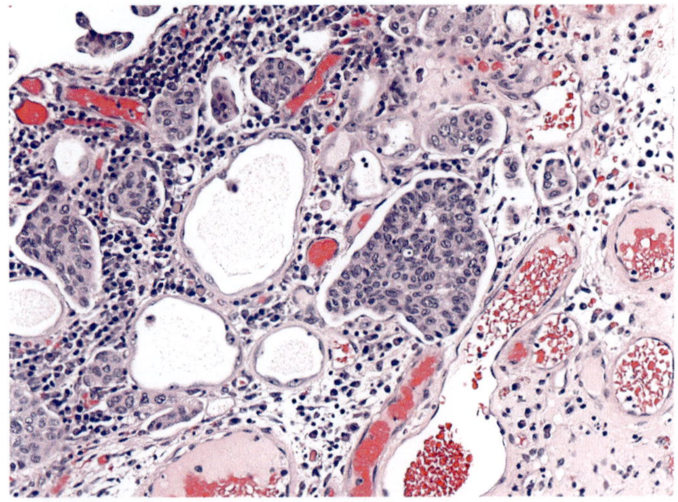

Figure 7.57 — Invasive high-grade urothelial carcinoma with adjacent nephrogenic adenoma, histologic section. Variably-sized carcinoma nests are showing lamina propria invasion with the typical "clefting" artifact. Lamina propria is chronically inflamed with vascular-like, dilated tubules with peritubular hyalinization lined by hobnail cells typical of nephrogenic adenoma. The nephrogenic adenoma most likely developed secondary to previous instrumentation, transurethral resection, or biopsy of the tumor. Invasion into lamina propria is staged as pT1. It is the stage rather than the grade that dictates prognosis of urothelial carcinomas (H&E stain, high power).

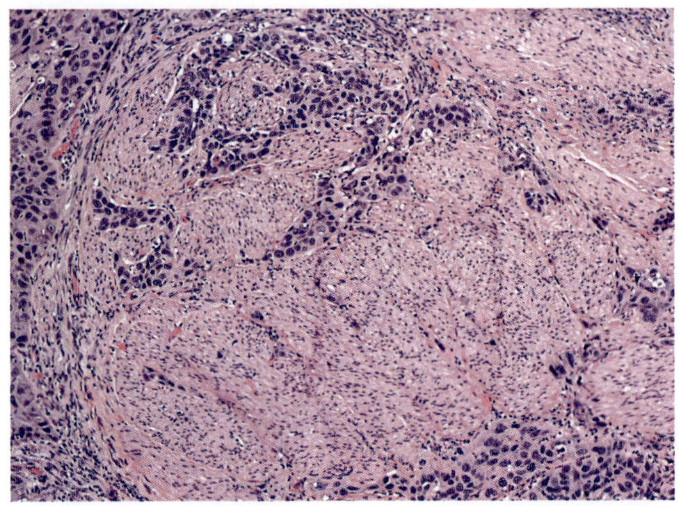

Figure 7.58 — Invasive high-grade papillary urothelial carcinoma invading the muscularis propria, histologic section. Nests and cords of urothelial carcinoma invade the muscle bundles. Invasion of the muscularis propria is pT2 stage and an indication for cystectomy (H&E stain, high power).

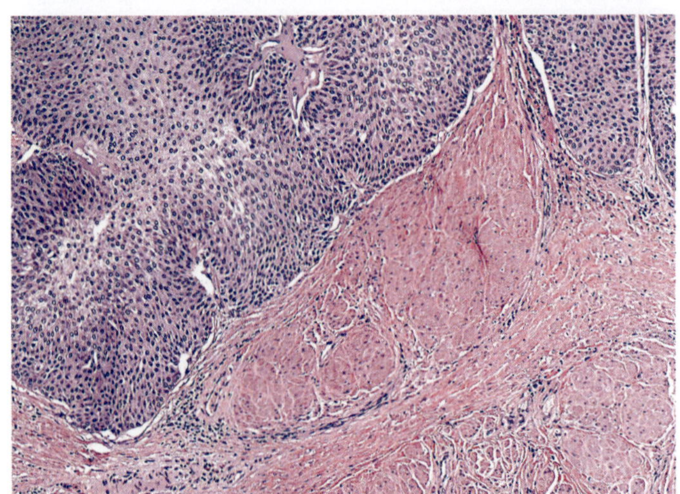

Figure 7.59 — Invasive low-grade urothelial carcinoma, histologic section. Only a small number of low-grade urothelial carcinomas ever invade. This low-grade papillary urothelial carcinoma invades with a broad front and had reached the muscularis propria (H&E stain, medium power).

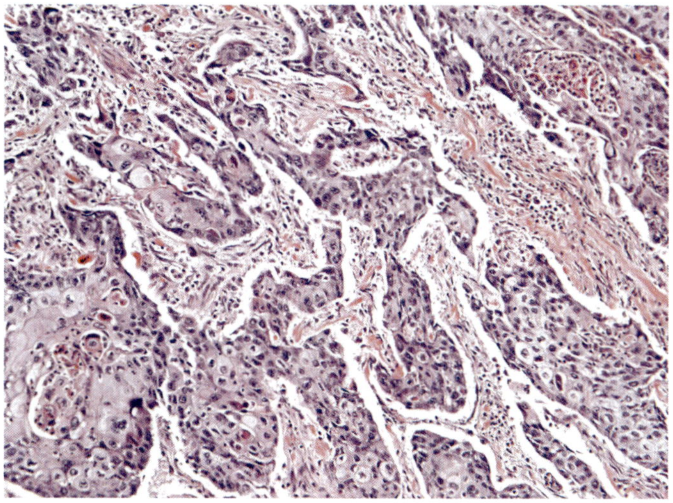

Figure 7.60 — Invasive high-grade urothelial carcinoma with squamous differentiation, histologic section. Squamous differentiation is very common in urothelial carcinomas and is seen in approximately 60 percent of the cases. The diagnosis "squamous cell carcinoma" should be reserved for pure squamous cell carcinoma. Squamous differentiation is implied when there is keratin pearl formation, intercellular bridging, or single cell keratinization (H&E stain, medium power).

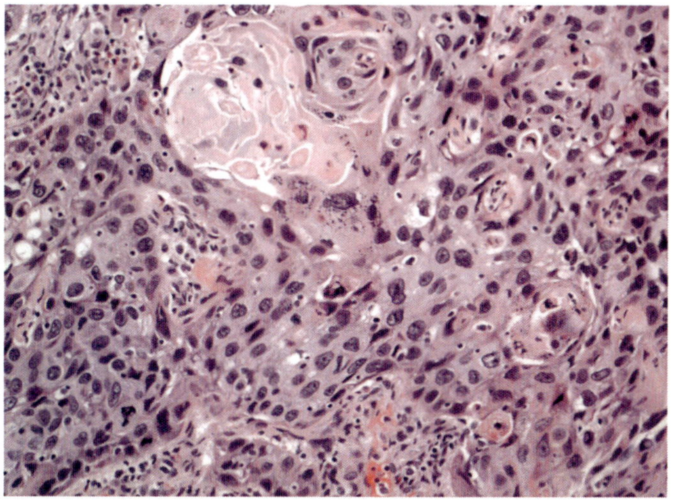

Figure 7.61 — Invasive high-grade urothelial carcinoma with squamous differentiation, histologic section. This example of squamous differentiation in urothelial carcinoma, in addition to keratin pearl formation, also shows development of a granular cell layer. Knowledge of these features of the primary neoplasm may prove helpful in recognizing the primary site for a metastatic carcinoma (H&E stain, high power).

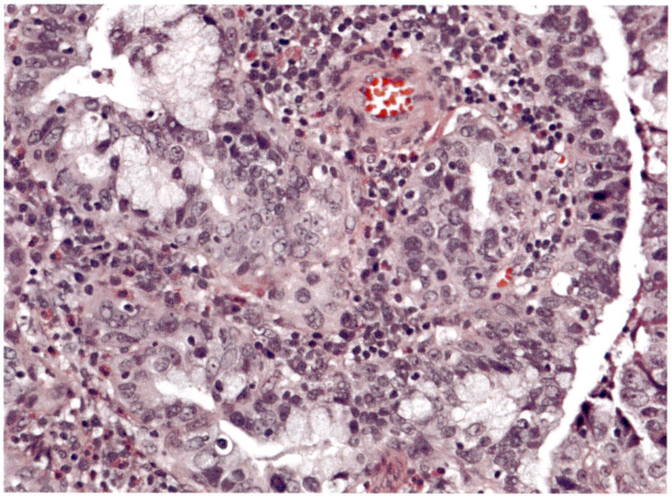

Figure 7.62 — Invasive high-grade urothelial carcinoma with glandular differentiation, histologic section. In addition to some urothelial carcinomas showing gland-like lumina, divergent differentiation towards gland formation or signet-ring cell features may also be seen. Glandular differentiation is seen in 10 percent of urothelial carcinomas. It has not been proven that having squamous or glandular differentiation significantly alters the behavior of the primary neoplasm. Some studies suggest such divergent differentiation means poor response to radiation or chemotherapy; these studies, however, have not yet been clinically proven (H&E stain, medium power).

Figure 7.63 — Invasive high-grade urothelial carcinoma with mucinous features, histologic section. Nests of invasive carcinoma float in mucin lakes. Some cells contain intracytoplasmic mucin (H&E stain, medium power).

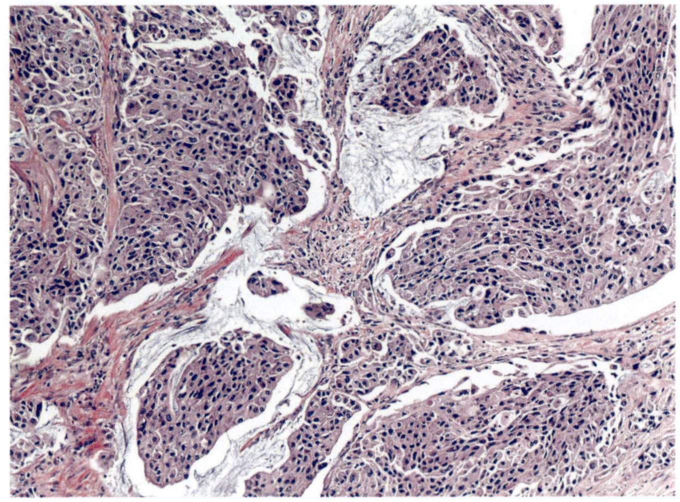

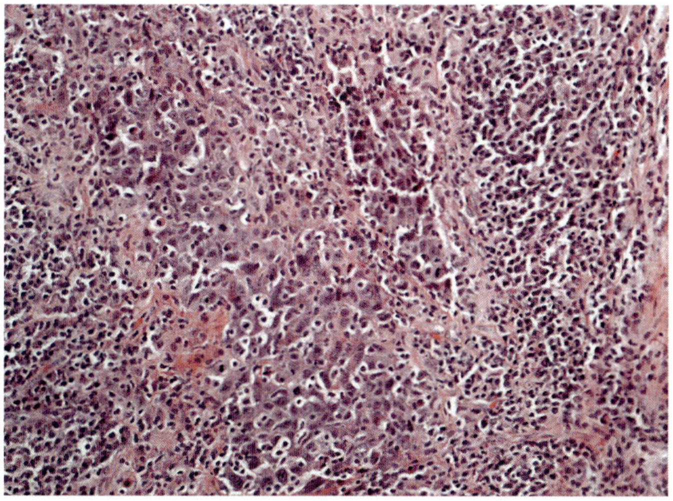

Figure 7.64 — Lymphoepithelioma-like urothelial carcinoma, histologic section. As the name implies, this rare variant of urothelial carcinoma resembles the undifferentiated nasopharyngeal carcinoma of the head and neck, which is also known as lymphoepithelioma. The epithelial component comprises large cells with pale eosinophilic cytoplasm, vesicular nuclei with clumped chromatin, and prominent nucleoli. The cells are arranged in a syncytial pattern surrounded and infiltrated by intense chronic inflammatory infiltrates. The inflammation sometimes obscures the epithelial component, making the diagnosis difficult. No association with EBV has been elicited (H&E stain, medium power).

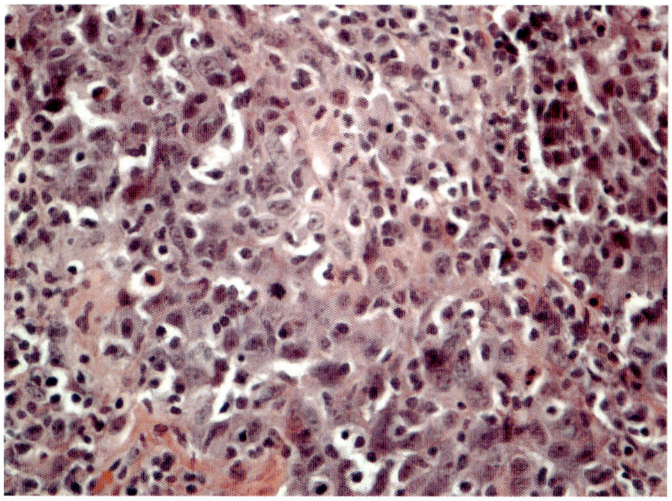

Figure 7.65 — Lymphoepithelioma-like urothelial carcinoma, histologic section. A mitotic figure is evident in the epithelial component. The cytoplasmic membranes of the malignant epithelial cells are indistinct. Differential diagnosis for this carcinoma is with lymphoma and conventional urothelial carcinoma with brisk inflammatory response. This variant can occur in pure form or mixed with conventional urothelial carcinoma. When in pure form the prognosis is slightly better and in some cases responds to chemotherapy (H&E stain, high power).

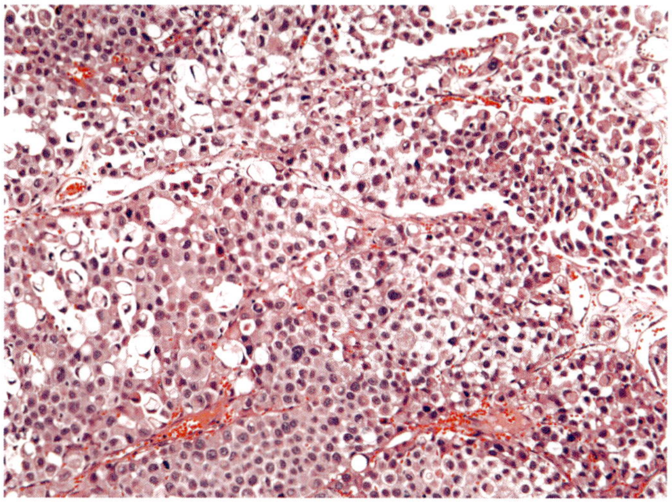

Figure 7.66 — Undifferentiated urothelial carcinoma with signet-ring cell and plasmacytoid features, histologic section. Urothelial carcinoma with plasmacytoid features only rarely has pure histology. More often it is mixed with conventional urothelial carcinoma or has been noted with micropapillary and nested features. The malignant cells resemble plasma cells with eosinophilic cytoplasm and eccentric nuclei, which are hyperchromatic with clumped chromatin. Intracytoplasmic vacuoles are present in some cells, consistent with focal signet-ring cell features. Cells are dyscohesive and arranged in sheets or nests in a loose myxoid stroma (H&E stain, medium power).

Figure 7.67 — Undifferentiated urothelial carcinoma with signet-ring cell and plasmacytoid features, histologic section. This image of urothelial carcinoma with plasmacytoid features shows a solid growth pattern, nuclear pleomorphism, and brisk mitoses. Plasmacytoid urothelial carcinomas are considered aggressive tumors with poor prognosis. The differential diagnosis includes plasmacytoma. Occasional positivity with CD138, a marker for plasma cells, has been noted in these tumors, however cytokeratin immunostains strongly highlight the malignant cells of plasmacytoid urothelial carcinoma (H&E stain, medium power).

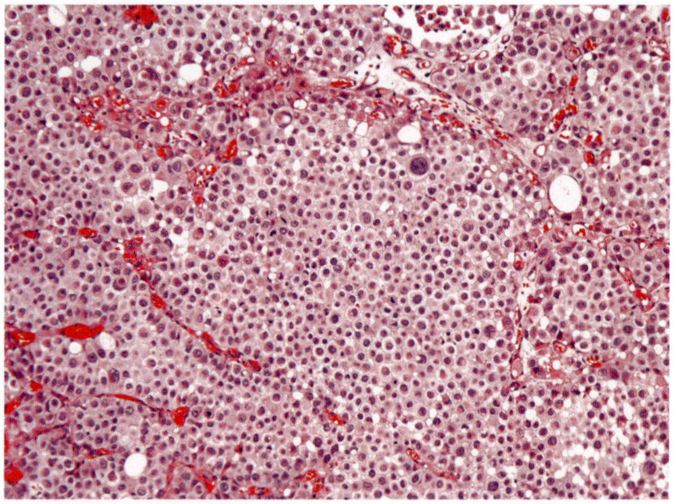

Figure 7.68 — Plasmacytoid urothelial carcinoma, histologic section. The cells of this variant are dyscohesive, and although they have eccentric nuclei and amphophilic cytoplasm, the nuclei lack the clumped chromatin of plasma cells (H&E stain, high power).

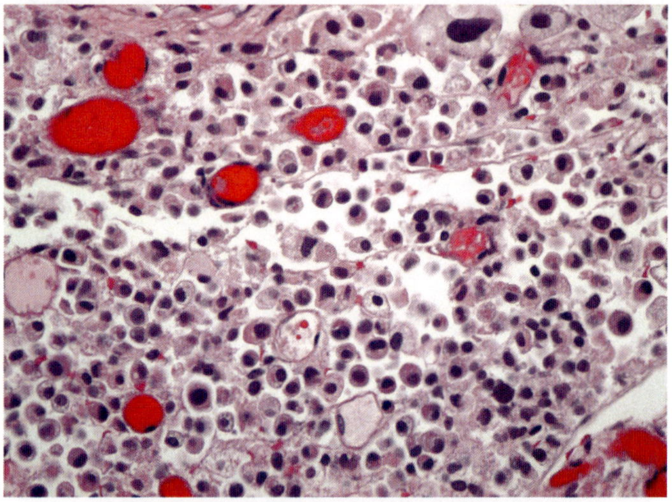

Figure 7.69 — Plasmacytoid urothelial carcinoma highlighted by cytokeratin, histologic section. Strong positivity with pancytokeratin is seen in the tumor cells (CK immunostain, low power).

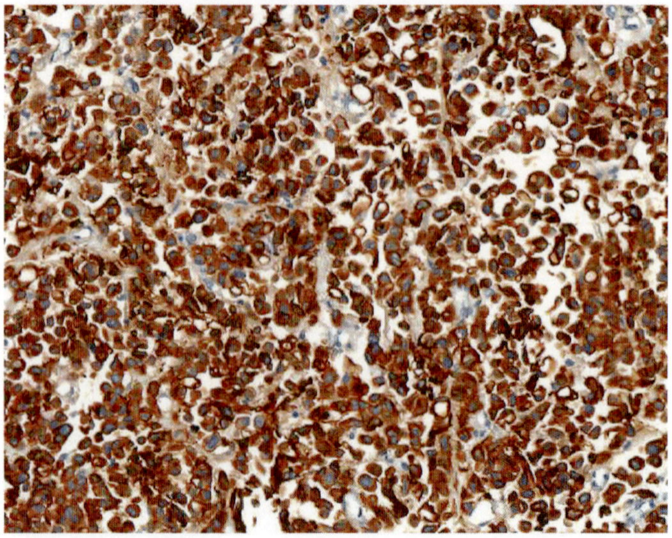

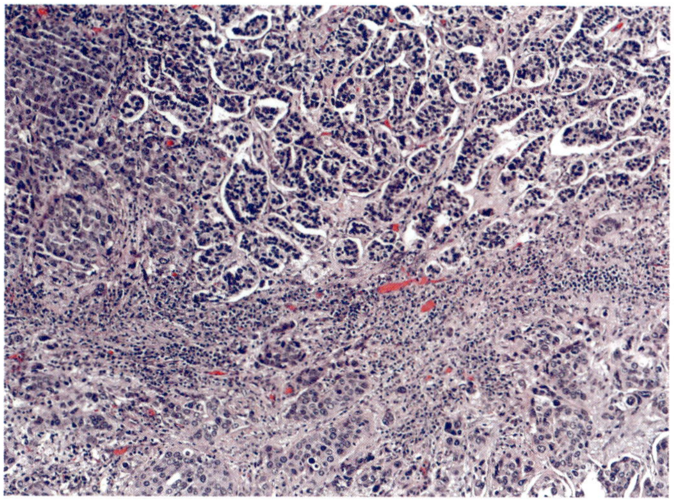

Figure 7.70 — Invasive micropapillary urothelial carcinoma, histologic section. This image shows invasive micropapillary carcinoma in the top half and invasive conventional urothelial carcinoma in the lower half of the field. The morphology of micropapillary carcinoma is similar to that seen in micropapillary carcinoma arising in the ovary. The invasive component makes small tight nests that reside in lacunar spaces. There may be scant myxoid stroma seen and other times there is no stroma or desmoplastic response to the invading carcinoma. The cells comprising the invading nests are usually small and have hyperchromatic nuclei. In cases where micropapillary carcinoma is a component of conventional urothelial carcinoma, it should be quantified as a percentage of the entire tumor (H&E stain, low power).

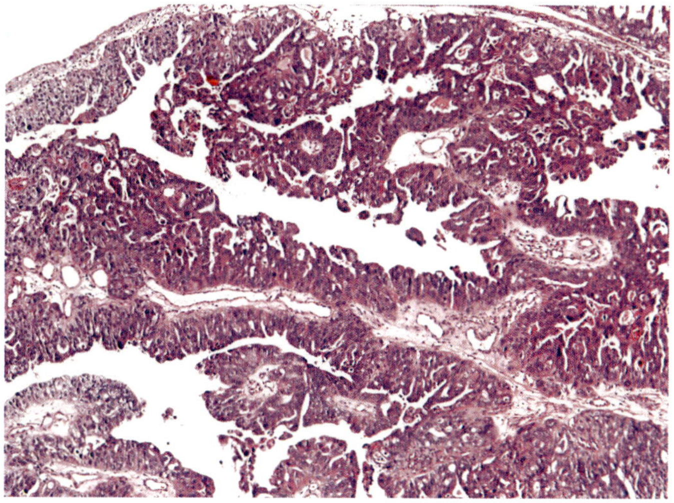

Figure 7.71 — Noninvasive micropapillary urothelial carcinoma, histologic section. On the surface noninvasive micropapillary carcinoma forms small filiform structures and papillae, usually without fibrovascular cores. The architecture of the noninvasive component may be quite complex, as seen in the image (H&E stain, low power).

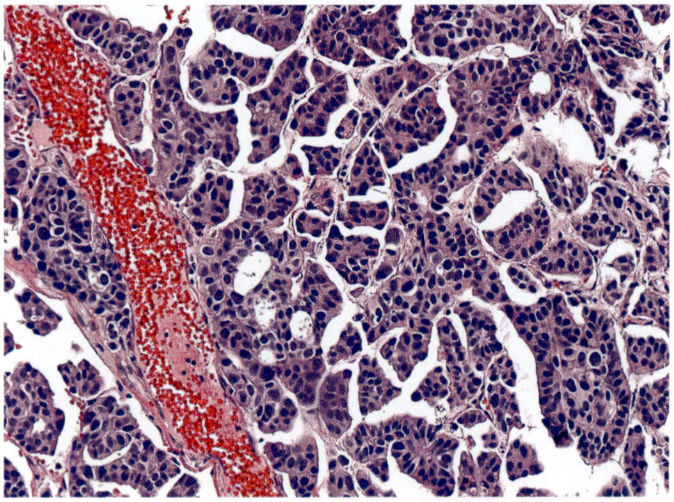

Figure 7.72 — Noninvasive micropapillary urothelial carcinoma, histologic section. A majority of micropapillary carcinomas are myoinvasive at the time of initial diagnosis. These are considered aggressive variants and are frequently associated with lymphovascular invasion. The five- and ten-year survival rates are 51 percent and 24 percent, respectively. The image shows the angulated nests in lacunar spaces with little intervening stroma. The architecture of these carcinomas mimics lymphovascular invasion. Utilization of immunohistochemistry for endothelial cells (CD31 and D2-40) to definitively identify lymphatic invasion proves helpful (H&E stain, medium power).

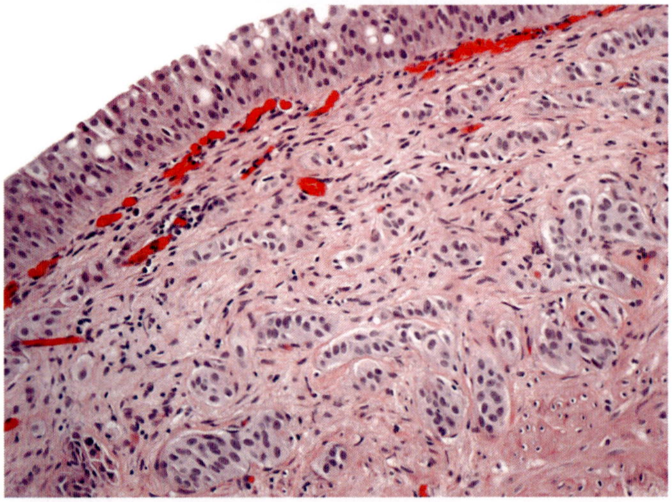

Figure 7.73 — Invasive nested variant of urothelial carcinoma, histologic section. This urothelial carcinoma shows bland, low-grade morphology and grows in small, ovoid nests. This variant has not been noted to be associated with a surface in situ lesion. The differential diagnosis, especially in a small biopsy specimen, includes florid proliferation of von Brunn's nests. Unlike von Brunn's nests, those of the nested variant of urothelial carcinoma are irregular in size and shape and are haphazardly arranged. The nuclei appear enlarged and may have prominent nucleoli (H&E stain, high power).

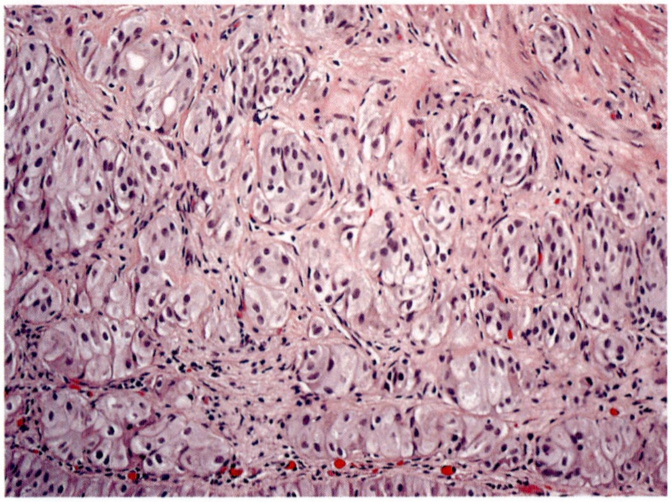

Figure 7.74 — Invasive nested variant of urothelial carcinoma, histologic section. Despite their innocuous appearance, these neoplasms present at a higher clinical stage and behave more aggressively, often myoinvasive at the time of diagnosis. The stromal response is in the form of edema and inflammation. A desmoplastic reaction is not seen around these tumors. Other differential diagnoses include paraganglioma and nephrogenic adenoma, especially when there are tubule formations (H&E stain, high power).

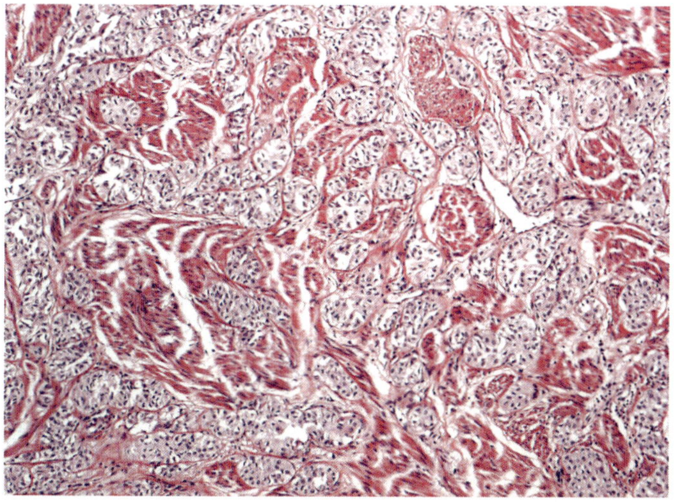

Figure 7.75 — Nested variant of urothelial carcinoma with muscle invasion, histologic section. Deep invasion of the muscularis propria is seen in this image. Note the bland morphology of the invading carcinoma (H&E stain, medium power).

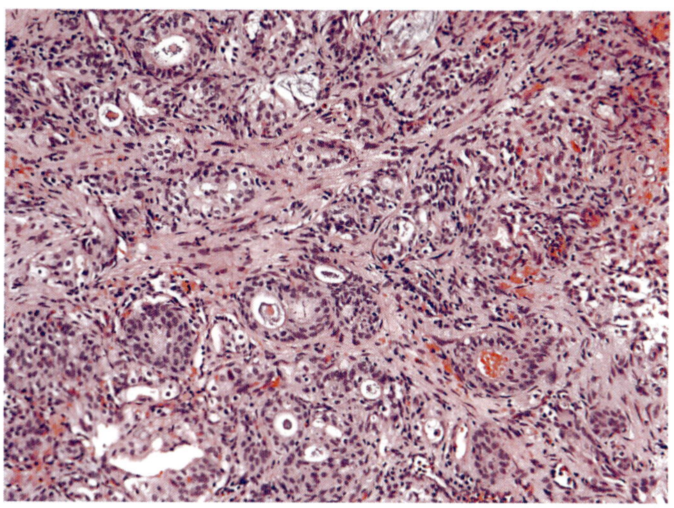

Figure 7.76 — Nested variant of urothelial carcinoma with tubules, histologic section. Sometimes a nested variant may show tubule formation within the nests. These may be seen focally or could be more widespread. The tubules may be lined by cuboidal or columnar cells. The morphology remains low grade. As seen in the image, the stroma is usually inflamed. The irregular invasive appearance helps with arriving at the correct diagnosis of carcinoma (H&E stain, medium power).

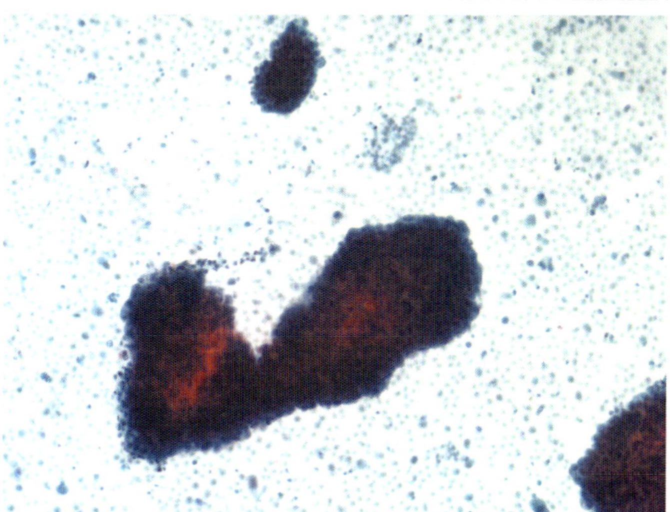

Figure 7.77 — High-grade papillary urothelial carcinoma, instrumented urine. Large fragments of urothelium with supporting fibrovascular stalks are indicative of a papillary lesion. However, the grading of the lesion must be interpreted using higher magnification. Numerous single degenerated cells are present in the background (Papanicolaou stain, medium power).

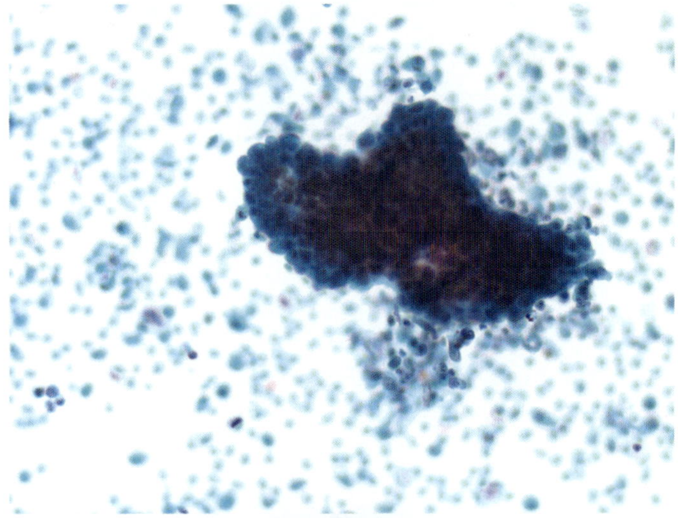

Figure 7.78 — High-grade papillary urothelial carcinoma, instrumented urine. Surrounding this fragment of urothelium are numerous individual cells, both nucleolated and anucleate, suggesting a tremendous amount of cellular shedding and degeneration. The individual cells within the fragment have high N/C ratios and are large and hyperchromatic, all indicative of a high-grade lesion (Papanicolaou stain, medium power).

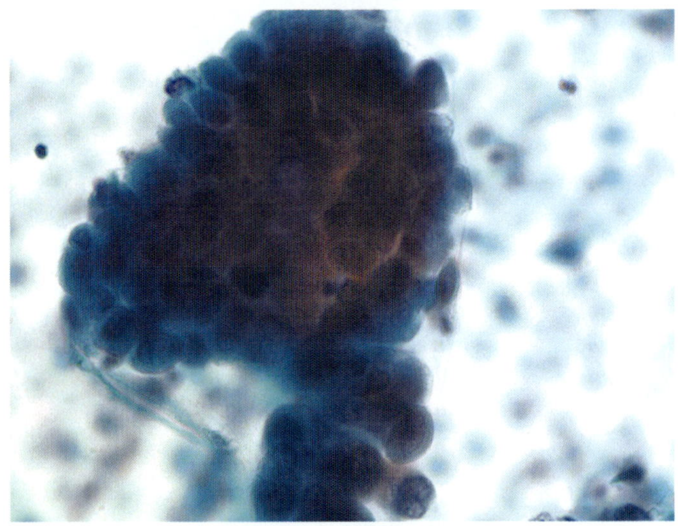

Figure 7.79 — High-grade papillary urothelial carcinoma, instrumented urine. High magnification will confirm the morphologic details of large cells with high N/C ratios, hyperchromatic nuclei, occasional prominent nucleoli, and irregular nuclear outlines for a diagnosis of high-grade urothelial carcinoma (Papanicolaou stain, high power).

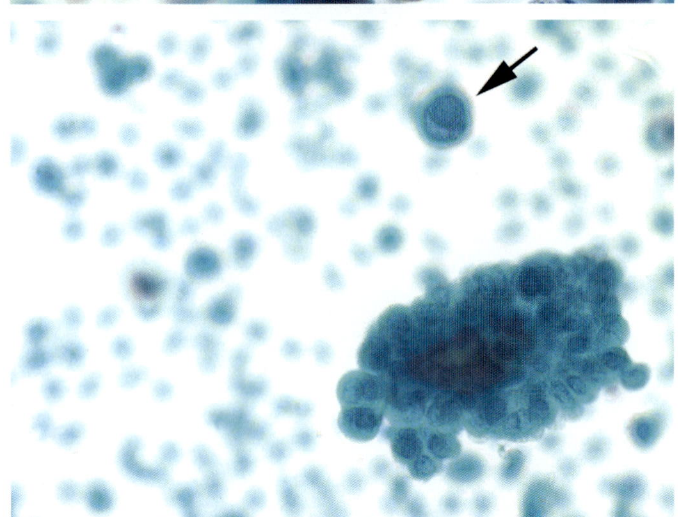

Figure 7.80 — High-grade papillary urothelial carcinoma, instrumented urine. Not only will fragments of urothelium have cells with characteristics of high-grade carcinoma, but individual cells are the norm in such samples. They are more easily identified as high-grade (arrow) and should be searched for in a sample if the suggestion of that diagnosis is made but not confirmed by the fragments of tissue (Papanicolaou stain, high power).

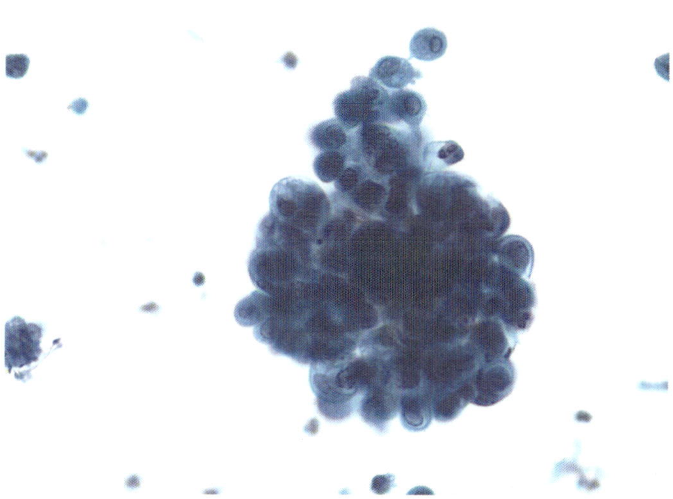

Figure 7.81 — High-grade papillary urothelial carcinoma, instrumented urine. Cytoplasmic differentiation manifested by vacuoles, or squamous opacity should not dissuade the diagnosis of urothelial carcinoma. Such differentiation is characteristic of high-grade lesions (Papanicolaou stain, high power).

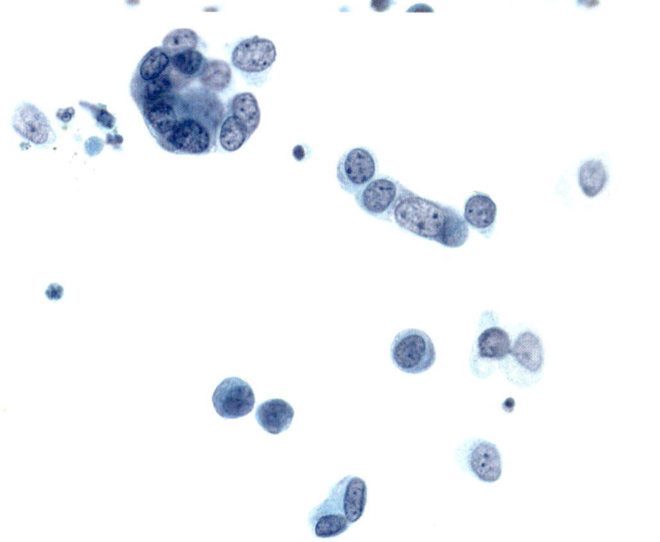

Figure 7.82 — High-grade papillary urothelial carcinoma, voided urine. Individual cells and small groups of cells are more frequently seen than large fragments in high-grade lesions. The clean background suggests absence of invasion (Papanicolaou stain, medium power).

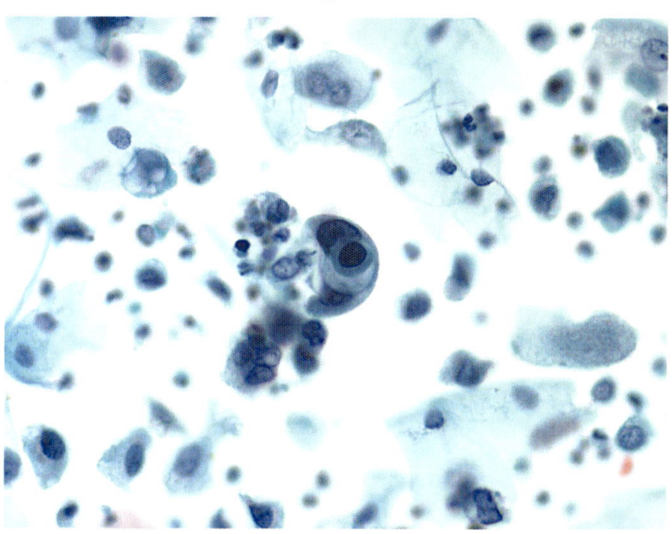

Figure 7.83 — High-grade papillary urothelial carcinoma, voided urine. This crescent-shaped fragment has demarcated cytoplasmic boundaries, varying from opaque cytoplasm to vacuoles, which suggests squamous differentiation. High grade is obvious, based on the size of the nuclei and the chromatin pattern. Urothelial carcinoma can have features of both squamous and glandular cells (Papanicolaou stain, medium power).

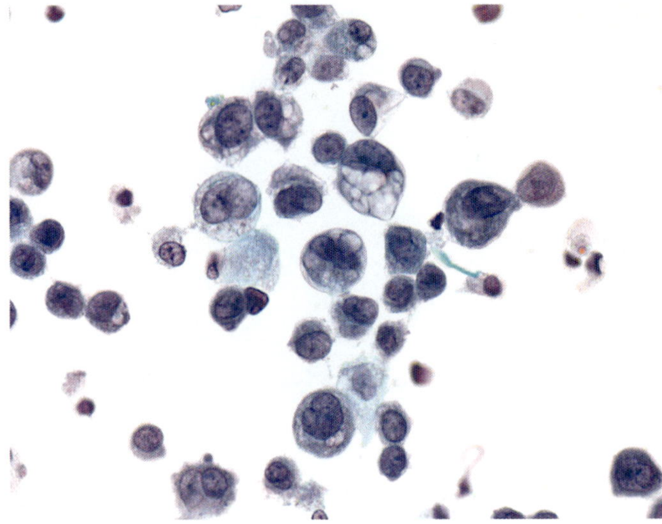

Figure 7.84 — High-grade papillary urothelial carcinoma, voided urine. The vacuoles in the cytoplasm of these cells suggest a glandular lesion. However, the individuality of the cells is unusual if an adenocarcinoma is truly the source. Unless suggested by history or presence of another primary lesion, high-grade urothelial carcinoma is the most likely diagnosis (Papanicolaou stain, high power).

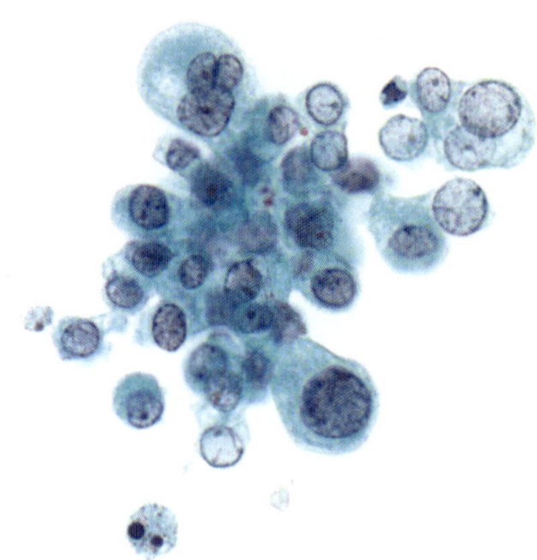

Figure 7.85 — High-grade papillary urothelial carcinoma, voided urine. Cells within the same sample will vary from low grade to high grade based on their morphologic characteristics. As usual, the cells with the most malignant characteristics form the basis for the grading of the sample (Papanicolaou stain, medium power).

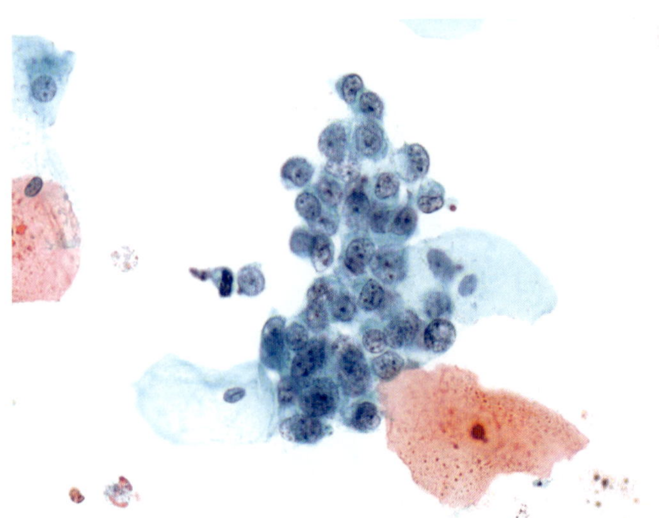

Figure 7.86 — High-grade papillary urothelial carcinoma, voided urine. While the features of high-grade urothelial carcinoma are usually considered to be variability in nuclear chromatin and cell size, occasionally the cellular monotony may suggest a low-grade lesion. However, the size of the nuclei when compared to the size of an intermediate squamous nucleus is considerably larger, and therefore should imply the diagnosis of high-grade carcinoma. Also, the presence of nucleoli in such large cells with high N/C ratios is consistent with a high-grade diagnosis (Papanicolaou stain, medium power).

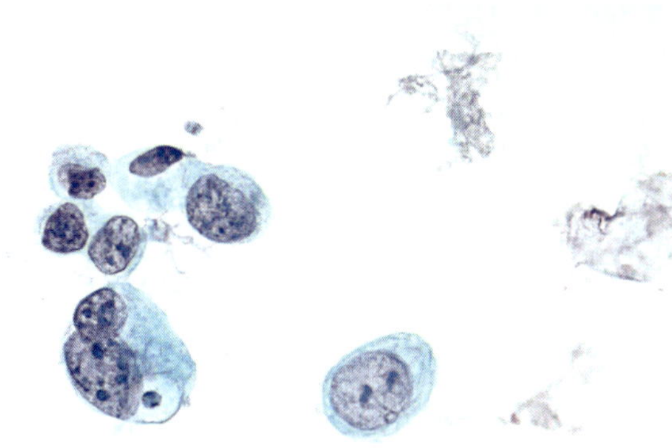

Figure 7.87 — High-grade papillary urothelial carcinoma, voided urine. Cells that are binucleate with unequal size are immediately characterized as malignant. All of the cells within this photograph have characteristics of a very high-grade urothelial carcinoma (Papanicolaou stain, high power).

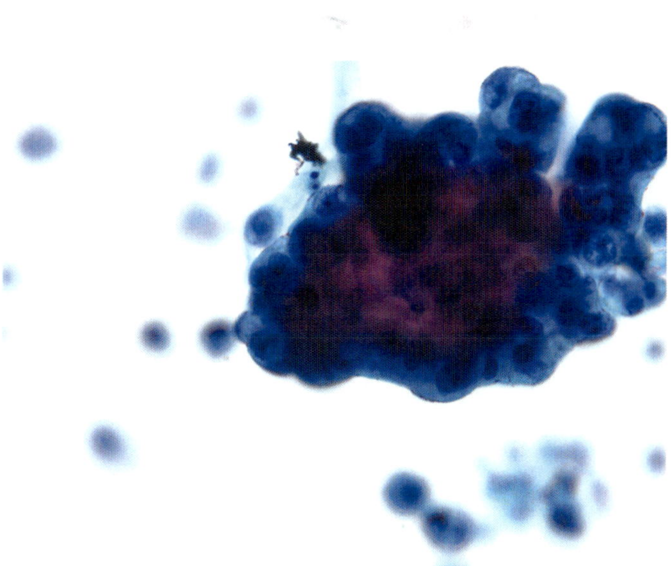

Figure 7.88 — High-grade papillary urothelial carcinoma, instrumented urine. Three dimensional fragments of high-grade urothelium suggest a papillary lesion even though a fibrovascular stalk is not present. Within this fragment are large and ugly nuclei with prominent nucleoli. Vacuolization is simply a variation in the differentiation of the cell line (Papanicolaou stain, high power).

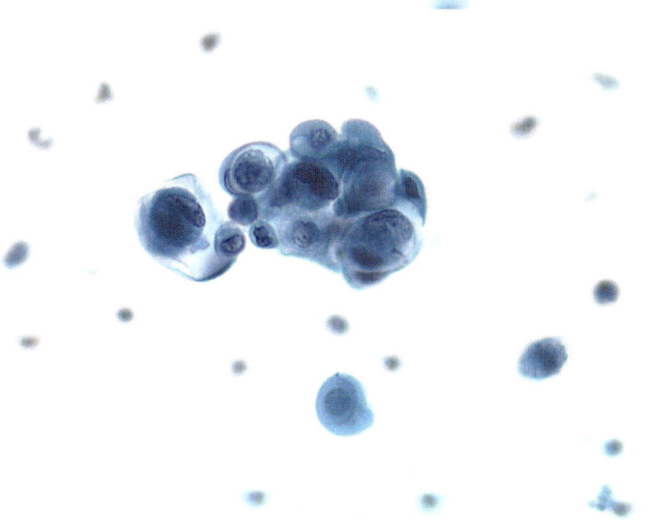

Figure 7.89 — High-grade papillary urothelial carcinoma, instrumented urine. This high-grade urothelial carcinoma displays "ball and claw" groupings that are characteristic of squamous differentiation. In addition, most of the cells have opaque cytoplasm and very sharply defined cytoplasmic boundaries as well as cell separation, all squamous features. Unless the entire malignant population of cells in the sample displays squamous differentiation, the most likely diagnosis is a high-grade urothelial carcinoma (Papanicolaou stain, high power).

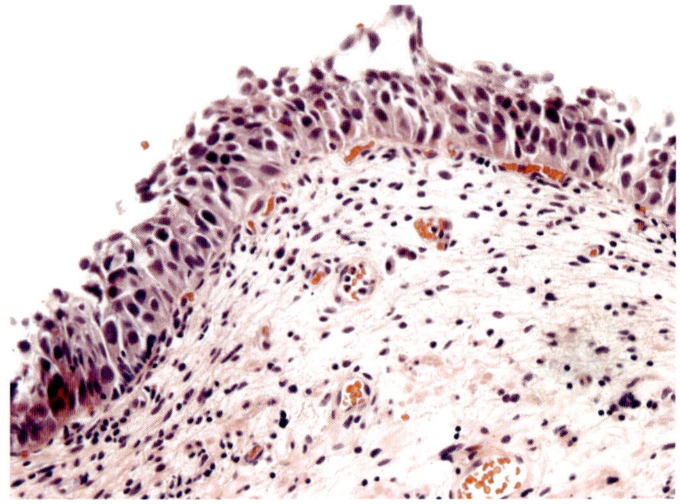

Figure 7.90 — Flat urothelial carcinoma in situ (CIS), histologic section. CIS is a high-grade precursor lesion to invasive urothelial carcinoma. By definition, it is urothelial carcinoma confined to the mucosa. In general, CIS has cellular crowding, loss of polarity, increased N/C ratios, nuclear pleomorphism, increased mitoses and dyscohesiveness. The image depicts the loss of polarity with cellular crowding and hyperchromasia of the nuclei. The surface appears to lose cells due to lack of cohesiveness (H&E stain, medium power).

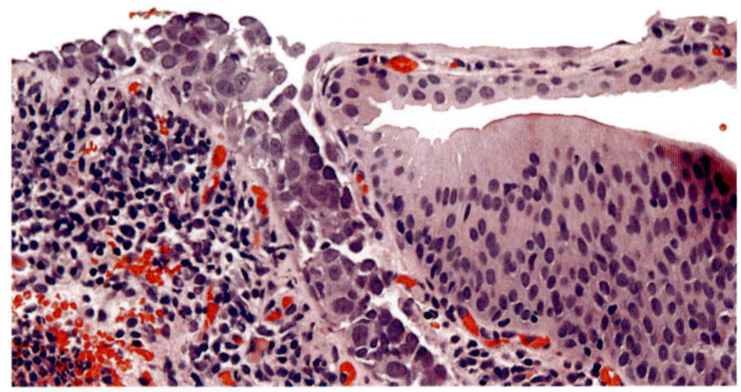

Figure 7.91 — Flat urothelial CIS with normal adjacent urothelium, histologic section. In comparison with the normal urothelium on the right, CIS nuclei are at least twice the size, with disorganization, nuclear membrane irregularities, prominent nucleoli, and dyscohesive nature. An excellent reference is the ever-present stromal lymphocyte; normal urothelial nuclei are two to three times the size of the lymphocyte, while CIS nuclei are four to five times larger (H&E stain, medium power).

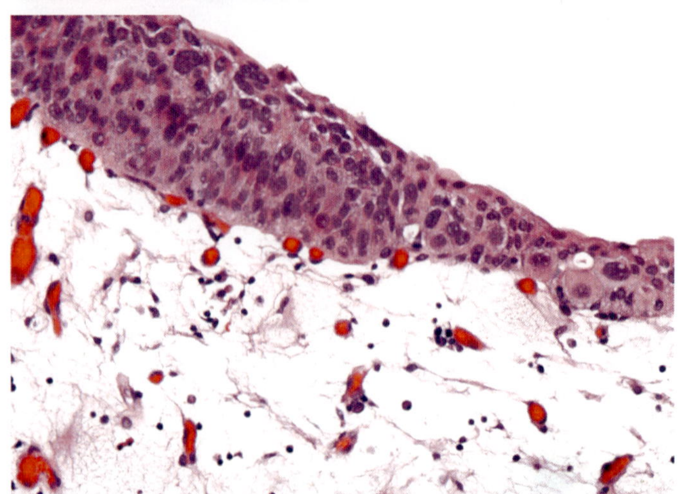

Figure 7.92 — Flat urothelial CIS, histologic section. The mucosa involved by CIS may be thin due to loss of layers, completely denuded, hyperplastic, or of normal thickness. The histologic diagnosis of CIS does not require full thickness dysplasia. The presence of even few large hyperchromatic cells towards the surface, as seen in the image would suggest a diagnosis of CIS, (H&E stain, high power).

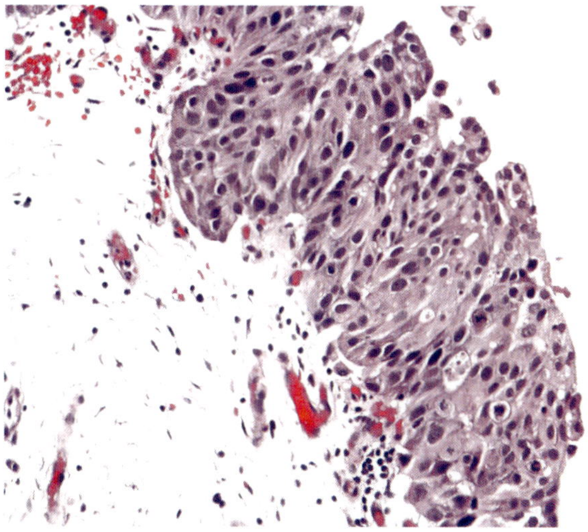

Figure 7.93 — Flat urothelial CIS, histologic section. This example of CIS shows increased mitoses and apoptosis, in addition to crowding, loss of polarity, hyperchromasia, and sloughing of the cells. Progression of CIS to invasive carcinoma occurs in up to 25 percent of patients. CIS is most often seen in association with high-grade papillary or invasive urothelial carcinoma (H&E stain, medium power).

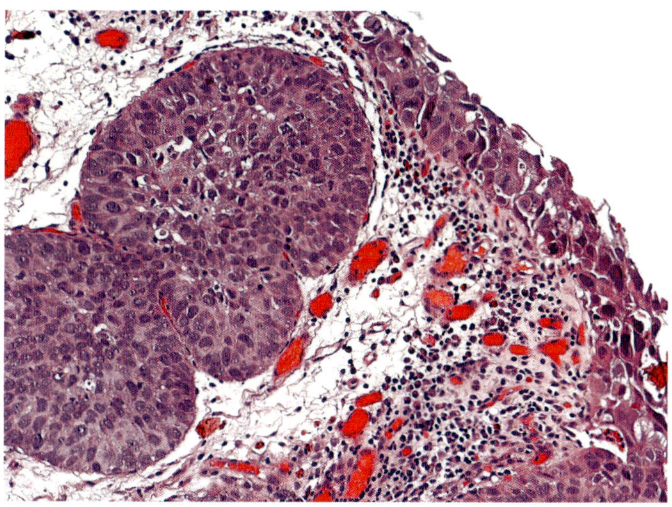

Figure 7.94 — Flat urothelial CIS, histologic section. CIS has involved a von Brunn's nest within lamina propria. This does not equate to invasion of the lamina propria, note the smooth edges of the von Brunn's nest with an intact basement membrane. The lamina propria underlying CIS is quite often inflamed and hypervascular, giving it the erythematous appearance visualized at cystoscopy (H&E stain, medium power).

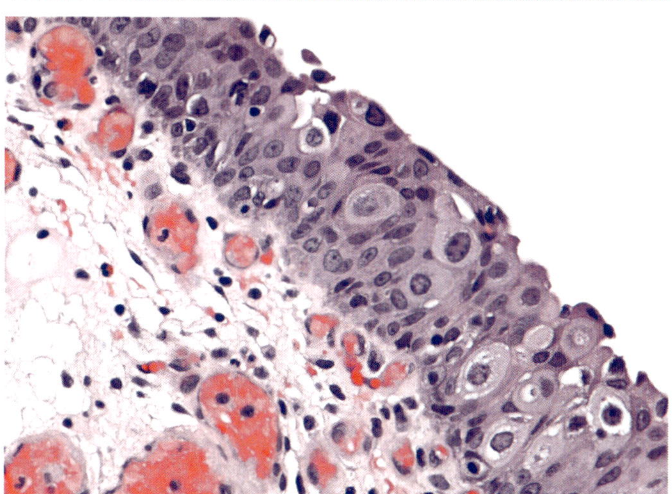

Figure 7.95 — Flat urothelial CIS with pagetoid spread, histologic section. CIS cells may cause cancerization of adjacent normal urothelium, as seen in the image. Single CIS cells are showing pagetoid spread within the benign urothelium. Lamina propria is congested and inflamed (H&E stain, high power).

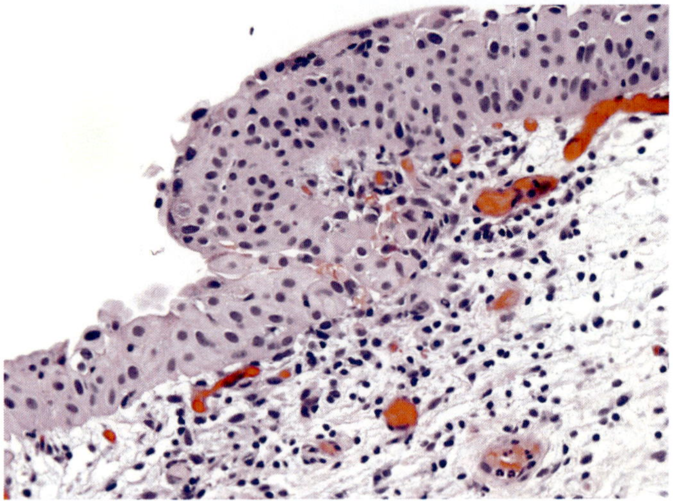

Figure 7.96 — Flat urothelial CIS with focus of early lamina propria invasion, histologic section. Flat CIS has broken through the basement membrane; small irregular nests and single nuclei are seen within the lamina propria, with slight clefting around the invading nests (H&E stain, high power).

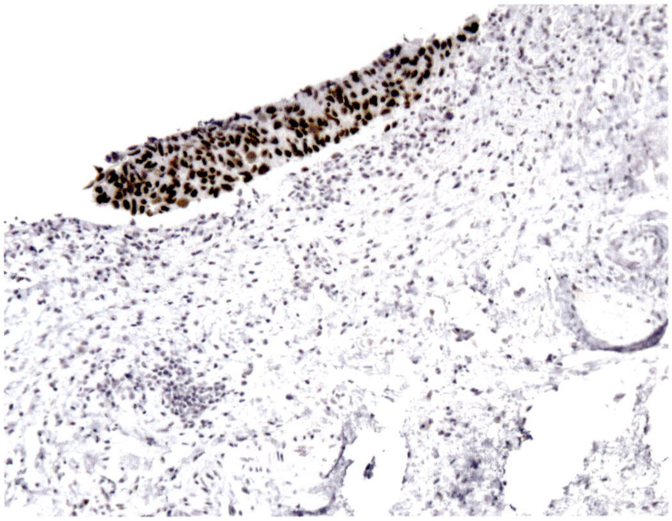

Figure 7.97 — Flat urothelial CIS highlighted by p53 immunostain, histologic section. CIS is thought to arise because of an early mutation or deletion in the cell cycle regulator, p53. CIS lesions often harbor p53 alterations (i.e., accumulation of p53 protein) and the malignant cells are strongly p53 immunoreactive (p53 immunostain, medium power).

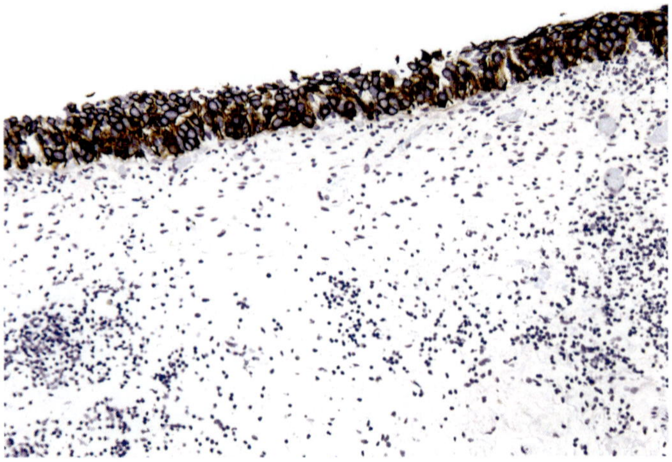

Figure 7.98 — Flat urothelial CIS with CK20 immunostain, histologic section. In normal urothelium, only the umbrella cell layer is selectively CK20 positive. However, when the mucosa is involved by CIS, the entire thickness of the urothelium is highlighted by a strong immunolabeling to CK20 (CK20 immunostain, medium power).

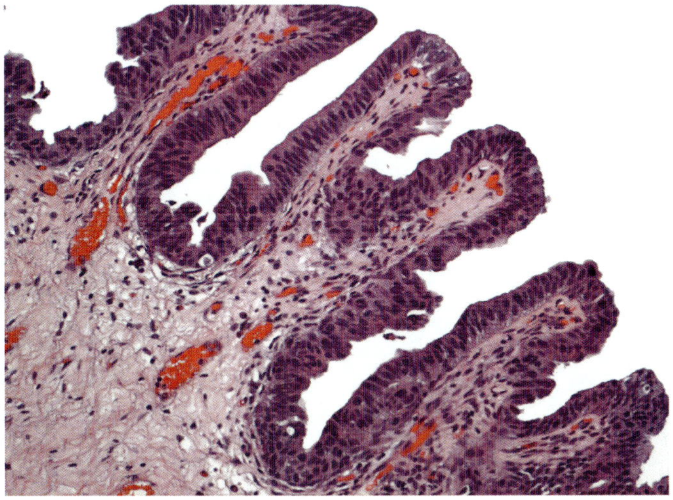

Figure 7.99 — Flat urothelial CIS with glandular differentiation, histologic section. This lesion, when it involves the bladder, is most often not accompanied by invasive adenocarcinoma, hence the term "in situ adenocarcinoma," (a term not currently preferred). Noninvasive urothelial carcinoma with glandular differentiation has also been associated with infiltrating urothelial carcinoma, small-cell carcinoma, and micropapillary urothelial carcinoma. The latter two portend a bad prognosis. Morphologically, noninvasive urothelial carcinoma with glandular differentiation has the appearance of high-grade dysplasia seen in adenomatous polyps of the bowel. There are elongated, hyperchromatic, pseudostratified nuclei with increased mitoses (H&E stain, high power).

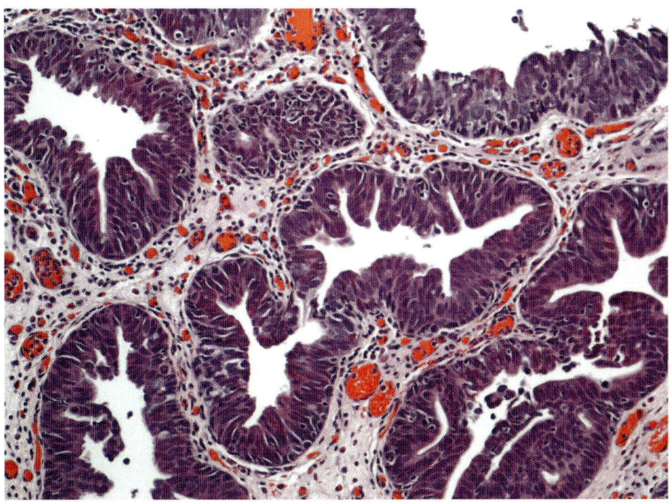

Figure 7.100 — Noninvasive urothelial carcinoma with glandular differentiation and flat CIS, histologic section. Noninvasive urothelial carcinoma with glandular differentiation seen in the lower half of the image is accompanied by flat CIS on the surface. Note the stratification of elongated hyperchromatic nuclei lining the gland-like spaces in the lamina propria (H&E stain, high power).

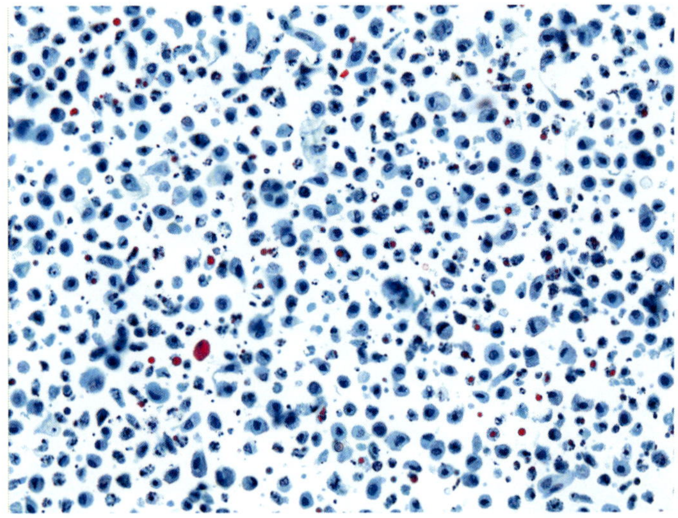

Figure 7.101 — Flat urothelial CIS, voided urine. In contrast to high-grade papillary carcinoma, with its fragments of tissue, samples from a flat CIS characteristically contain single cells. Occasional small groupings may be seen, but the predominant cell type is single and may have definite squamous features such as tadpole cytoplasmic tails and opaque cytoplasm (Papanicolaou stain, low power).

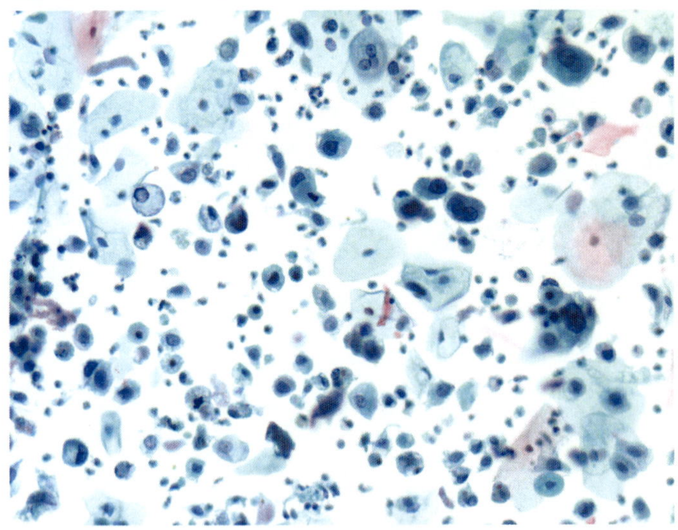

Figure 7.102 — Flat urothelial CIS, voided urine. The size of the lesion, and the sampling method, voided versus washing, will determine the numbers of abnormal cells in the sample. Although most high-grade urothelial carcinomas shed abundant cells, careful search is sometimes needed and even a few cells with high-grade characteristics should be sufficient to at least suggest the diagnosis if not confirm it (Papanicolaou stain, medium power).

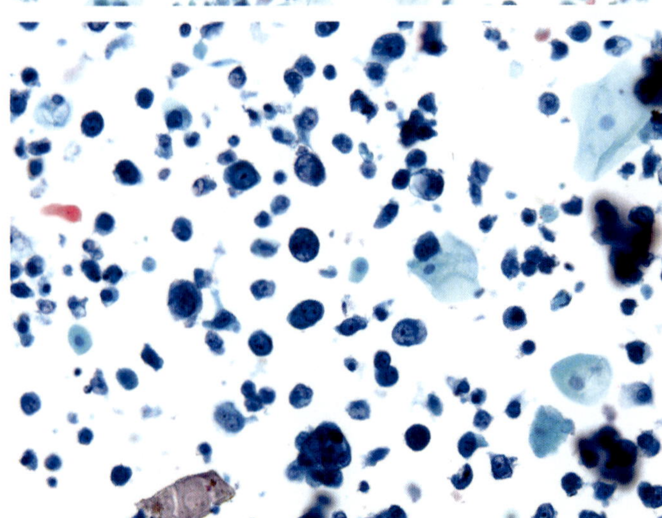

Figure 7.103 — Flat urothelial CIS, voided urine. The classic picture of flat CIS of the urinary bladder is a clean background, implying lack of invasion, and single, large, highly abnormal cells. This photograph is prototypical (Papanicolaou stain, medium power).

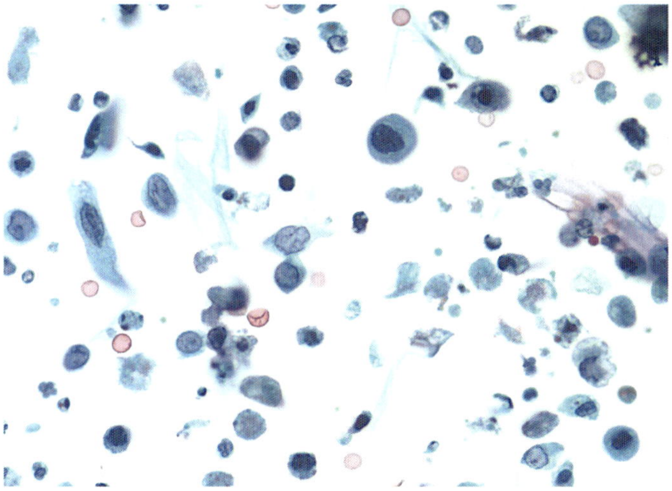

Figure 7.104 — Flat urothelial CIS, voided urine. Although the classic nuclear appearance of a high-grade lesion is hyperchromatic, pale nuclear chromatin may be seen, and so long as the large size and abnormal shape are present in a cell with a high N/C ratio, the diagnosis can still be made. Usually, however, mixtures of these cell types will be seen as well as mixtures of cell size with varying degrees of degeneration, as in this sample. Despite the amount of cytoplasmic fragmentation and occasional red blood cells, the background can still be interpreted as "clean" due to lack of necrotic debris, thus implying absence of invasion (Papanicolaou stain, medium power).

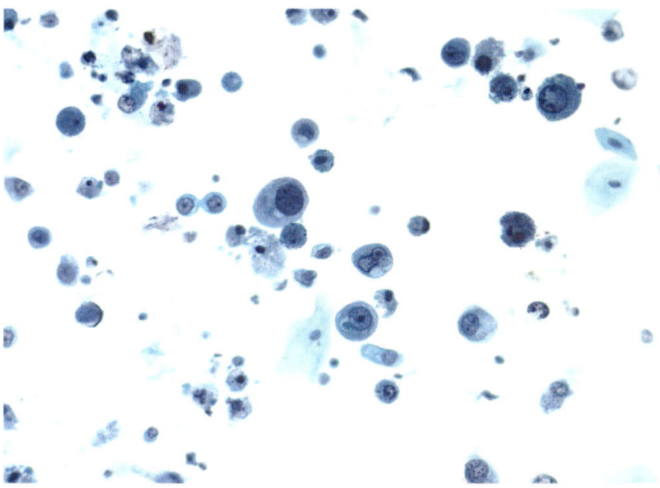

Figure 7.105 — Flat urothelial CIS, voided urine. The range of cell size in a flat CIS of the bladder is impressive. Along with the classic large cells, smaller cells can be found that will still originate in the tumor and should be looked for and appreciated, since occasionally this will be the only cell type in a sample, especially from a voided urine (Papanicolaou stain, medium power).

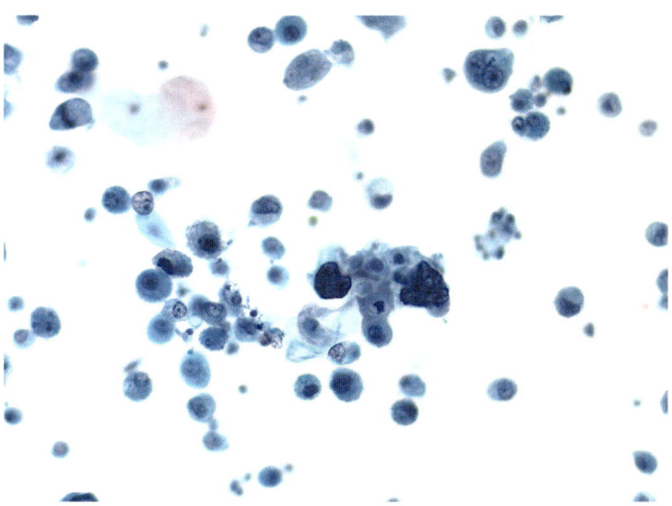

Figure 7.106 — Flat urothelial CIS, voided urine. Extreme hyperchromasia and degeneration of the nuclear chromatin may suggest polyoma virus infection in cells of a CIS. However, the nuclear shape variation is diagnostic of carcinoma and should not be confused with simply a viral infection. Notwithstanding, polyoma virus can infect cancer cells (see Figures 4.7–4.13; Papanicolaou stain, medium power).

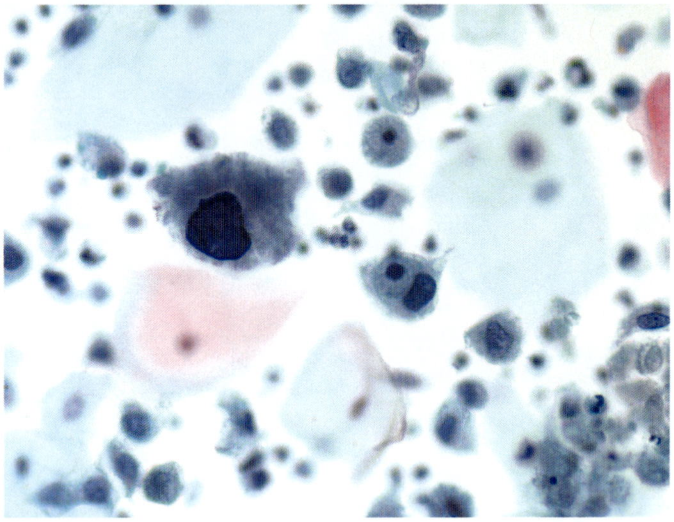

Figure 7.107 — Flat urothelial CIS, voided urine. High-grade urothelial carcinoma does not necessarily have to have cells with a high N/C ratio. Simply the size of the nucleus and the overall size of the cell can be sufficient to indicate a high grade (Papanicolaou stain, high power).

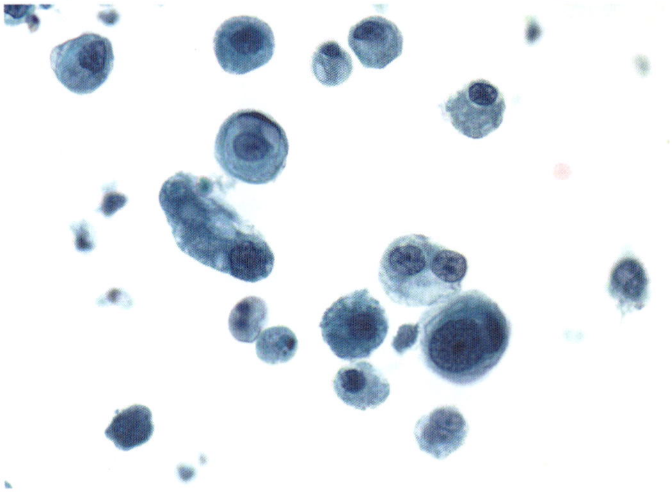

Figure 7.108 — Flat urothelial CIS, voided urine. Within these samples of a high-grade urothelial carcinoma can be cytoplasmic features of both squamous and glandular cells. This is an indication of the multipotential of this particular cell line (Papanicolaou stain, high power).

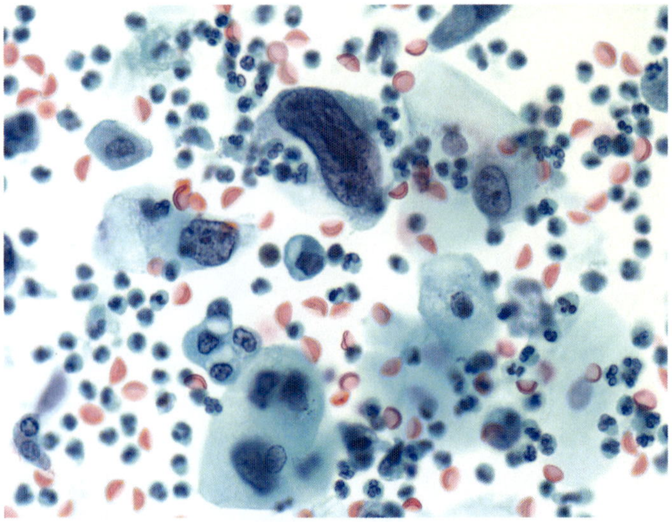

Figure 7.109 — Flat urothelial CIS, voided urine. Very bizarre cells within a sample might suggest origin in another site, as most high-grade urothelial carcinomas have a consistent range of cell size. If the urothelial carcinoma has been radiated or is very inflamed as in this sample, the morphologic changes may be very dramatic (Papanicolaou stain, high power).

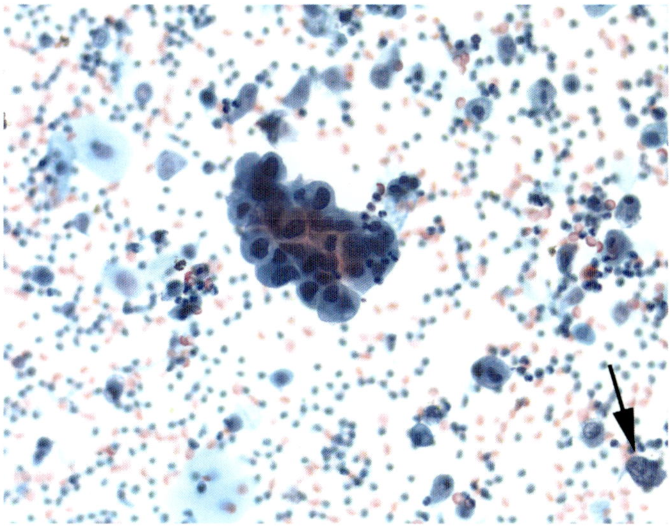

Figure 7.110 — Flat urothelial CIS, voided urine. Within a sample of a flat CIS, there may be fragments of urothelium that are of lesser grade, especially if the specimen has been catheterized. The cells in the center of this photograph have N/C ratios that are lower than would be anticipated for a high-grade lesion. However, at the lower right hand corner of the field is a large cell with a very high N/C ratio, characteristic of a high-grade lesion (arrow). Careful search of the entire sample is essential for an accurate diagnosis (Papanicolaou stain, medium power).

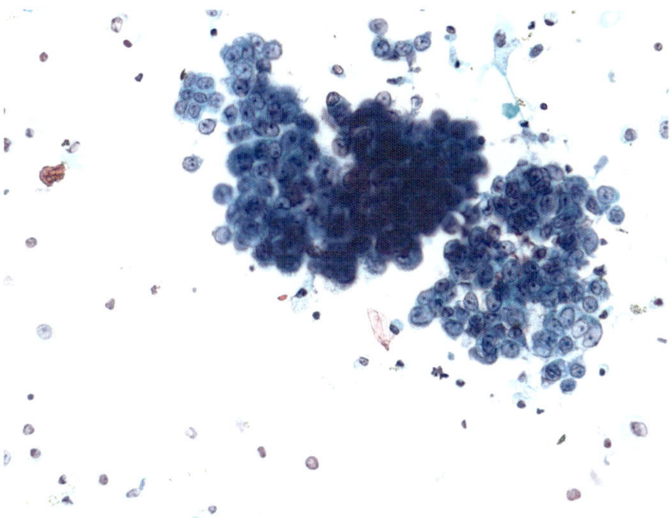

Figure 7.111 — Flat urothelial CIS, instrumented urine. Mostly cohesive cells are clustered in fragments that on initial examination are uniform and suggest a low grade. However, the N/C ratios are very high, nucleoli are prominent, and compared with the size of the occasional red cells or lymphocytes in the background, the cells are very large. This should be diagnosed as a high-grade lesion, despite the misleading feature of uniform cells within the lesion (Papanicolaou stain, medium power).

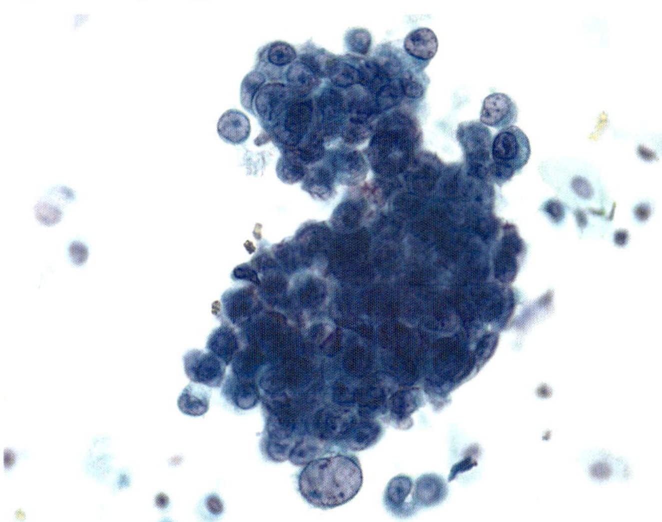

Figure 7.112 — Flat urothelial CIS, instrumented urine. A dense fragment of tissue contains large cells with almost no cytoplasm and unevenly textured chromatin. The variable size, mostly large, and the disorganized arrangement of these cells are characteristics of a high-grade lesion. This may represent a papillary lesion, although if the sample was obtained by catheter or bladder washing, this would explain the presence of a large fragment (Papanicolaou stain, high power).

Figure 7.113 — Flat urothelial CIS, instrumented urine. Samples obtained by catheterization may contain cells from the depths of the epithelium as well as the surface. This is in contrast to samples where the cells are spontaneously exfoliated and therefore will be isolated rather than in tissue fragments. Knowing the method of sample collection is essential to proper interpretation of the cells present (Papanicolaou stain, high power).

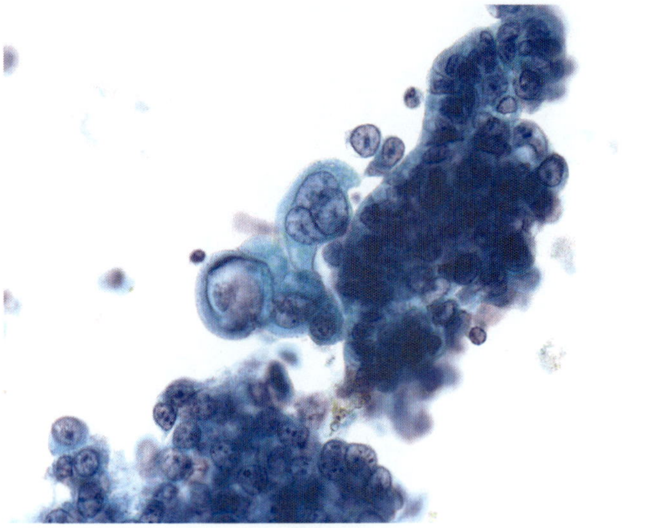

Figure 7.114 — Flat urothelial CIS, voided urine. A strip of epithelium contains densely packed large cells when compared with the nucleus of the superficial squamous cell alongside the tissue fragment. There is no question that this is a high-grade lesion. Depending upon the sample collection, one can interpret this fragment as either from a papillary lesion if spontaneously exfoliated, or simply a flat CIS if catheterized (Papanicolaou stain, high power).

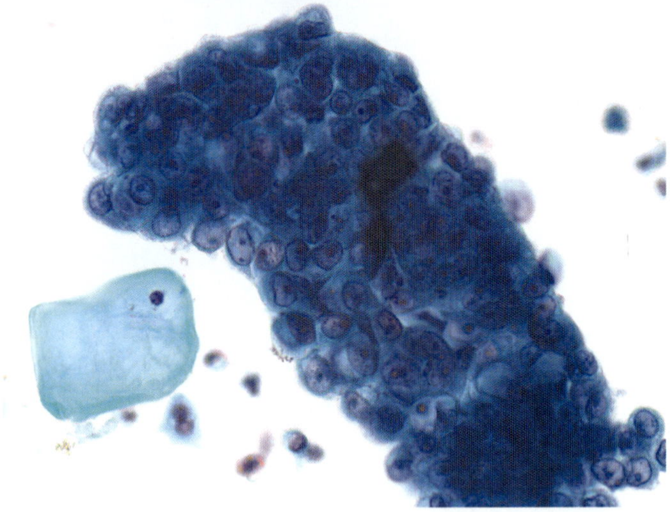

Figure 7.115 — Flat urothelial CIS, instrumented urine. Flat CIS tends to disaggregate easily. Therefore, even when a sample has been obtained by catheterization, tissue fragments will appear loose with spacing in between the cells. Some of this also may be due to squamous differentiation, which tends to have less cellular cohesion than adenocarcinoma. Mitoses are readily seen (arrows). The cytomorphology of each of the cells within this sample is characteristic of a high-grade lesion, despite whatever cytoplasmic differentiation is seen (Papanicolaou stain, medium power).

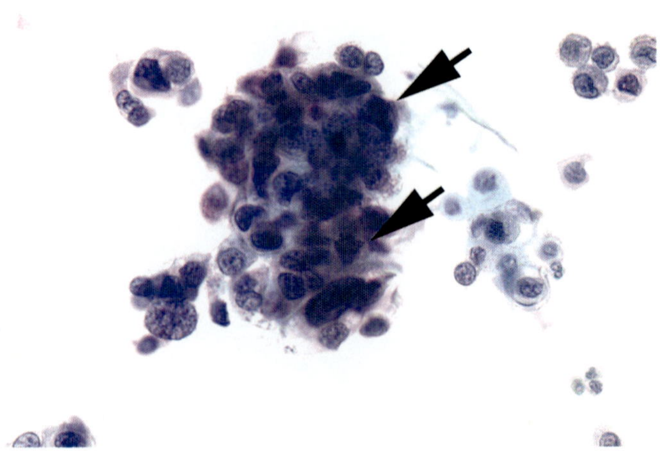

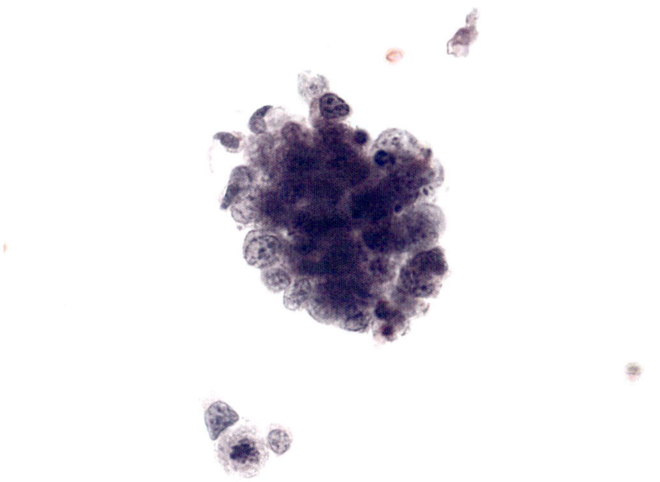

Figure 7.116 — Flat urothelial CIS, instrumented urine. Carcinoma in-situ can be quite degenerated on the surface of the lesion, and this should not deter the diagnosis of a high-grade lesion if the nuclear characteristics are present. At least an interpretation of "suspicious for a high-grade carcinoma" is important for the clinician (Papanicolaou stain, high power).

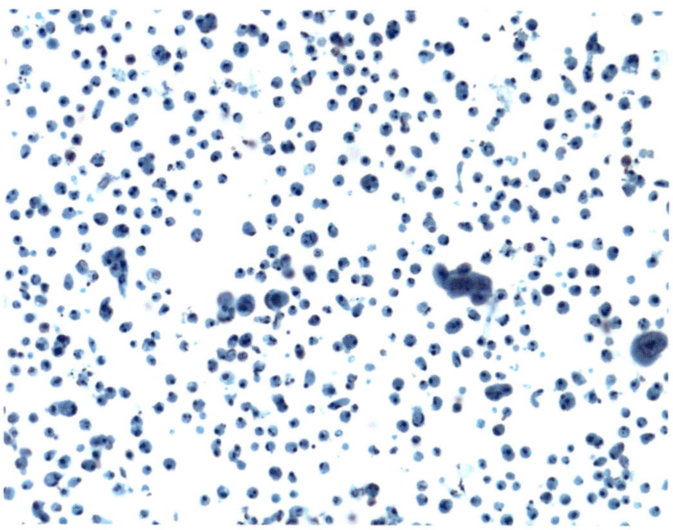

Figure 7.117 — Urothelial carcinoma in an ileal loop (neobladder), voided urine. During cystectomy, a loop of large or small intestine is turned into a pouch to capture the urine from the kidneys. The appearance of the cells within the enteric pouch, either ileal loop or neobladder, are essentially the same (see Figures 3.45–3.46). Careful search for new or residual tumor in urine is essential for appropriate management of the patient. Even on low power, the tumor cells can be identified. Higher power inspection is important for verification (Papanicolaou stain, low power).

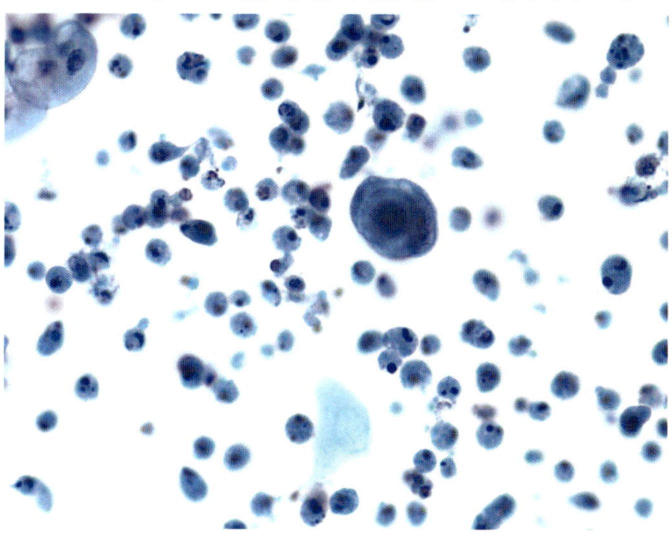

Figure 7.118 — Urothelial carcinoma in an ileal loop (neobladder), voided urine. The majority of lesions that occur in the ureters and renal pelvises after cystectomy for high-grade urothelial carcinoma are also high grade. The identification of these cells within an enteric pouch is usually simple, although the scarcity of cells can present a difficult screening task (Papanicolaou stain, medium power).

Figure 7.119 — Urothelial carcinoma in an ileal loop (neobladder), voided urine. Some enteric pouches continue to produce abundant mucus that can obscure cellular elements and make identification of abnormal cells difficult. Search for markedly atypical cells is imperative (Papanicolaou stain, low power).

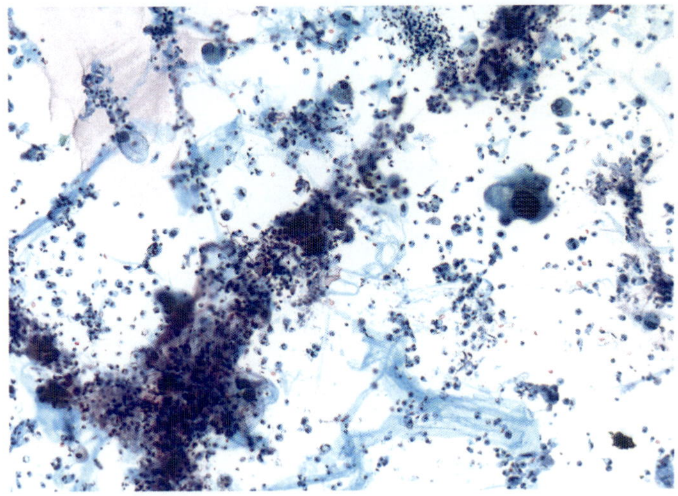

Figure 7.120 — Urothelial carcinoma in an ileal loop (neobladder), voided urine. Careful search of the sample in the previous photograph yielded single enlarged cells with features of high-grade carcinoma. This immediately implies a new lesion either within one of the ureters or one of the renal pelvises (Papanicolaou stain, medium power).

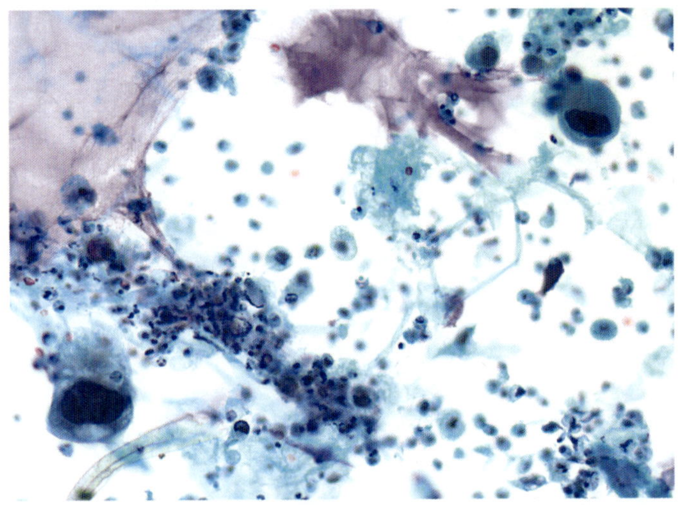

8

Uncommon Primary Neoplasms

- Squamous Cell Carcinoma
- Small-Cell Carcinoma
- Adenocarcinoma
- Other Neoplasms

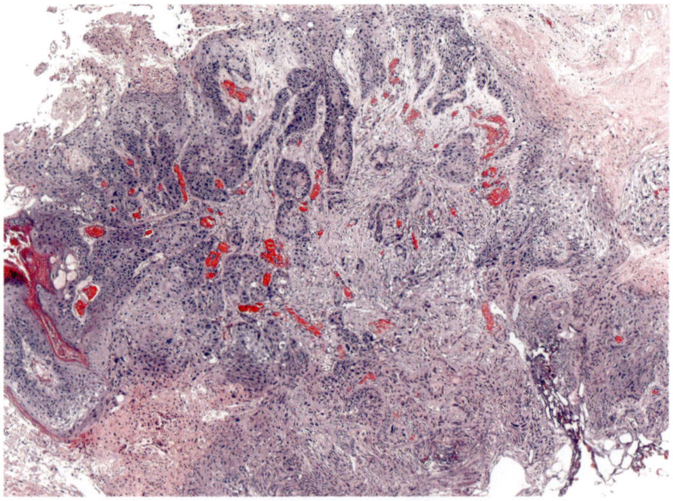

Figure 8.1 — Squamous cell carcinoma of the bladder, histologic section. Transurethral resection of bladder tumor (TURBT) showing well-differentiated squamous cell carcinoma with keratinization. Note the surface has extensive keratinaceous debris, which on cystoscopy appears as necrotic material. The stroma around the invasive component is desmoplastic. Grossly, these tumors are sessile and ulcerated (H&E stain, low power).

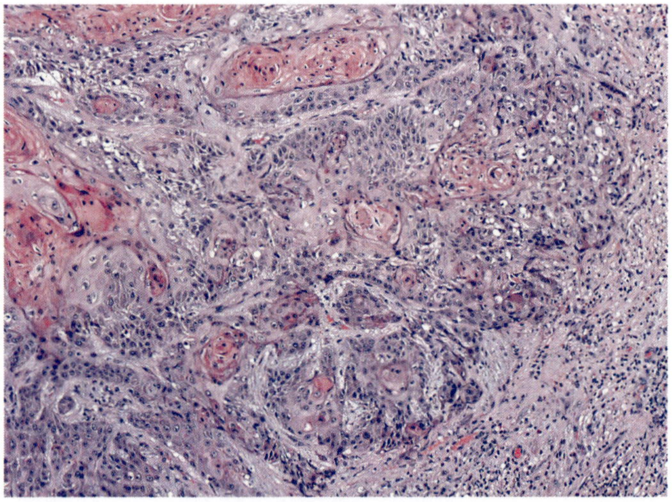

Figure 8.2 — Squamous cell carcinoma of the bladder, histologic section. Pure squamous cell carcinoma is rare and accounts for 5 percent of bladder carcinomas, more commonly urothelial carcinoma has squamous differentiation. In regions where schistosomiasis of the bladder is endemic, squamous cell carcinoma accounts for up to 75 percent of the bladder cancers. Severe recurrent chronic inflammation and bladder calculi are other risk factors. The image shows invasive keratinizing squamous cell carcinoma with irregular nests and keratin pearl formation. The stroma surrounding the nests is desmoplastic and inflamed (H&E stain, medium power).

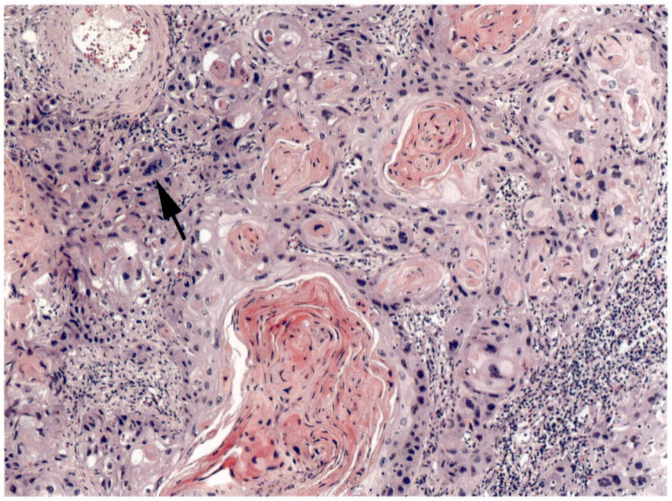

Figure 8.3 — Squamous cell carcinoma of the bladder, histologic section. Cellular pleomorphism is evident in irregular nests with keratin pearls and inflamed stroma. An atypical mitosis is seen (arrow). Squamous cell carcinoma is usually diagnosed at a relatively advanced stage than urothelial carcinoma, hence it has a poorer prognosis. Adjacent mucosa quite often has keratinizing squamous metaplasia, which is considered a risk factor (H&E stain, high power).

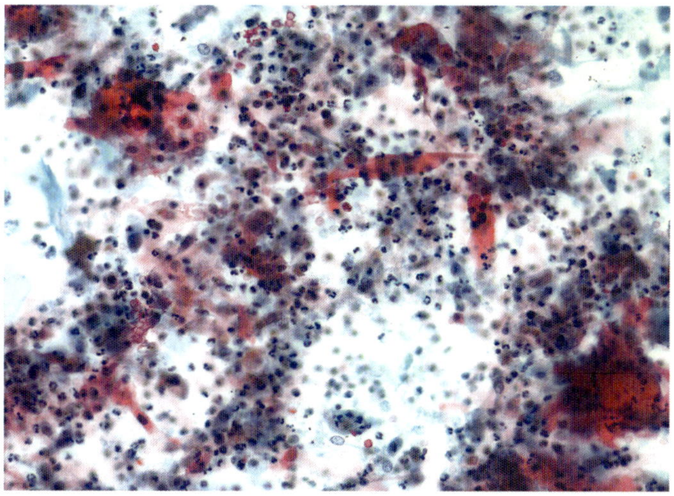

Figure 8.4 — Squamous cell carcinoma of the bladder, voided urine. Squamous carcinomas of the bladder are unusual in the North American continent as they are usually caused by one of the *Schistosoma* parasites. When they do occur, they are characteristically the same as any other squamous cell carcinoma in the body, that is, they display keratinized cytoplasm with hyperchromatic nuclei. The photograph here displays those kinds of cells in a background of acute inflammation and degeneration (Papanicolaou stain, low power).

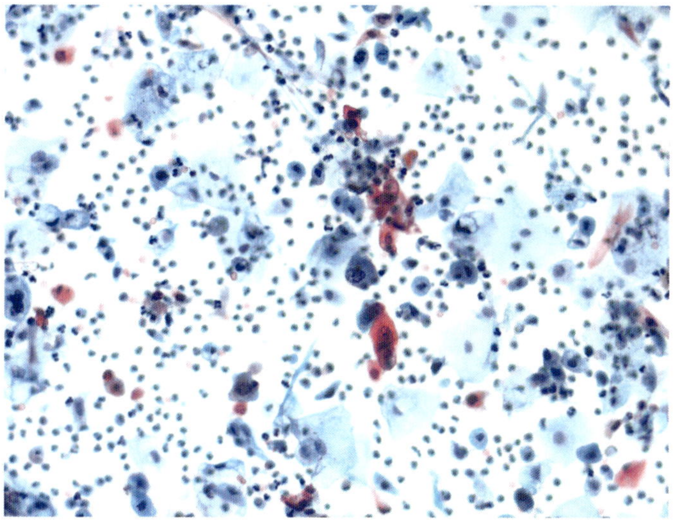

Figure 8.5 — Squamous cell carcinoma of the bladder, voided urine. Squamous cells in urinary cytology are not always indicative of a squamous lesion. The nuclear criteria must be present in the vast majority of the cells, that is, hyperchromasia, irregular nuclear outlines and coarse chromatin, and a definitely squamous cytoplasm (Papanicolaou stain, low power).

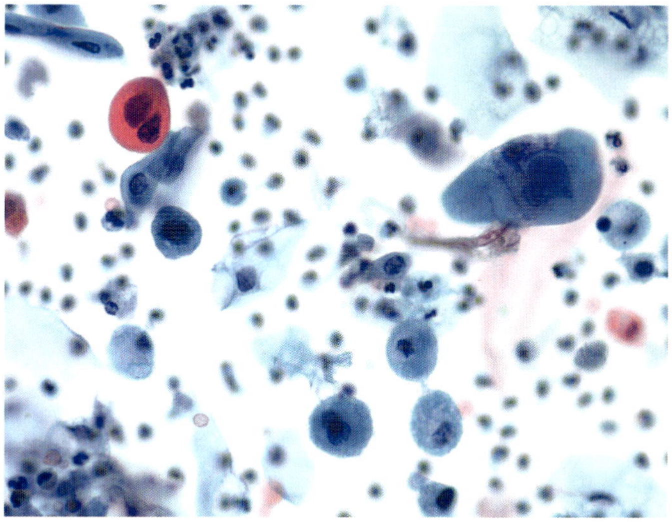

Figure 8.6 — Squamous cell carcinoma of the bladder, voided urine. Closer inspection of the sample from the previous figure demonstrates squamous cytoplasm in many of the cells, some of which are keratinized, and most of which have hyperchromatic nuclei (Papanicolaou stain, high power).

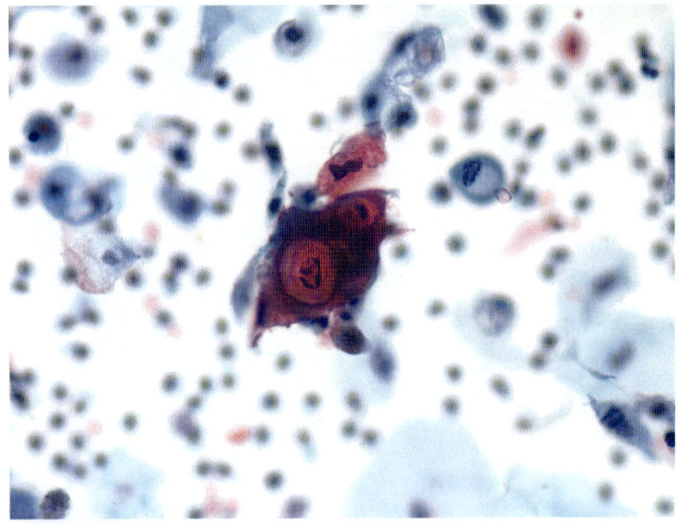

Figure 8.7 — Squamous cell carcinoma of the bladder, voided urine. Characteristic features of squamous carcinoma are universal, including concentric rings of cytoplasm surrounding a degenerated karyopyknotic nucleus, and keratinization of cytoplasm of other cells. While squamous differentiation can be seen in any high-grade urothelial carcinoma, when the majority of the cells displays squamous differentiation, then a squamous lesion must be considered (Papanicolaou stain, high power).

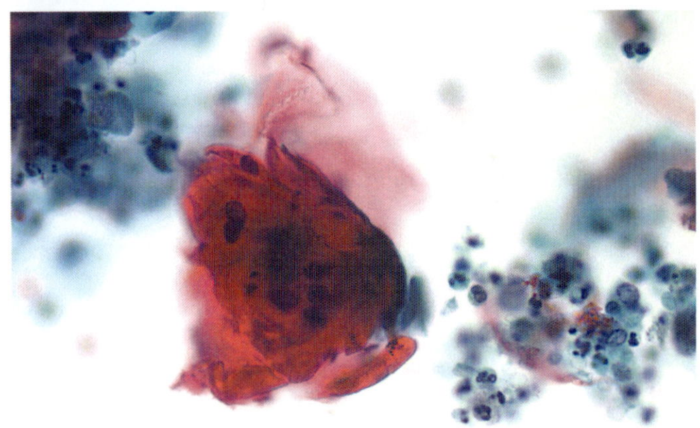

Figure 8.8 — Squamous cell carcinoma of the bladder, voided urine. Well-differentiated squamous cells may occur in urothelial carcinoma samples, but when binucleation and hyperchromasia are present, a well-differentiated squamous carcinoma should be considered. Careful search for well-defined cancer cells is mandatory. Bladder biopsy should follow when a lesion is suspected (Papanicolaou stain, high power).

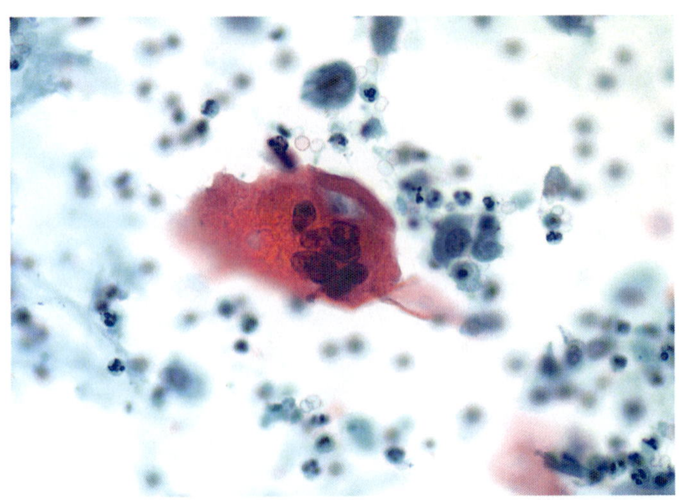

Figure 8.9 — Squamous cell carcinoma of the bladder, voided urine. Multinucleated squamous epithelial cells might be misinterpreted as giant histiocytes, but the orangeophilia of the cytoplasm is clearly from a keratinized lesion (Papanicolaou stain, high power).

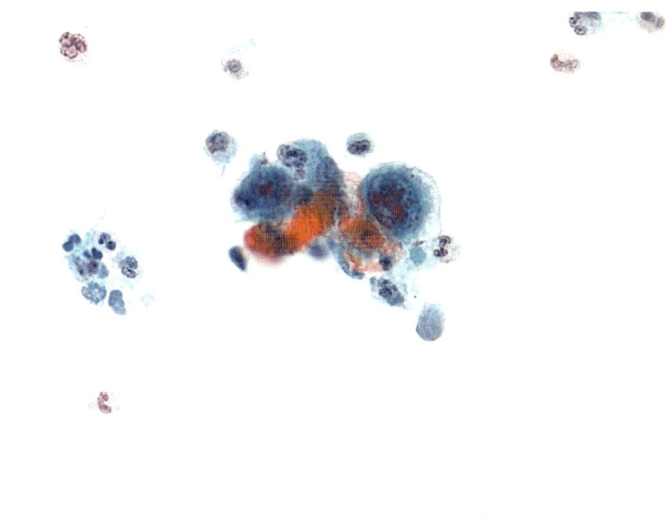

Figure 8.10 — Squamous cell carcinoma of the bladder, voided urine. Not all cancer cells in a squamous lesion need be keratinized in order to categorize it as a squamous cell carcinoma. Moderately and poorly differentiated squamous carcinomas may also be seen within the bladder (Papanicolaou stain, high power).

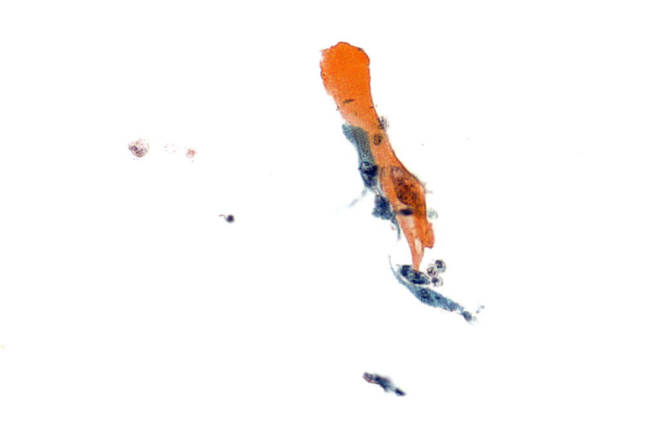

Figure 8.11 — Squamous cell carcinoma of the bladder, voided urine. Classic squamous cancer cells are rarely found in the bladder, but when they are, they are definitely dramatic and diagnostic (Papanicolaou stain, medium power).

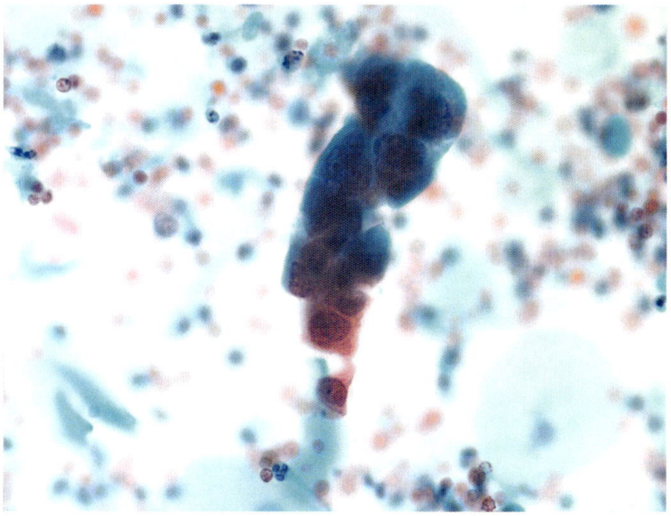

Figure 8.12 — Squamous cell carcinoma of the bladder, voided urine. Within this dislodged fragment are cells displaying both keratinized and nonkeratinized cytoplasm. The overall appearance of each of the cells is that of a metaplasia, and while most of them are obviously urothelial, the squamous differentiation is manifested by the keratinized cells. The final diagnosis was a squamous cell carcinoma based on the rest of the sample (Papanicolaou stain, high power).

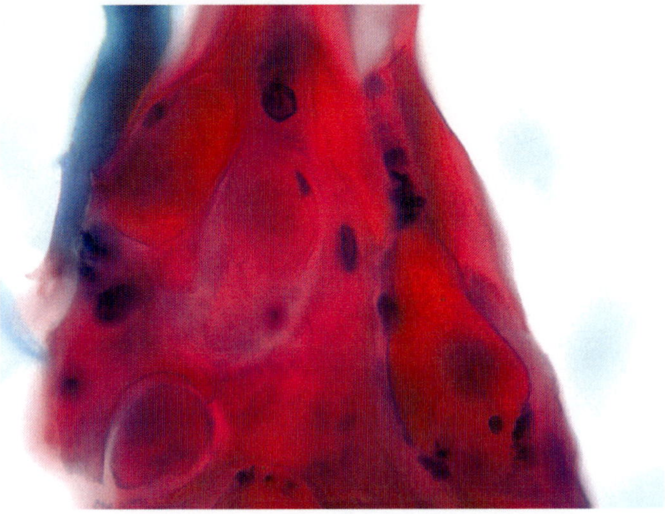

Figure 8.13 — Squamous cell carcinoma of the bladder, voided urine. Distinctly keratinized cells with variable nuclear shapes distinguish a well-differentiated squamous carcinoma (Papanicolaou stain, high power).

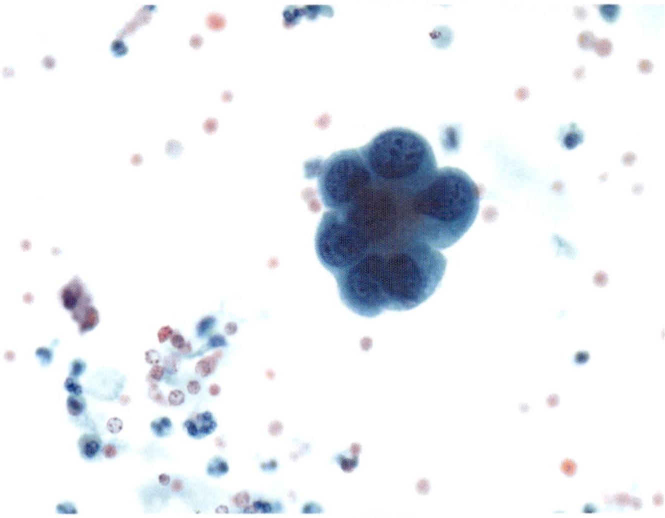

Figure 8.14 — Squamous cell carcinoma of the bladder, voided urine. Among the cells found in a sample from a high-grade carcinoma with squamous differentiation will be nonkeratinized cells, a criterion commonly found in the classic high-grade urothelial carcinoma. The distinction of squamous carcinoma is made based on the entire sample, when the preponderance of cells displays squamous differentiation (Papanicolaou stain, high power).

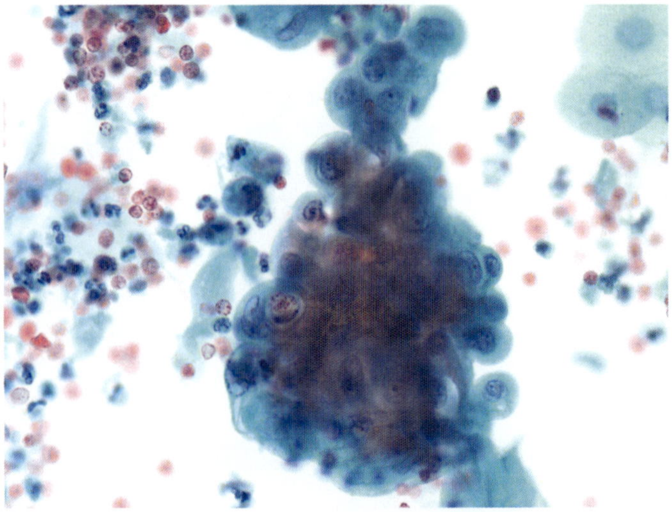

Figure 8.15 — Squamous cell carcinoma of the bladder, voided urine. Even though this particular group of cells appears the same as other high-grade urothelial carcinoma cells, the final diagnosis was squamous cell carcinoma, based on the majority of cells in the sample and the tissue biopsies (Papanicolaou stain, high power).

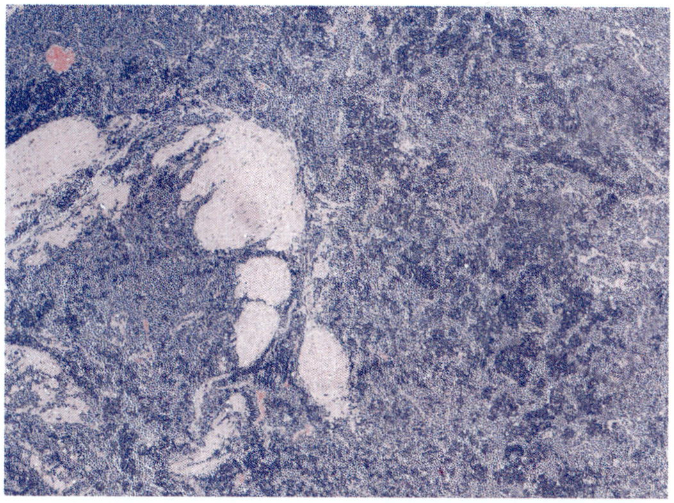

Figure 8.16 — Small-cell carcinoma of the bladder, histologic section. Diffuse involvement of the bladder wall is seen by small-cell carcinoma infiltrating around bundles of muscularis propria. Primary small-cell carcinoma of the bladder presents at a higher stage and may be widely disseminated at or soon after the time of diagnosis with regional lymph node, visceral, brain, and bone metastases (H&E stain, low power).

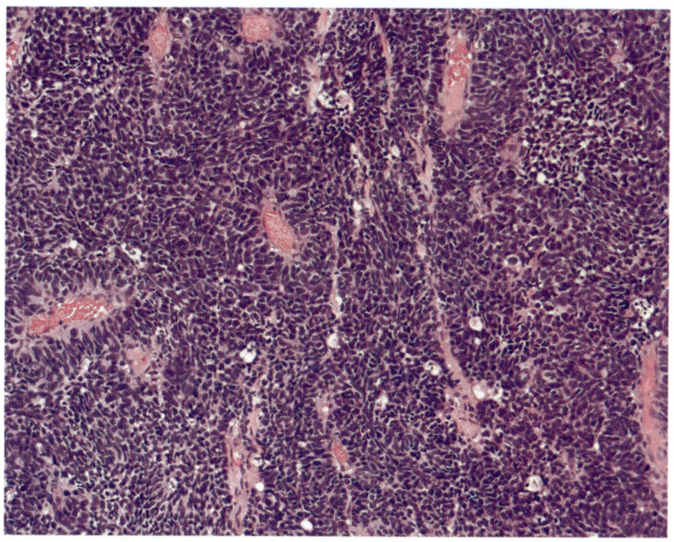

Figure 8.17 — Small-cell carcinoma of the bladder, histologic section. Small-cell carcinoma of bladder is morphologically indistinct from pulmonary and small-cell carcinomas arising at other sites. Tumor cells usually grow in a sheetlike fashion, the nuclei are large and hyperchromatic with granular chromatin and inconspicuous nucleoli, nonoverlapping, and molded to each other. The cytoplasm is scant. Areas of geographic necrosis are common. Recognition of small-cell carcinoma is significant, as this diagnosis has therapeutic and prognostic implications (H&E stain, low power).

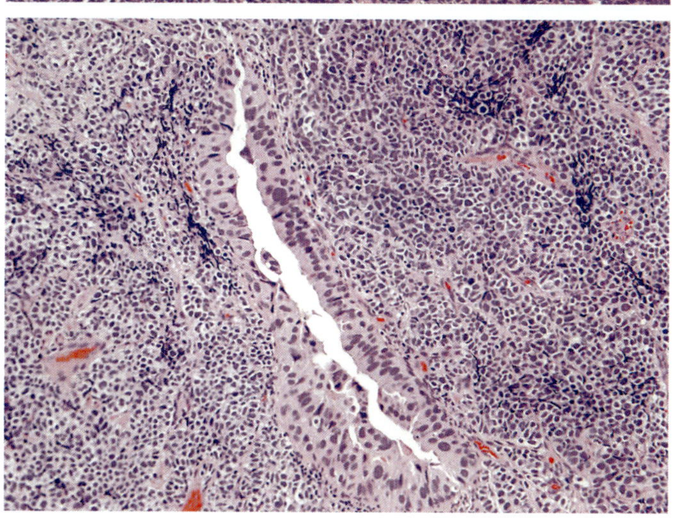

Figure 8.18 — Small-cell carcinoma of the bladder with urothelial carcinoma, histologic section. About half of bladder small-cell carcinomas have an associated urothelial carcinoma, adenocarcinoma, squamous cell carcinoma, or sarcomatoid carcinoma component. Pure small-cell carcinomas of the bladder occasionally have surface urothelial CIS or adenocarcinoma in situ (H&E stain, medium power).

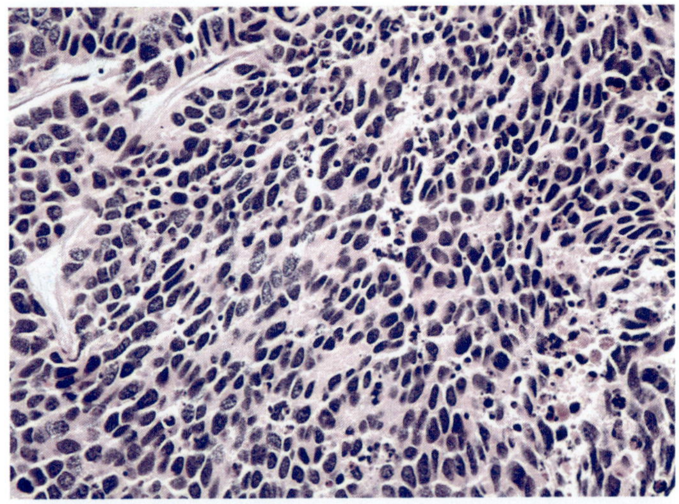

Figure 8.19 — Small-cell carcinoma of the bladder, histologic section. Brisk mitoses and apoptotic bodies with areas of necrosis are common in small-cell carcinoma as seen in this image. Main differential diagnosis is from lymphomas, where immunohistochemical stains for CD45, cytokeratin, synaptophysin, and chromogranin help cinch the diagnosis. Thyroid transcription factor 1 (TTF1) stains a significant number of bladder small-cell carcinomas as well as those from other sites (H&E stain, medium power).

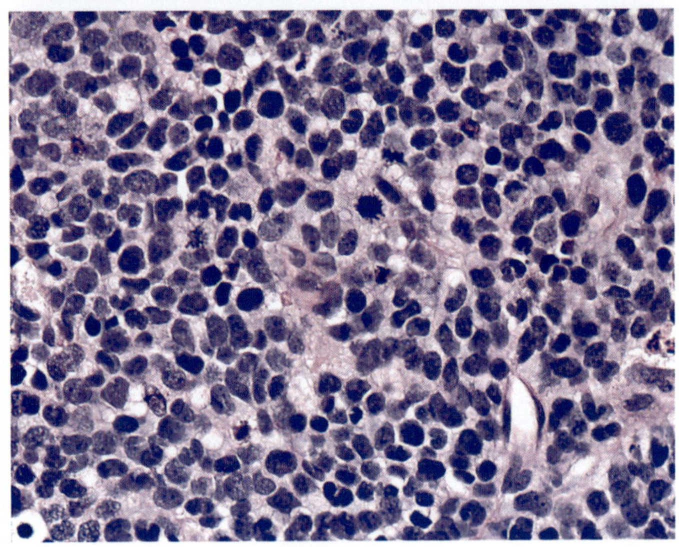

Figure 8.20 — Small-cell carcinoma of the bladder, histologic section. Increased mitoses, scant cytoplasm, and hyperchromatic nuclei are all typical features of small-cell carcinoma. Bladder small-cell carcinomas can sometimes produce paraneoplastic syndromes, with hypercalcemia and ectopic ACTH production (H&E stain, high power).

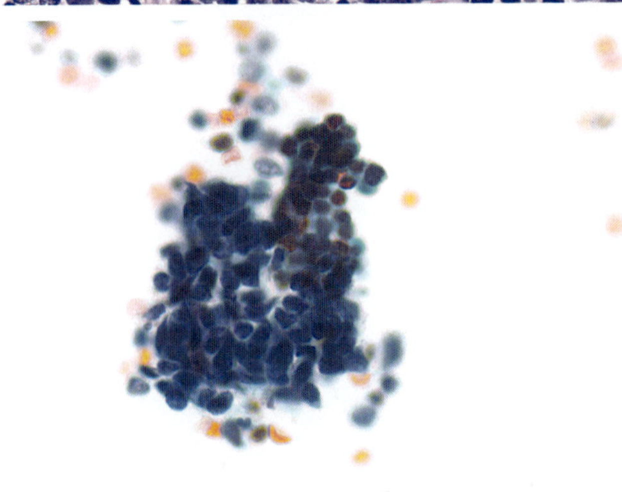

Figure 8.21 — Small-cell carcinoma of the bladder, voided urine. Small-cell carcinomas present with the same characteristics in the bladder as anywhere else in the body. They may originate in the bladder, prostate, uterine cervix, or be metastatic from a distant site. A large fragment displays hyperchromatic nuclei with scant cytoplasm, and nuclear molding (Papanicolaou stain, high power).

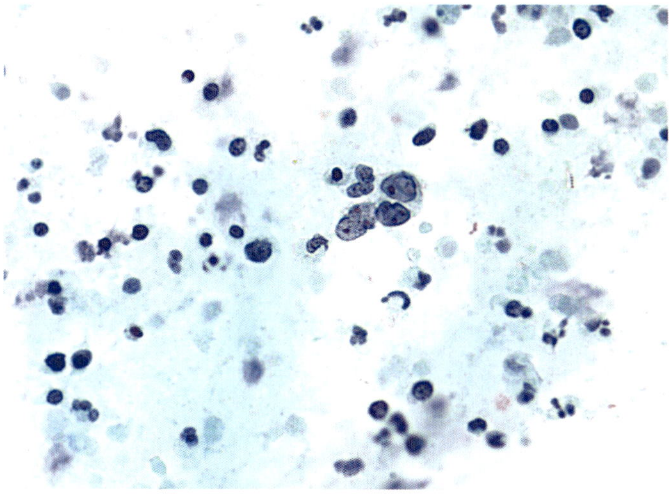

Figure 8.22 — Small-cell carcinoma of the bladder, voided urine. The contrast between the lymphocytes in the background and the tumor cells in the center is dramatic, and in fact the tumor cells are really not so "small." These "small cells" are unusual in that they have prominent nucleoli. Distinguishing these cells from a poorly-differentiated adenocarcinoma is possible only by careful appreciation of the rest of the sample, and may in fact rely on immunohistochemistry (Papanicolaou stain, high power).

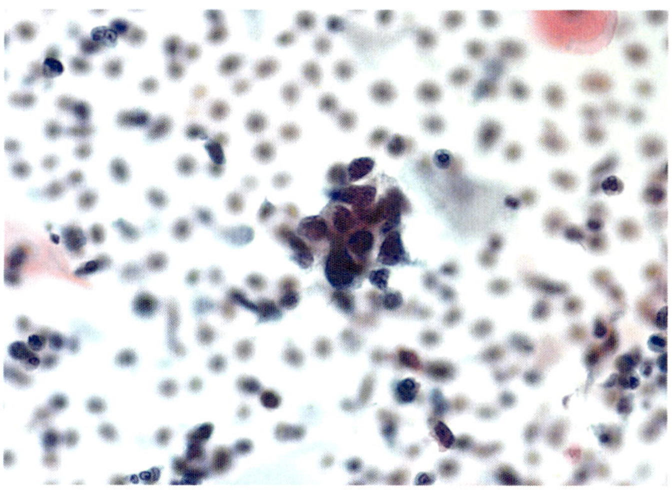

Figure 8.23 — Small-cell carcinoma of the bladder, voided urine. In liquid preparations, the focal plane may not accommodate all of the cells at once. The group in the center of the photograph is distinctly from a small-cell carcinoma; this diagnosis is based on the quality of the nuclear chromatin and the nuclear molding (Papanicolaou stain, high power).

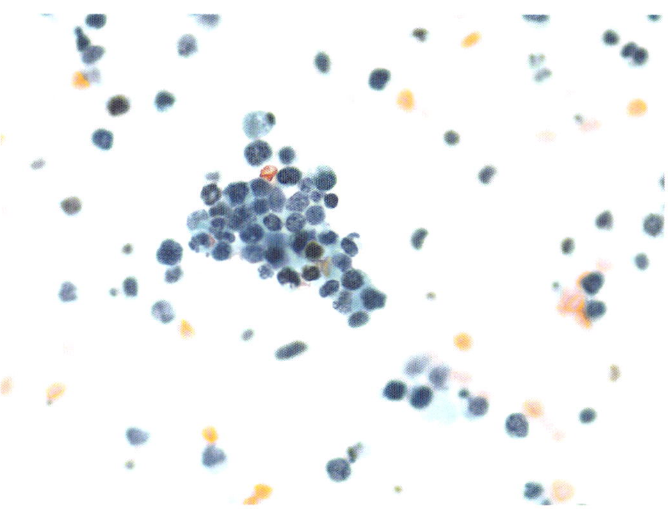

Figure 8.24 — Small-cell carcinoma of the bladder, voided urine. Not all cells from a small-cell carcinoma are small, and variation in size may be seen, as in this group. Apoptotic bodies are a prominent feature of this class of tumors (Papanicolaou stain, medium power).

Figure 8.25 — Small-cell carcinoma of the bladder, voided urine. Tandem arrangement or single file grouping is characteristic of small-cell carcinoma anywhere in the body. However, certain adenocarcinomas, such as from the breast, can also present with the same configuration. But, the nuclear chromatin of a small-cell carcinoma is homogeneous and finely granular, usually without nucleoli, whereas the chromatin of an adenocarcinoma will be more delicate and open, with prominent nucleoli (Papanicolaou stain, medium power).

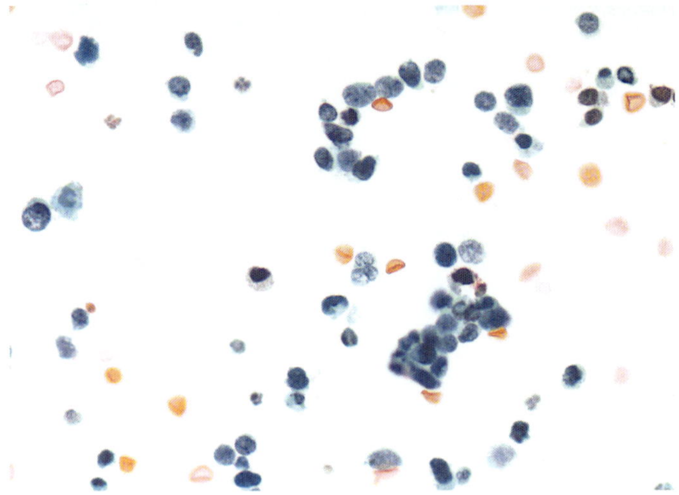

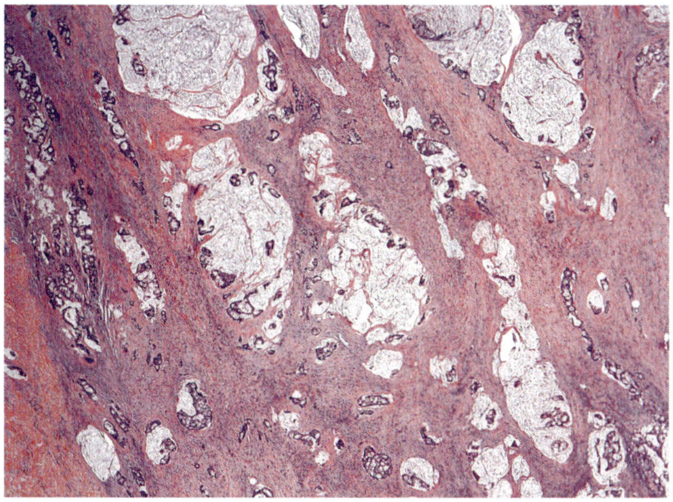

Figure 8.26 — Urachal mucinous adenocarcinoma, histologic section. The urachus extends from the bladder dome to the umbilicus. In approximately 30 percent of cases, embryonic remnants remain within the urachus. The lining, which is urothelial, can undergo glandular metaplasia. Carcinomas arising in the urachus are usually adenocarcinomas. These resemble colonic adenocarcinomas and are commonly mucinous as seen in the image. Pools of mucin dissect through the muscle layers, and adenocarcinoma glands float within the mucin (H&E stain, medium power).

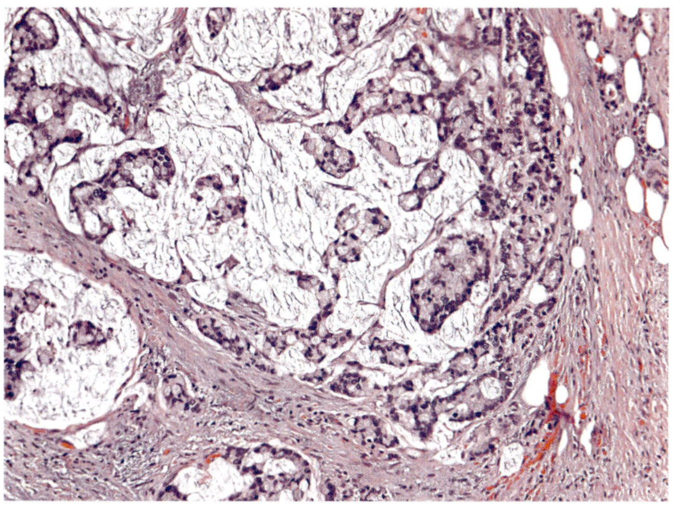

Figure 8.27 — Urachal mucinous adenocarcinoma, histologic section. Moderately differentiated mucinous adenocarcinoma of the urachus. The floating glands form a cribriform pattern; cells lining the malignant glands have intracytoplasmic mucin. Differential diagnosis includes primary bladder adenocarcinoma and metastatic adenocarcinoma from the bowel. There should be no in situ lesion on the bladder surface, and the urachal carcinoma should be located within the bladder wall at the dome. Partial cystectomy can be done for urachal tumors with removal of the median umbilical ligament and the umbilicus (H&E stain, medium power).

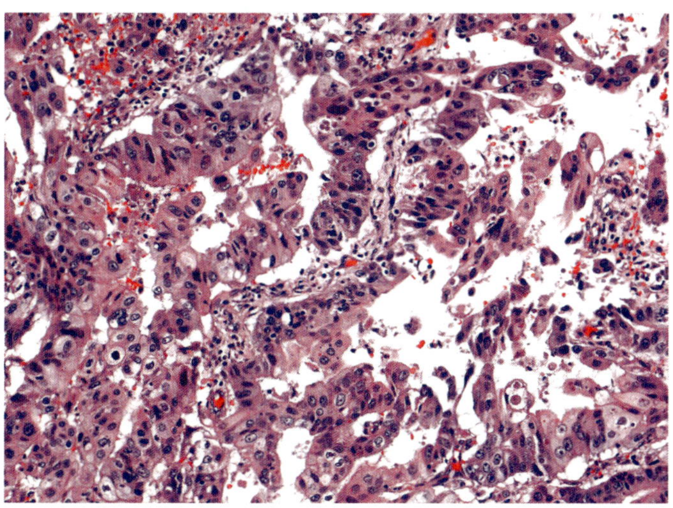

Figure 8.28 — Urachal adenocarcinoma, histologic section. A nonmucinous urachal adenocarcinoma is shown here. Note the similarities to enteric adenocarcinoma with elongated nuclei and dark cytoplasm. This carcinoma demonstrates fairly prominent pleomorphism and formed a large mass undermining the bladder urothelium extending outside the bladder. There was no in situ lesion or intestinal metaplasia identified within the bladder mucosa (H&E stain, medium power).

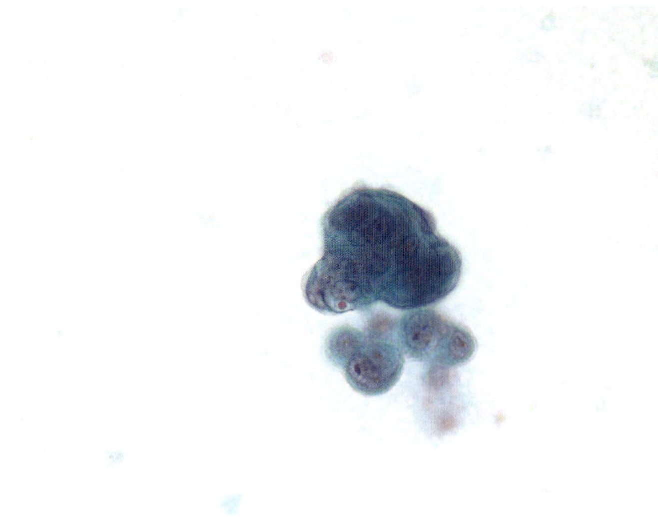

Figure 8.29 — Adenocarcinoma of the bladder, voided urine. Glandular differentiation in urothelial cells may be distinguished from true adenocarcinomas by the nuclear characteristics. Adenocarcinomas have a more delicate nuclear chromatin and prominent red nucleoli, whereas urothelial cells with glandular differentiation have nuclei with coarser chromatin and variable nuclei, usually dark blue (Papanicolaou stain, high power).

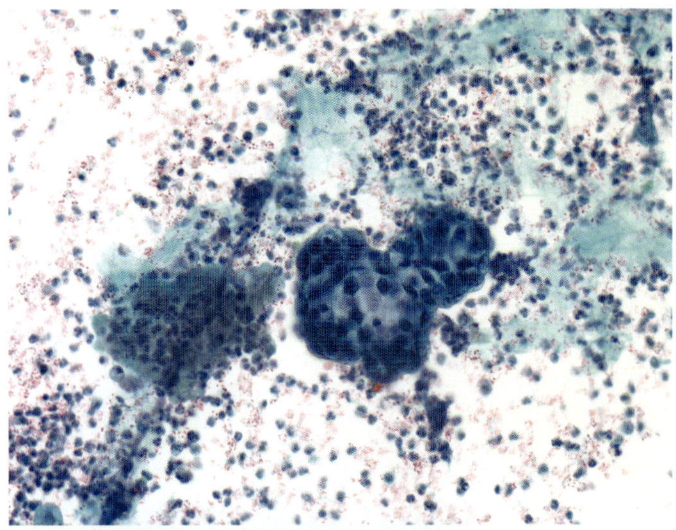

Figure 8.30 — Adenocarcinoma of the bladder, voided urine. Adenocarcinomas in urine have the same characteristics as adenocarcinomas in other body cavity fluids, that is, these cell groups present as three-dimensional clusters that have rounded up (Papanicolaou stain, medium power).

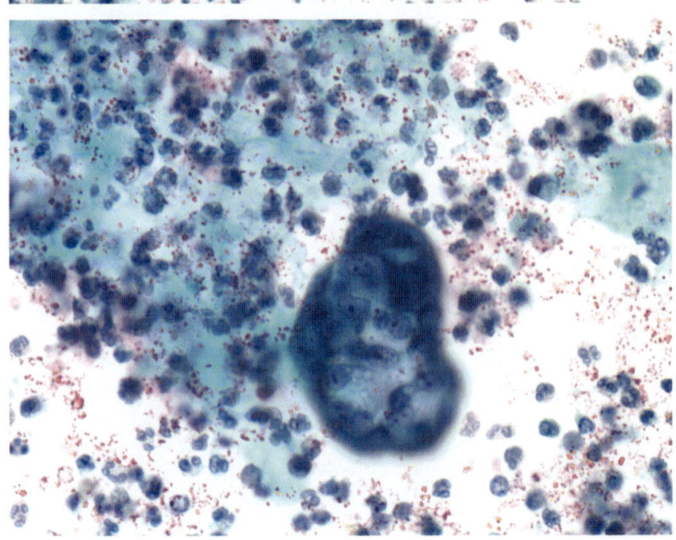

Figure 8.31 — Adenocarcinoma of the bladder, voided urine. True gland formation can be appreciated in tissue fragments that have rounded up so that the center of the fragment is hollow, and the outer boundaries of the tissue fragment are very smooth (Papanicolaou stain, medium power).

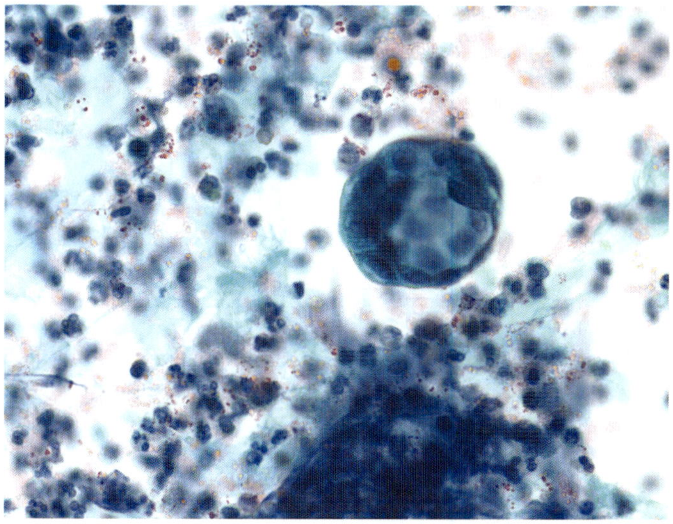

Figure 8.32 — Adenocarcinoma of the bladder, voided urine. Even with small groups of cells, the smooth outer boundary and hollow core can be appreciated. Urothelial cells with cytoplasmic glandular differentiation do not display these floating glands (Papanicolaou stain, medium power).

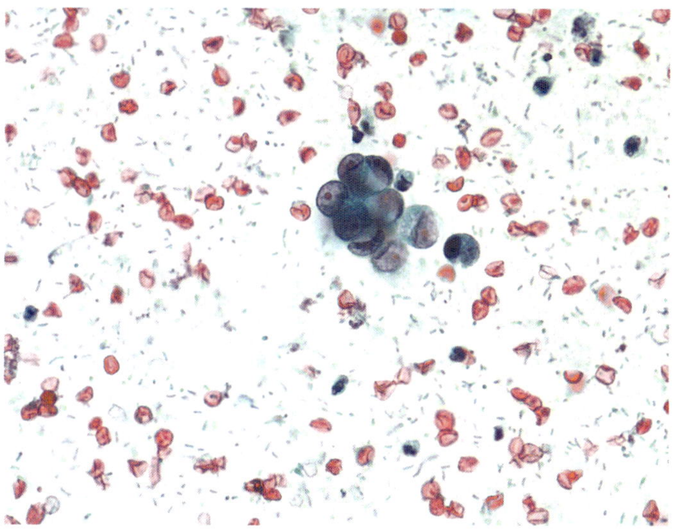

Figure 8.33 — Adenocarcinoma of the bladder, voided urine. This small group of cells is clearly different from urothelial carcinoma with glandular differentiation. Here the nuclei are eccentrically placed and distinguished by prominent red nucleoli. The site of origin cannot be determined by morphology alone, as these could also originate in the prostate or some other primary site (Papanicolaou stain, medium power).

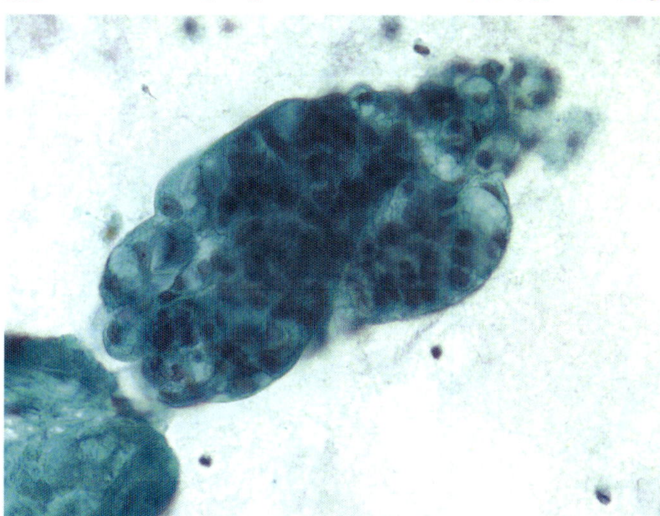

Figure 8.34 — Adenocarcinoma of the bladder, voided urine. While the final diagnosis in this patient was adenocarcinoma, the cytomorphology is difficult to identify as distinct from glandular differentiation in a urothelial cancer. Not every case will be clear cut (Papanicolaou stain, high power).

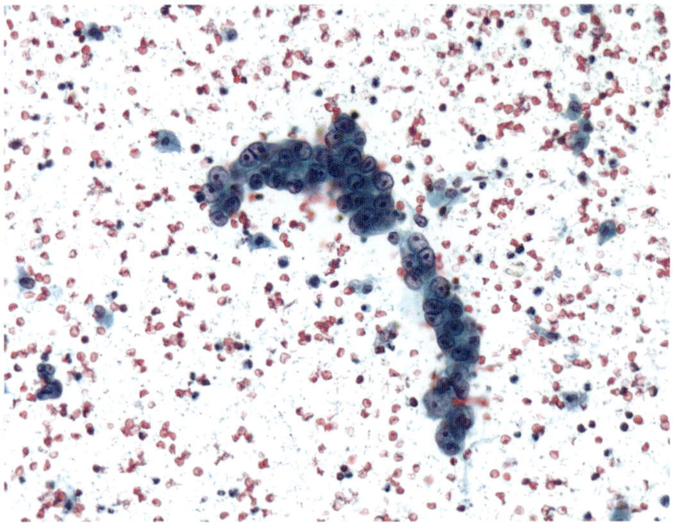

Figure 8.35 — Adenocarcinoma of the bladder, voided urine. An unusual presentation, these cells could be mistaken for a renal tubular epithelial cast at first glance. However, they are very well preserved in contrast to the usual degenerative changes in renal tubular epithelial cells. Also, the nuclear characteristics, prominent red nucleoli and delicate chromatin, are distinct from benign cells from the renal tubules. Microacini are also appreciated within this string of cancer cells (Papanicolaou stain, medium power).

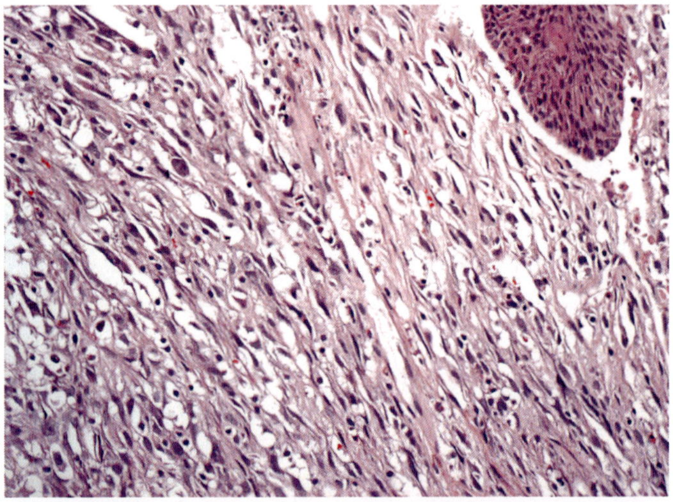

Figure 8.36 — Sarcomatoid carcinoma of the bladder with squamous cell carcinoma, histologic section. This is a biphasic tumor with malignant spindle cell, and epithelial components; a synonym for this class of tumor is "carcinosarcoma." This image shows pleomorphic spindle cells in no particular arrangement and the right upper corner shows the associated squamous cell carcinoma. Sarcomatoid carcinoma is much more common than primary sarcoma of the bladder. The relative amount of the sarcomatoid component should be mentioned in the pathology report (H&E stain, medium power).

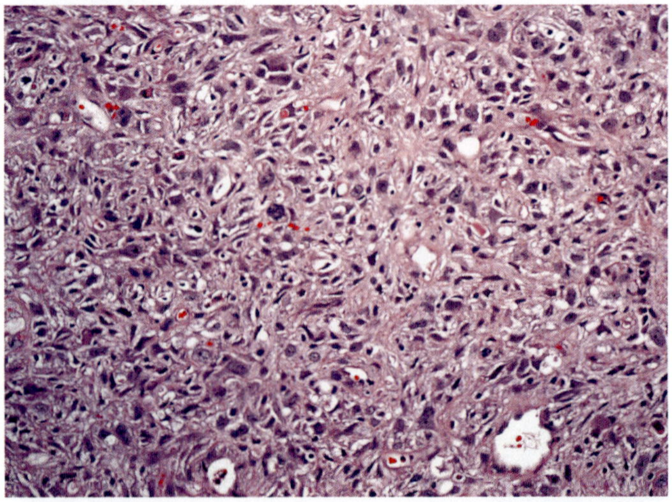

Figure 8.37 — Sarcomatoid carcinoma of the bladder, histologic section. This rare tumor is highly aggressive and presents at a high stage. This image shows the cellular pleomorphism and frequent mitoses. These tumors may have rhabdomyosarcomatous, chondrosarcomatous, or osteosarcomatous components. The associated epithelial malignancy may comprise urothelial, squamous, or small-cell carcinoma, or adenocarcinoma. Surface mucosa may have associated urothelial CIS. If there is no recognizable surface or invasive carcinoma component on routine stains, the diagnosis can be established by demonstrating epithelial differentiation immunohistochemically with p63 and high molecular weight cytokeratin as the most sensitive markers (H&E stain, medium power).

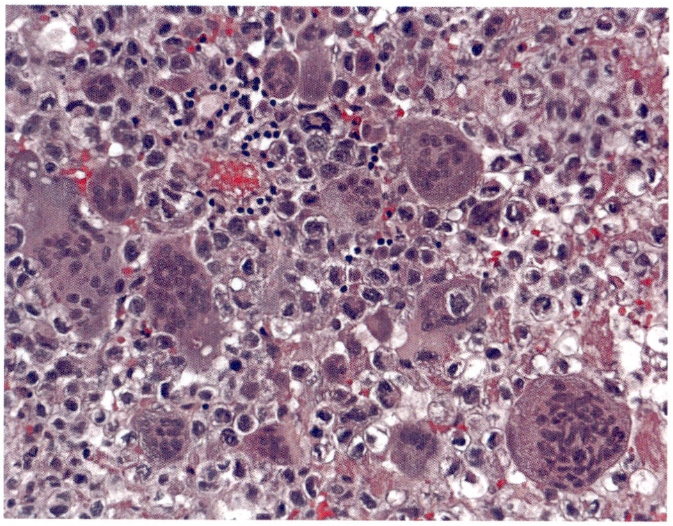

Figure 8.38 — Osteoclast-rich undifferentiated carcinoma of the bladder, histologic section. These rare tumors are considered aggressive variants of urothelial carcinoma with evenly distributed giant cells, resembling giant cell tumor of the bone. The giant cells are reactive and histiocytic in nature. The mononuclear cells are inconsistently reactive with antibodies to cytokeratins, EMA, S-100 protein, and actin (H&E stain, medium power).

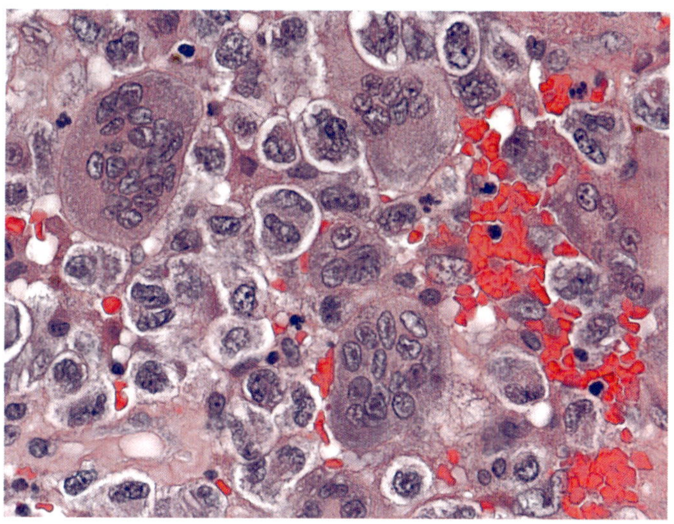

Figure 8.39 — Osteoclast-rich undifferentiated carcinoma of the bladder, histologic section. These tumors are biphasic with mixtures of oval mononuclear cells with vesicular nuclei, ample cytoplasm, and osteoclast-like giant cells arranged in sheets and nodules. Large areas of necrosis may be seen. Occasional areas of pools of blood may be present. Mitoses can be frequent. No bone or cartilage is present (H&E stain, high power).

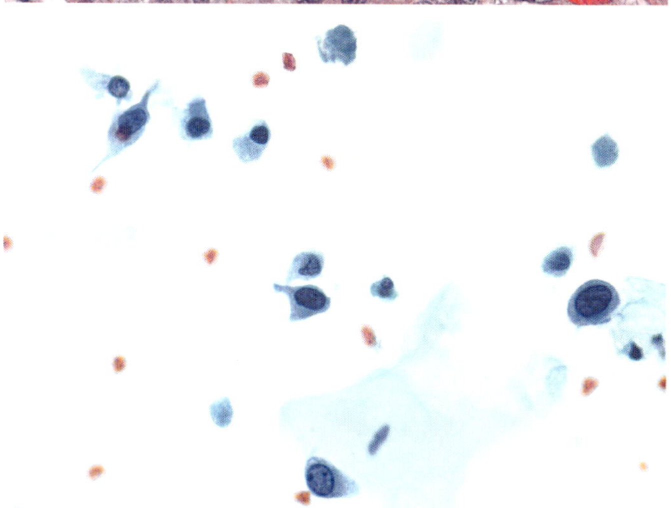

Figure 8.40 — Osteoclast-rich undifferentiated carcinoma of the bladder, voided urine. The final diagnosis in this patient was osteoclast-rich undifferentiated carcinoma. In this particular photograph, all that can be said is that malignant cells are present, and some actually resemble a high-grade urothelial carcinoma. Tissue biopsy is necessary for precise identification (Papanicolaou stain, medium power).

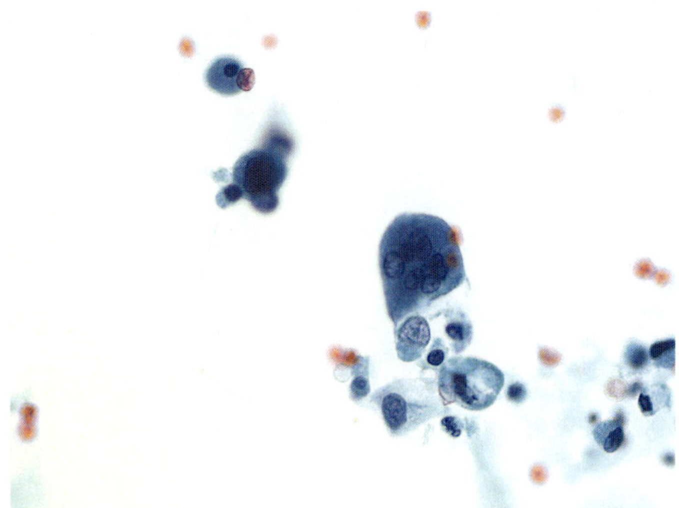

Figure 8.41 — Osteoclast-rich undifferentiated carcinoma of the bladder, voided urine. Accompanying the distinctly malignant cells in this sample are multinucleated cells that are not obviously histiocytes, since the cytoplasm is more opaque and homogeneous than that of typical histiocytes. The resemblance to osteoclasts is obvious, hence the name (Papanicolaou stain, high power).

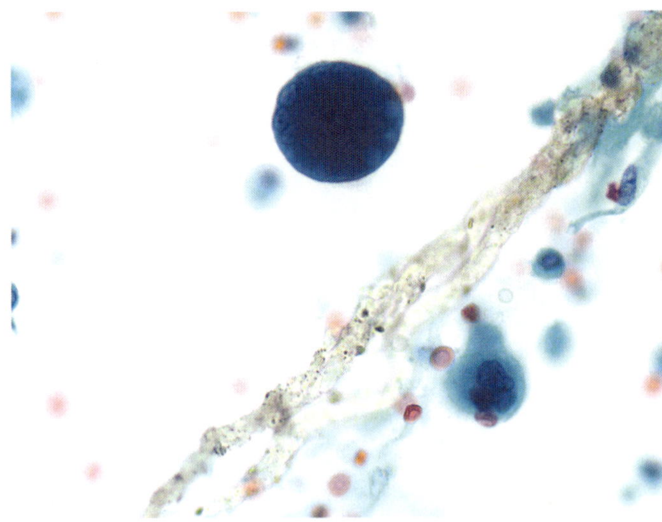

Figure 8.42 — Osteoclast-rich undifferentiated carcinoma of the bladder, voided urine. The mixture of cells within the sample, i.e., cells resembling a high-grade urothelial carcinoma but with aberrant cytoplasmic shapes and multi-nucleated cells, are indications of an unusual malignant tumor (Papanicolaou stain, medium power).

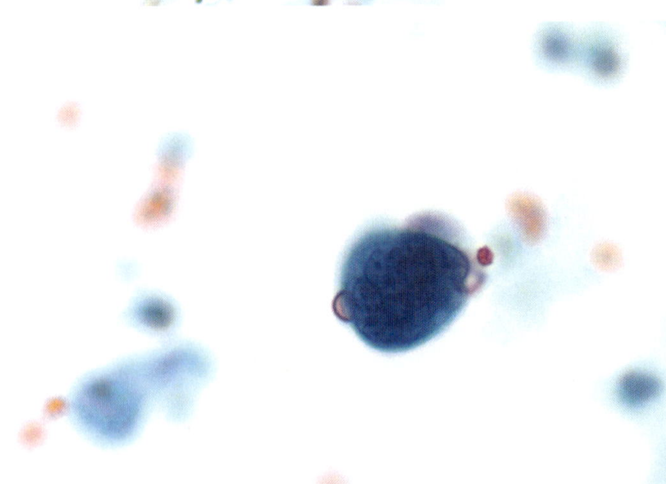

Figure 8.43 — Osteoclast-rich undifferentiated carcinoma of the bladder, voided urine. The nuclear presentation of the multinucleated cells varies between separate nuclei and amalgamation of multiple nuclei that have failed to separate (Papanicolaou stain, high power).

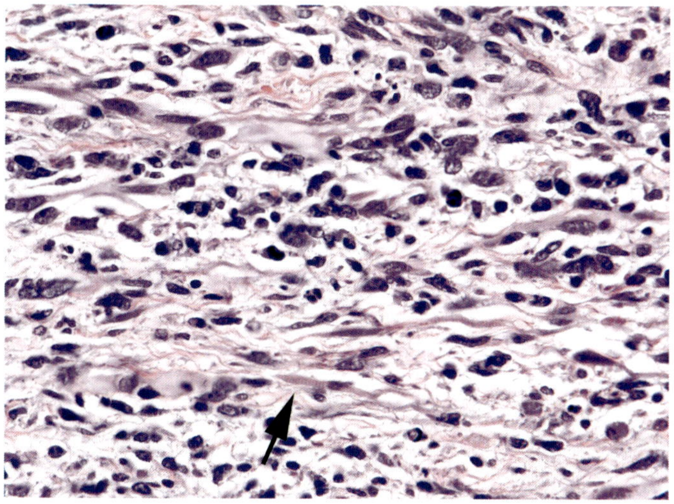

Figure 8.44 — Rhabdomyosarcoma of the bladder, histologic section. This image of embryonal rhabdomyosarcoma shows rhabdomyoblasts and strap cells with cross striations (arrow). Embryonal rhabdomyosarcomas of the bladder are more common in the pediatric age group. They may have an exophytic polypoid growth or may involve the bladder wall diffusely, the latter having worse prognosis. Combination of surgery and chemotherapy has improved prognosis (H&E stain, high power).

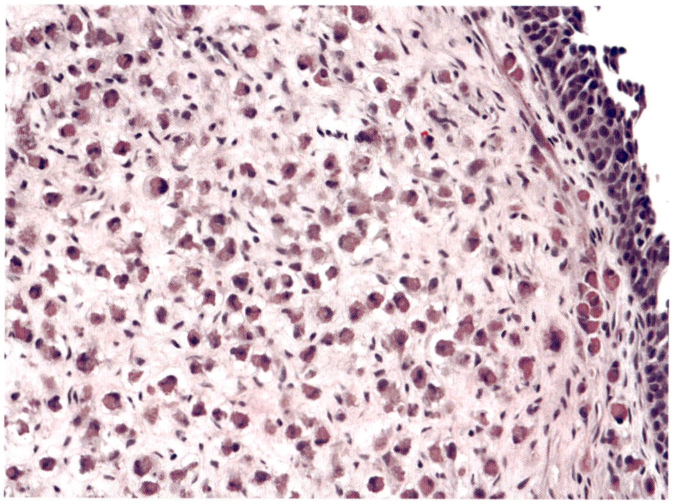

Figure 8.45 — Post-chemotherapy rhabdomyosarcoma of the bladder, histologic section. This treated rhabdomyosarcoma shows morphologic evidence of maturation in the form of increased numbers of rhabdomyoblasts. The overlying urothelium is intact (H&E stain, high power).

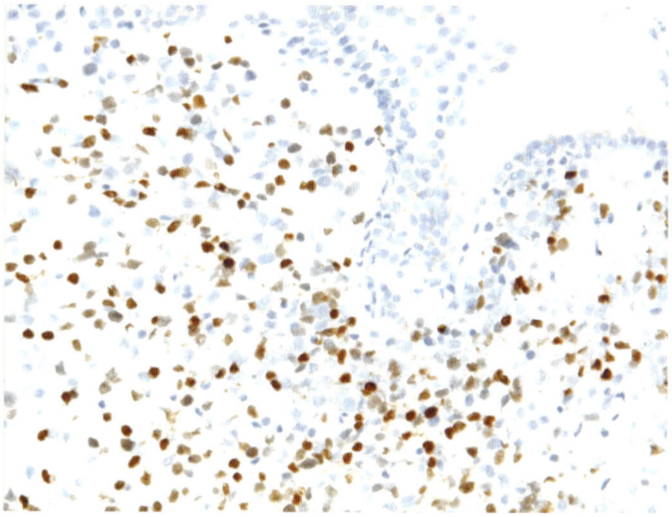

Figure 8.46 — Rhabdomyosarcoma of the bladder, histologic section. Malignant cells display strong immunolabeling with myogenin. Myogenin and MyoD1 are nuclear immunostains. Other immunoreactive stains include desmin, myoglobin, and vimentin (Myogenin immunostain, medium power).

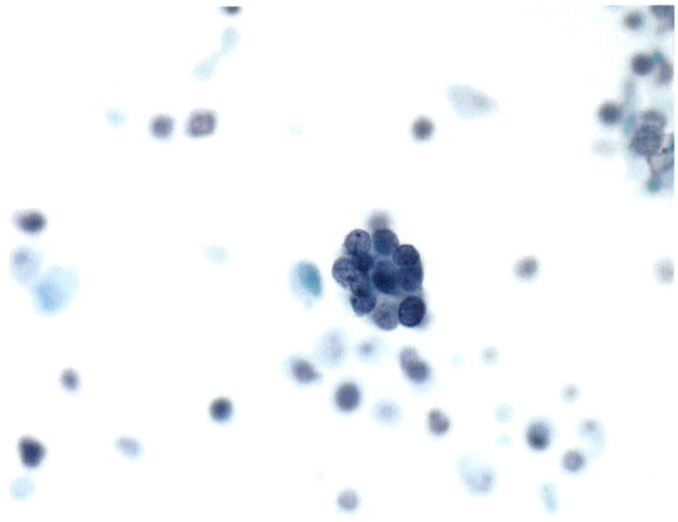

Figure 8.47 — Rhabdomyosarcoma of the bladder, voided urine. This cluster of very small cells might be interpreted as a small-cell undifferentiated carcinoma, but the characteristics of nuclear molding and homogeneous chromatin are absent. The sample was obtained from a young boy (Papanicolaou stain, medium power).

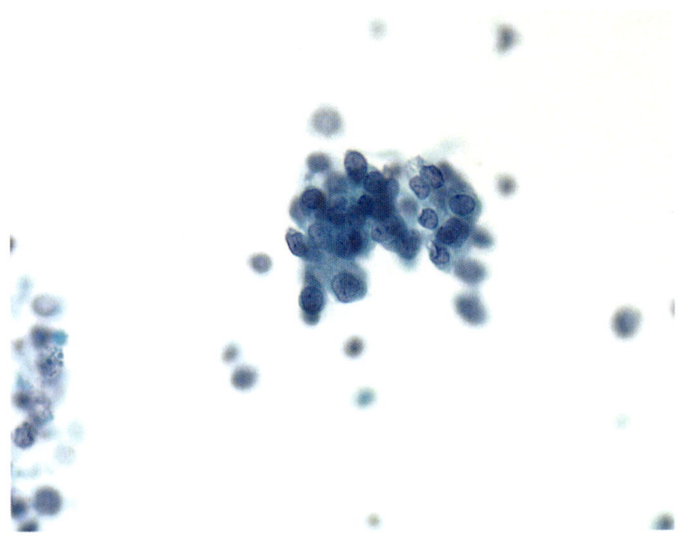

Figure 8.48 — Rhabdomyosarcoma of the bladder, voided urine. The variable amount of cytoplasm in these small cells also distinguishes them from the typical small-cell carcinoma. While these cells are clearly neoplastic and do not belong in the common group of epithelial bladder tumors, tissue studies with biomarkers are necessary for proper identification (Papanicolaou stain, low power).

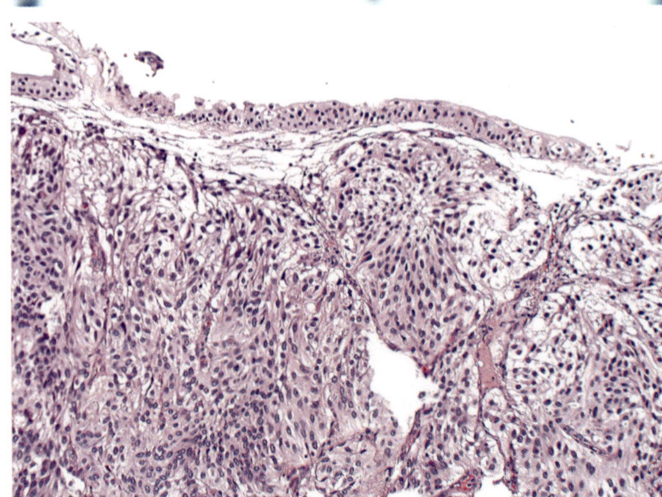

Figure 8.49 — Paraganglioma of bladder (bladder pheochromocytoma), histologic section. This is a rare lesion (<0.5 percent of bladder tumors) and 75 percent of the patients present with "micturition attacks" consisting of hypertension, palpitations, headaches, sweating, anxiety, and so forth upon filling or emptying of the bladder. There is a wide age range; size can be up to 10 cm and common locations are the trigone or the dome. The microscopic appearance is typical of paragangliomas elsewhere in the body with nesting of cells and plexiform capillary network investing the nests of cells in a Zellballen appearance. The cells have ovoid nuclei, with prominent nucleoli. The cytoplasm is amphophilic (H&E stain, low power).

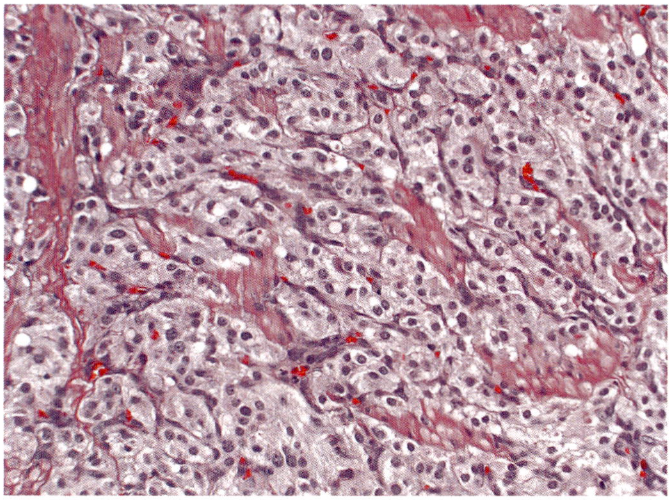

Figure 8.50 — Paraganglioma of bladder (bladder pheochromocytoma), histologic section. Paragangliomas may be seen infiltrating the muscularis propria as in this image. The surface urothelium may be ulcerated or intact. Hematuria is the second most common presenting symptom. Serum or urine catecholamine measurement confirms the diagnosis. The treatment for these tumors is transurethral resection or partial cystectomy (H&E stain, low power).

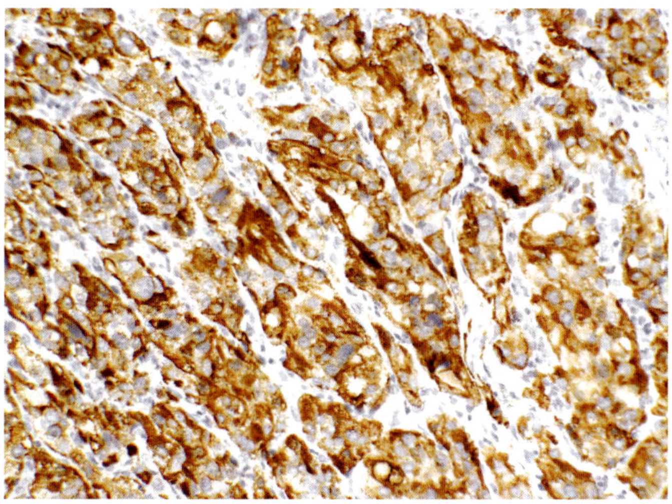

Figure 8.51 — Paraganglioma of bladder (bladder pheochromocytoma), histologic section. Bladder paraganglioma highlighted by synaptophysin immunostain. Other positive immunostains include chromogranin and NSE; S100 highlights the sustentacular cells present at the periphery of the cell nests. These lesions are negative for cytokeratins. The immunoprofile is helpful in differentiating it from urothelial carcinoma, which may show a nested appearance, however, these are positive for cytokeratins (CK7, CK20, and CK903; H&E stain, low power).

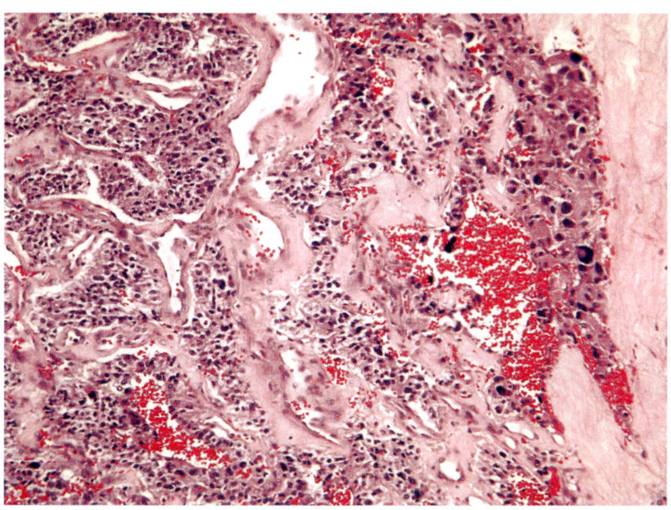

Figure 8.52 — Paraganglioma of bladder (bladder pheochromocytoma), histologic section. As seen in other endocrine tumors, there might be nuclear atypia in the form of bizarre shapes. This atypia is degenerative and smudgy in appearance, as seen towards the right of this image. The left side shows typical nested appearance with fibrous septa among the nests. These lesions may show focal hemorrhage and necrosis (H&E stain, low power).

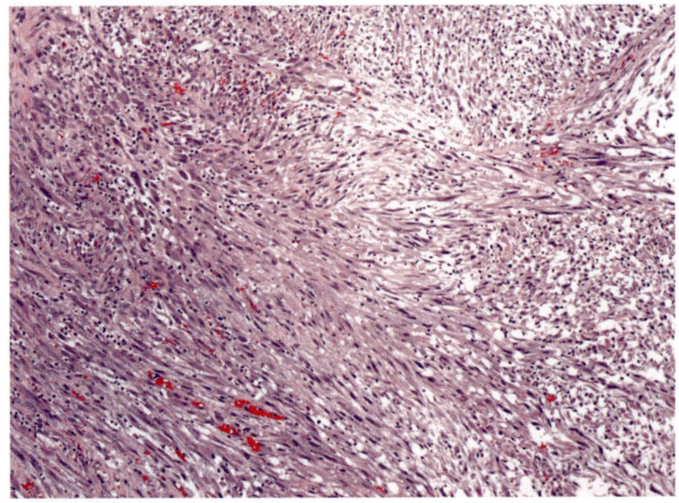

Figure 8.53 — Inflammatory myofibroblastic tumor (IMT) of the bladder, histologic section. IMT of the bladder is considered a neoplasm of uncertain malignant potential. Most of these lesions follow a benign course after transurethral resection. Close clinical follow-up is warranted rather than a radical procedure. IMTs comprise plump or elongated spindle cells that can be quite cellular, arranged in loose fascicles. There is a delicate capillary network with areas of edematous or myxoid stroma (H&E stain, low power).

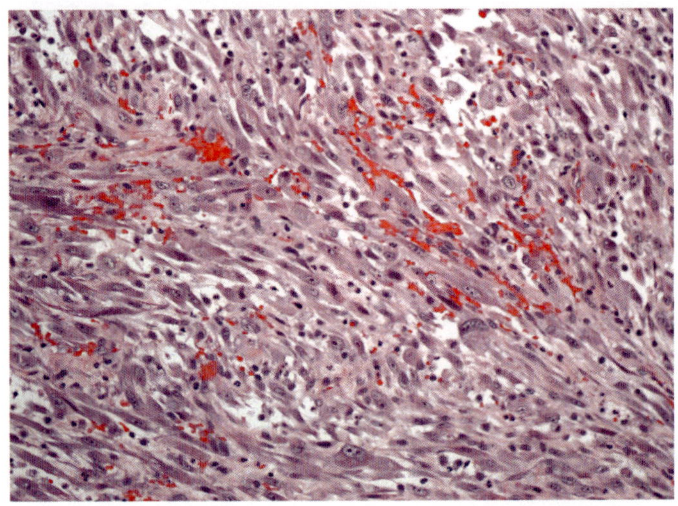

Figure 8.54 — Inflammatory myofibroblastic tumor (IMT) of the bladder, histologic section. The myofibroblastic cells of IMT have abundant eosinophilic cytoplasm, and there is a sprinkling of chronic and sometimes acute inflammatory cells within the lesion. The differential diagnosis includes leiomyosarcoma, rhabdomyosarcoma, and sarcomatoid carcinoma. In contrast to these malignancies, the nuclei are not hyperchromatic, and the cells have a tissue-culture-like appearance. Although frequent mitotic figures may be seen, atypical mitotic figures are absent. Extravasated RBCs are a frequent feature of these lesions (H&E stain, medium power).

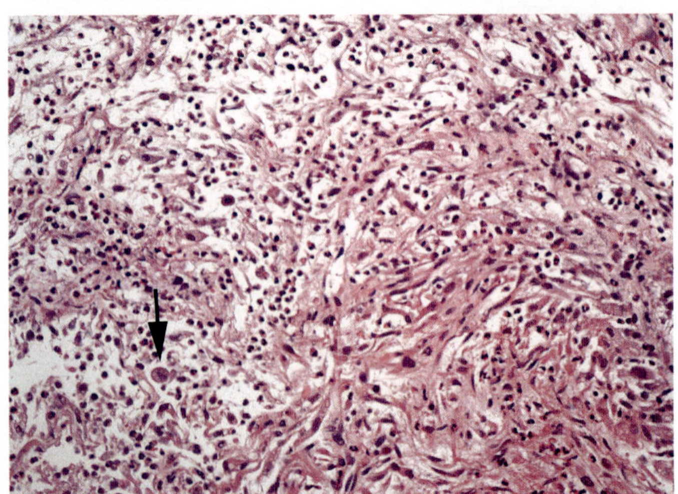

Figure 8.55 — Inflammatory myofibroblastic tumor (IMT) of the bladder, histologic section. Surface urothelium may become ulcerated and acute inflammation can be seen superficially. Chronic inflammatory infiltrates are usually present deep within the neoplasm. Lesions often have a myxoid stroma. Mitoses can be seen that are not atypical (arrow); (H&E stain, medium power).

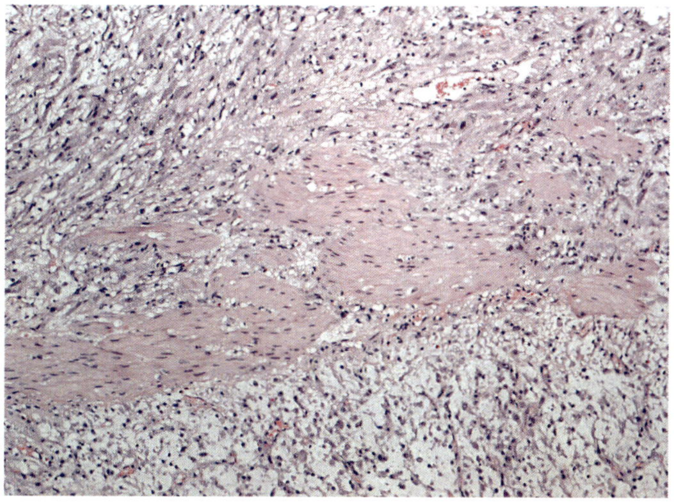

Figure 8.56 — Inflammatory myofibroblastic tumor (IMT) of the bladder, histologic section. IMTs infiltrate the bladder wall, focally destroying the muscularis propria, and can even extend into perivesicle adipose tissue (H&E stain, low power).

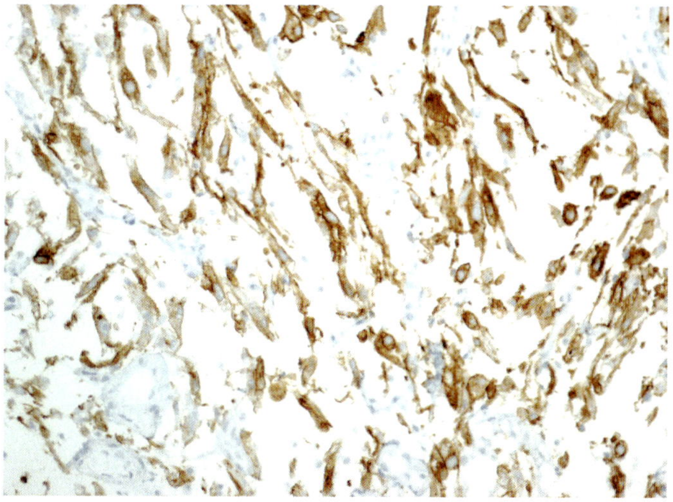

Figure 8.57 — Inflammatory myofibroblastic tumor (IMT) of the bladder, histologic section. Myofibroblasts displaying strong cytoplasmic immunolabeling with ALK1. Approximately 60 percent of bladder IMTs are immunoreactive to anaplastic lymphoma kinase 1 (ALK1 immunostain, medium power).

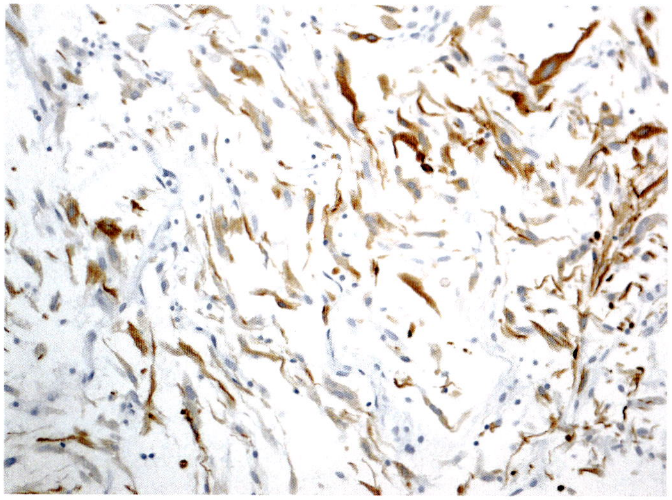

Figure 8.58 — Inflammatory myofibroblastic tumor (IMT) of the bladder, histologic section. In IMTs, the lesional myofibroblasts are also positive for cytokeratins. Other positive immunostains include actin and vimentin (CK immunostain, medium power).

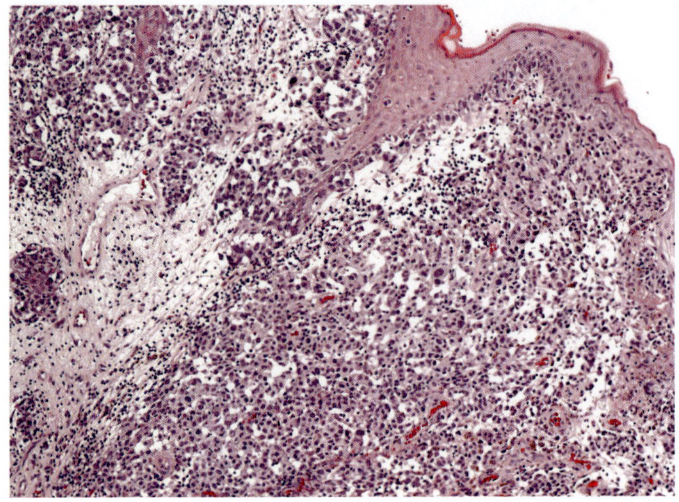

Figure 8.59 — Primary melanoma of the urethra, histologic section. The distal urethra is the site of primary melanoma, which is rare in the bladder. Urethral epithelium is seen associated with in situ and invasive melanoma. The malignant melanocytes have abundant pale eosinophilic cytoplasm with large nuclei and prominent nucleoli. Focally melanin pigment is identified. It is treated by complete urethrectomy with bilateral lymph node dissection (H&E stain, medium power).

9

Upper Urinary Tract Lesions

- Normal Urothelium
- Atypias
- Urothelial Neoplasms

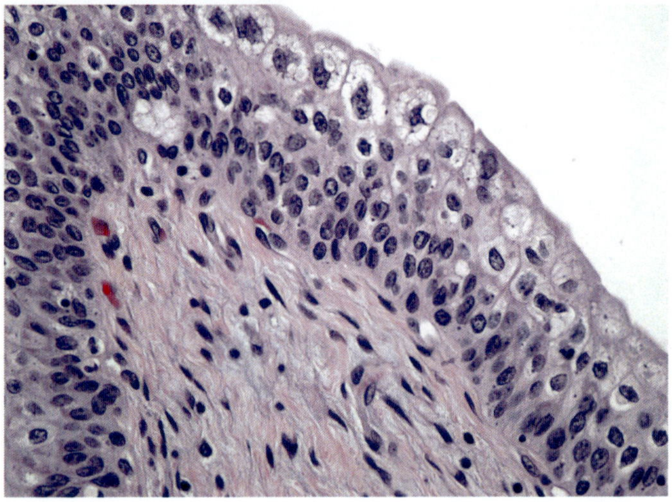

Figure 9.1 — Normal ureter urothelium, histologic section. Compared to the bladder the urothelium lining the upper urinary tract is three to four cell layers thick. In this high magnification of the ureter lining, the nuclei have the ovoid appearance with longitudinal grooves. The intact umbrella cell layer is quite spectacular with vacuolated cytoplasm and large nuclei. Some cells show binucleation and rounded luminal surface (H&E stain, high power).

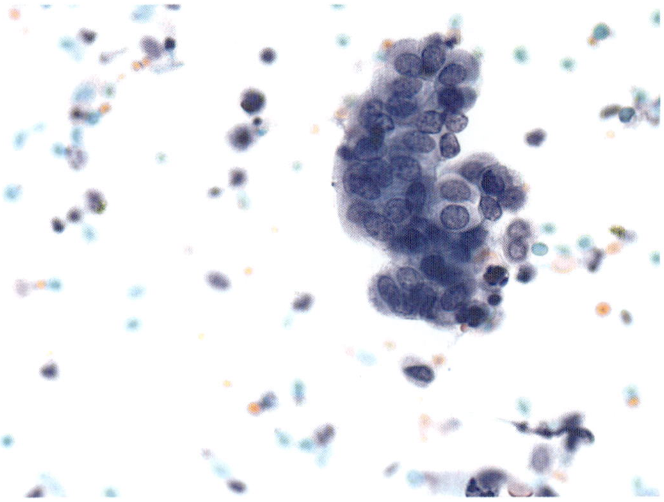

Figure 9.2 — Normal urothelial cells of the upper urinary tract, instrumented specimen. Cytologic samples from the upper urinary tract are always obtained by instrumentation when designated as upper tract. Therefore, an instrumentation artifact is to be expected. The distinction between true papillary lesions and fragments dislodged with a catheter is very difficult if not impossible. The assessment of the cytomorphology is much more important than deciding whether an instrumentation artifact or a papillary lesion is present. In this photograph, the nuclei are virtually all round, with some accentuation of the nuclear membrane and granularity of the nuclear chromatin. There is considerable inflammation in the background, most likely the cause of these minimal nuclear changes. N/C ratios are low, and the overall picture is one of a benign process (Papanicolaou stain, high power).

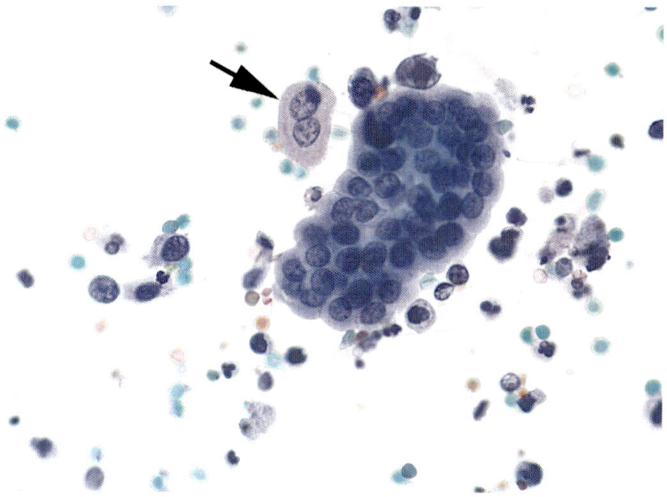

Figure 9.3 — Normal urothelial cells of the upper urinary tract, instrumented specimen. When deciding the presence or absence of atypia in a specimen, the normal umbrella cells constitute an internal control. In this photograph, the umbrella cell (arrow) has a somewhat granulated chromatin and thickened nuclear membrane, most likely due to the exuberant inflammation in the background. That would account for the nuclear changes within the tissue fragment. Those nuclei are round and surrounded by abundant vesicular cytoplasm. All features are that of a benign process (Papanicolaou stain, high power).

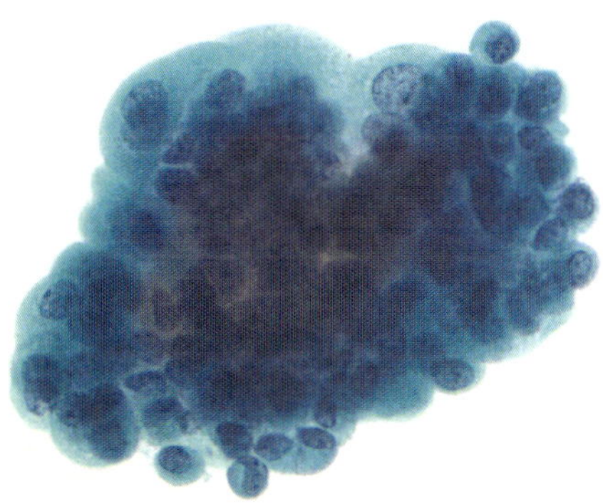

Figure 9.4 — Normal urothelial cells of the upper urinary tract, instrumented specimen. Careful inspection of fragments from the upper tract is necessary in order to see through the thickness produced by the instrumentation. This particular fragment is covered by umbrella cells and contains round basal cells with small nuclei (Papanicolaou stain, high power).

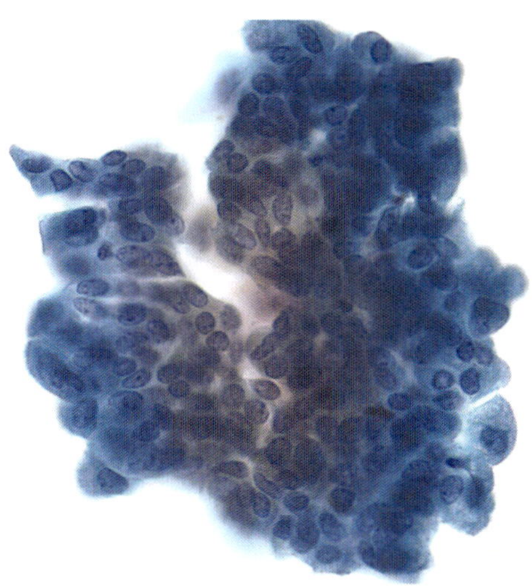

Figure 9.5 — Normal urothelial cells of the upper urinary tract, instrumented specimen. Very delicate cytoplasm and round nuclear shapes are characteristic of these umbrella cells from the upper tract. Despite a slight darkening of the nuclear chromatin, they are totally benign (Papanicolaou stain, high power).

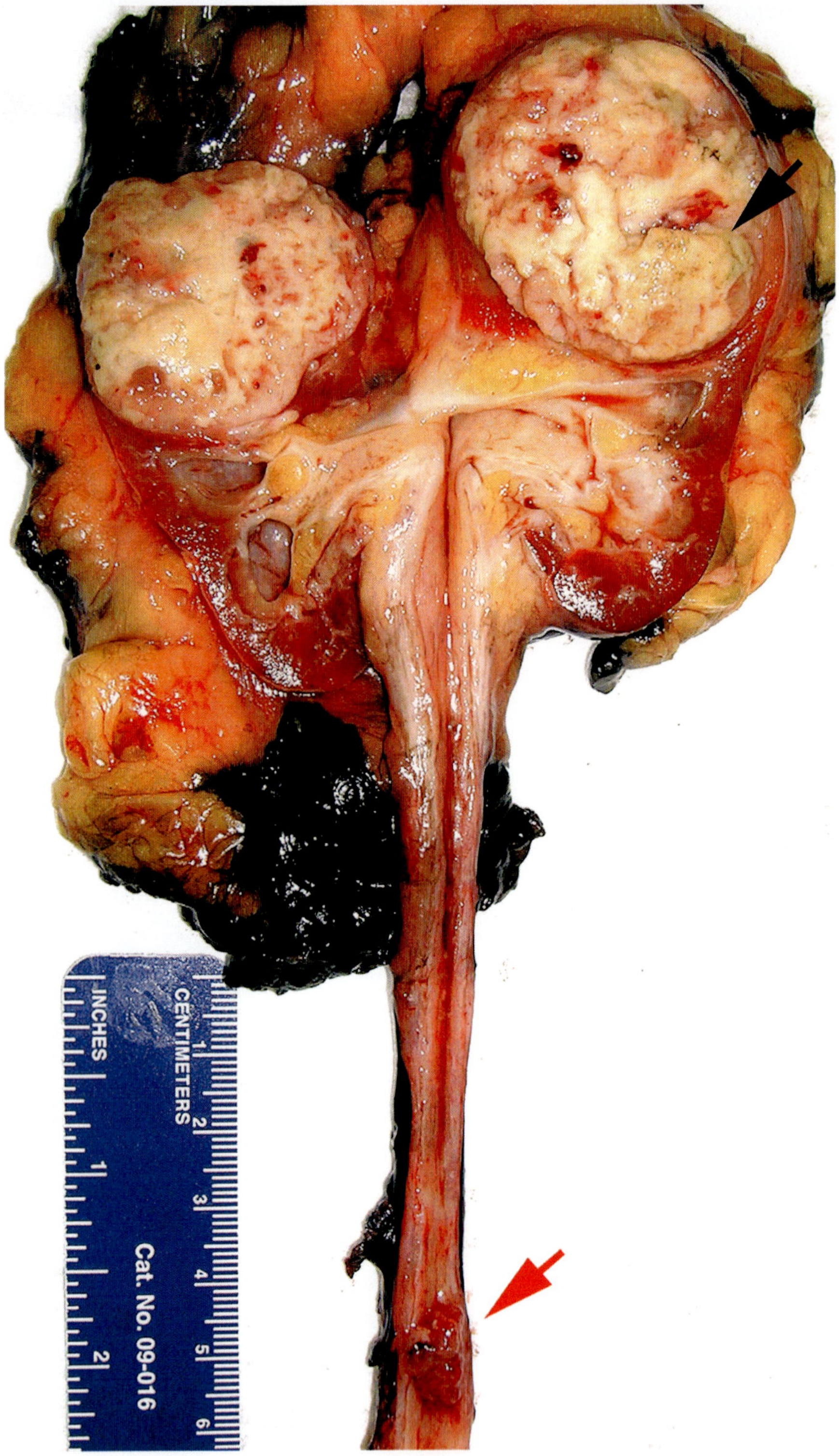

Figure 9.6 — Urothelial carcinoma, gross specimen. Nephroureterectomy specimen with multifocal urothelial carcinoma. The bivalved kidney has a large urothelial carcinoma with necrosis in the superior calyx (black arrow). The opened ureter also has urothelial carcinoma (red arrow). Patients who develop urothelial carcinoma can have multifocal disease involving the entire urinary tract. These lesions can arise synchronously or more commonly metachronously. Patients present with hematuria.

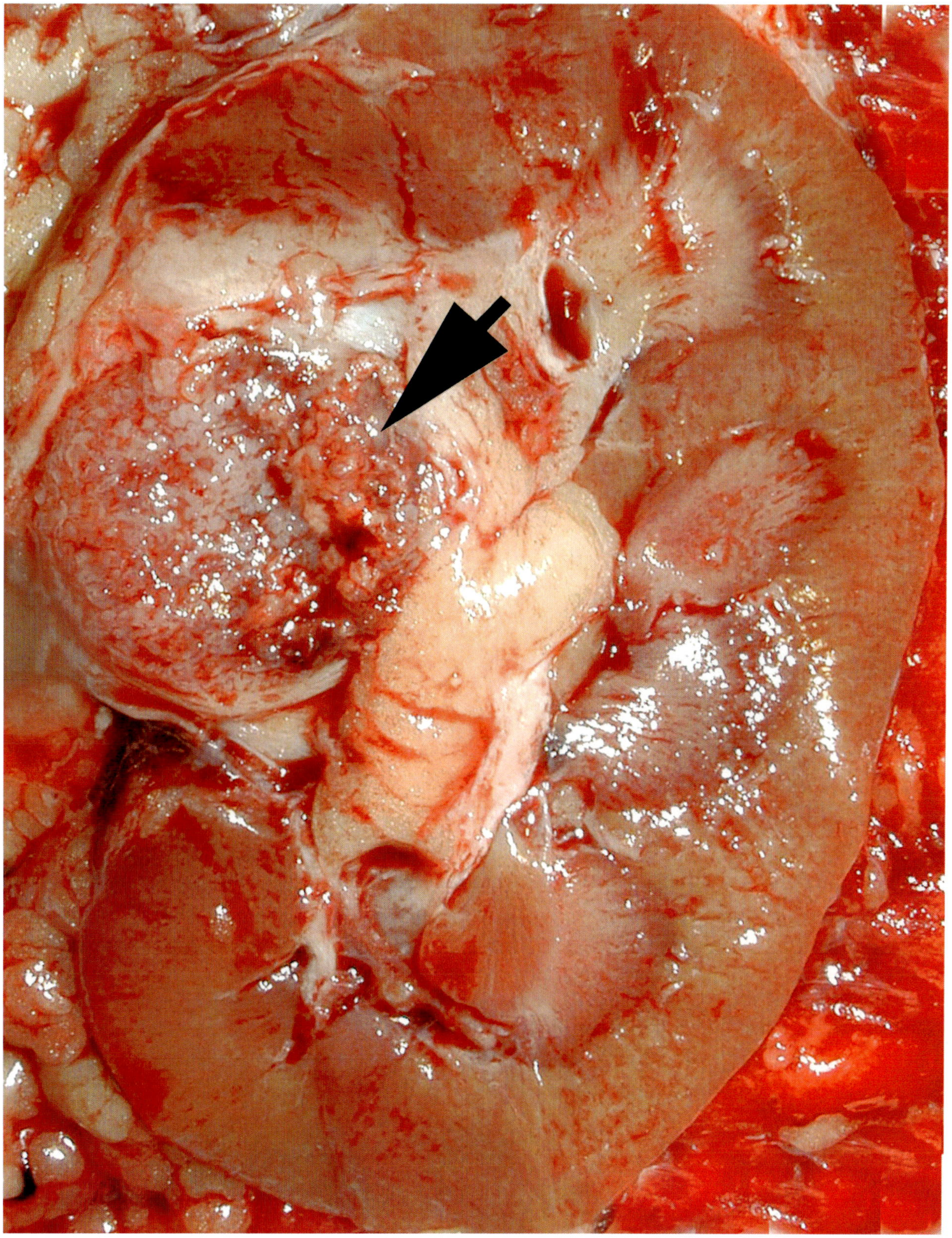

Figure 9.7 — Urothelial carcinoma, gross specimen. Nephrectomy specimen with papillary urothelial carcinoma. Renal pelvis is filled with a noninvasive papillary urothelial neoplasm (arrow). Prognosis of renal urothelial carcinoma depends on depth of invasion.

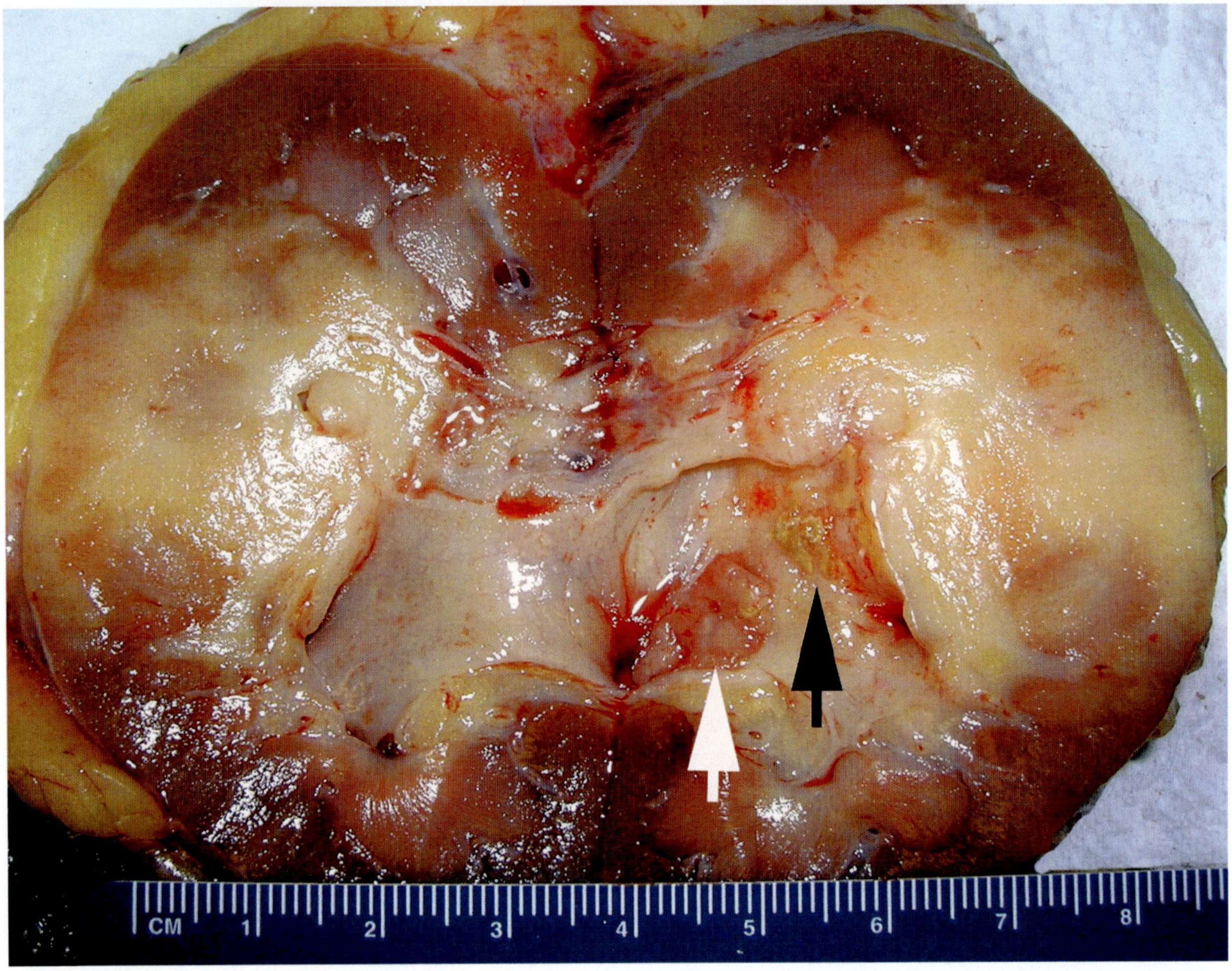

Figure 9.8 — Urothelial carcinoma, gross specimen. Nephrectomy specimen with infiltrating urothelial carcinoma. Bivalved kidney with ulcerated renal pelvis lesion (black arrow) and infiltrating high-grade urothelial carcinoma seen as the pale tan lesion in the mid-pole, involving the renal parenchyma, reaching up to the capsule (white arrow). Extension of urothelial carcinoma outside the kidney and coexisting bladder tumors are poor prognostic features.

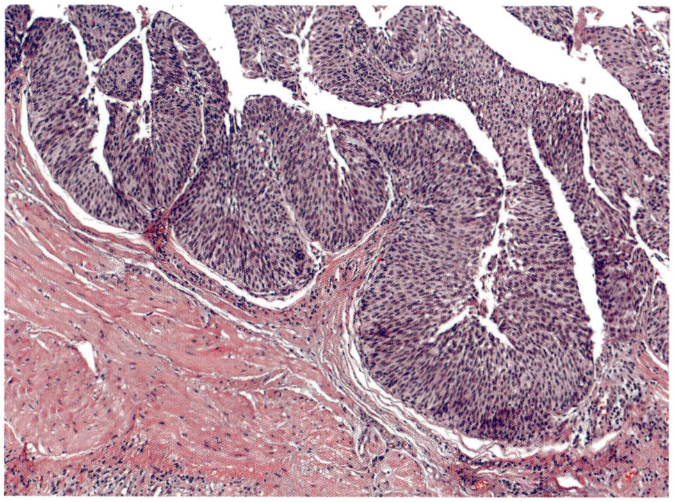

Figure 9.9 — Urothelial carcinoma of renal pelvis, histologic section. Section of renal pelvis with a low-grade papillary urothelial carcinoma growing exophytically. The basement membrane is intact. The urothelium has orderly arrangement with retained polarity and uniform cells. Renal urothelial carcinoma accounts for 7 percent of primary renal malignancies (H&E stain, low power).

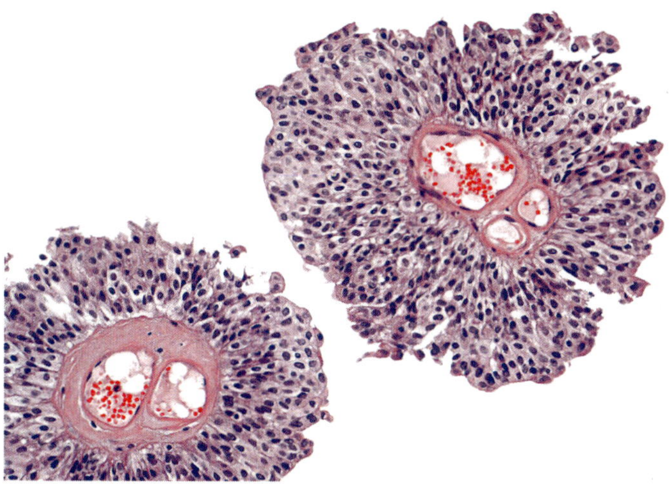

Figure 9.10 — Urothelial carcinoma of renal pelvis, histologic section. Low-grade papillary urothelial carcinoma. Well-formed fibrovascular cores are lined by uniform cohesive urothelial cells with relatively maintained polarity, with minimal cytological atypia (H&E stain, low power).

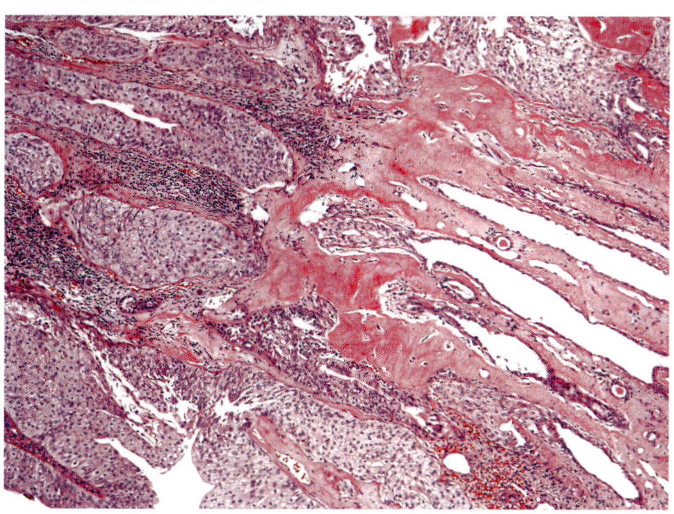

Figure 9.11 — Urothelial carcinoma of renal pelvis, histologic section. Low-grade papillary urothelial carcinoma extending down into the collecting ducts. Urothelial carcinoma of the renal pelvis and caliceal system can extend within the ducts and tubules of the medulla and cortex without invasion of the renal parenchyma. Such extension should still be considered noninvasive. The lesion has bland morphology with low nuclear to cytoplasmic ratio of the tumor cells (H&E stain, low power).

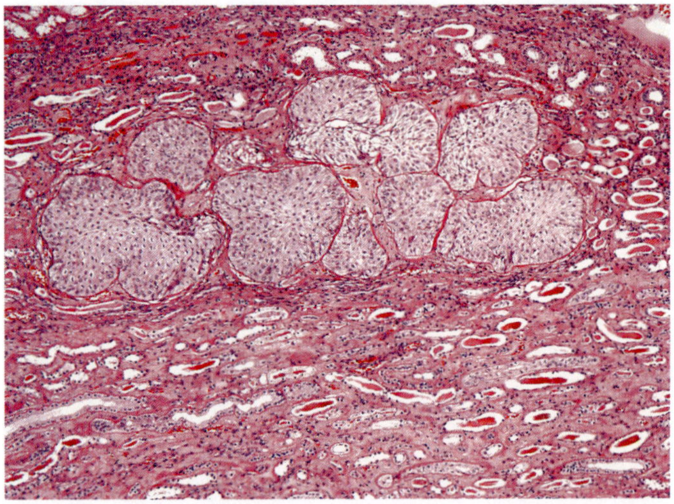

Figure 9.12 — Urothelial carcinoma of renal pelvis, histologic section. Low-grade urothelial carcinoma with renal tubular extension. Noninvasive urothelial carcinoma of the renal pelvis filling and expanding involved collecting ducts. Note the bland appearance of the carcinoma cells (H&E stain, low power).

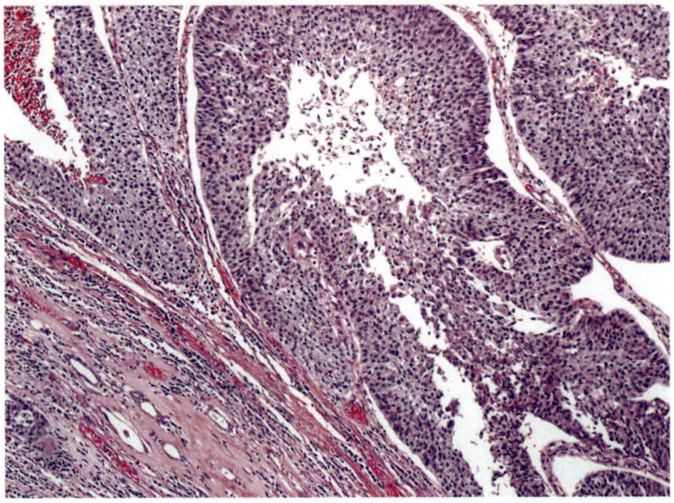

Figure 9.13 — Urothelial carcinoma of renal pelvis, histologic section. This section depicts exophytic growth of noninvasive high-grade papillary urothelial carcinoma. There is loss of polarity with dyscohesiveness of the tumor cells. Renal medulla is visible on the lower left side (H&E stain, low power).

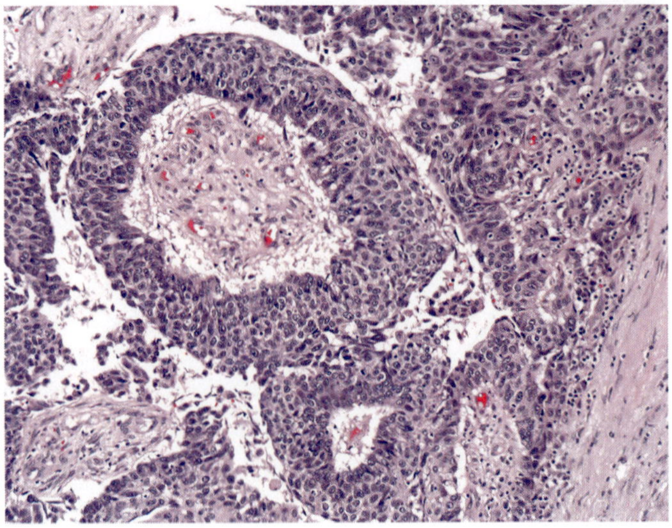

Figure 9.14 — Urothelial carcinoma of renal pelvis, histologic section. High-grade papillary urothelial carcinoma displays well-formed fibrovascular cores lined by cells with a high N/C ratio, clumped chromatin, prominent nucleoli, loss of polarity, and increased mitotic rate (H&E stain, low power).

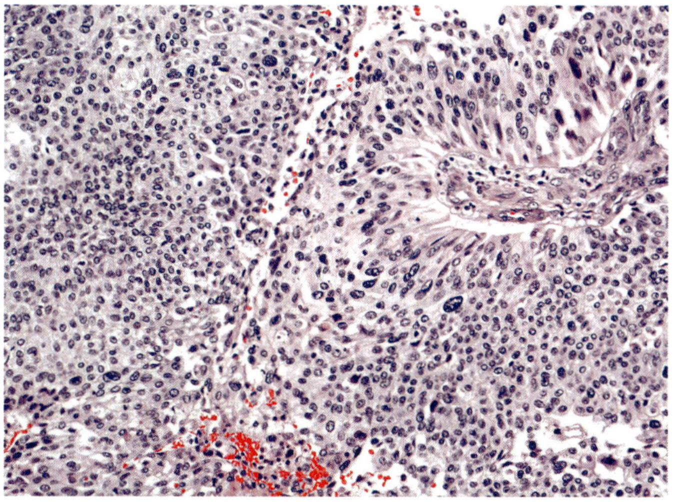

Figure 9.15 — Urothelial carcinoma of renal pelvis, histologic section. High-grade papillary urothelial carcinoma shows nuclear pleomorphism and increased mitoses (H&E stain, low power).

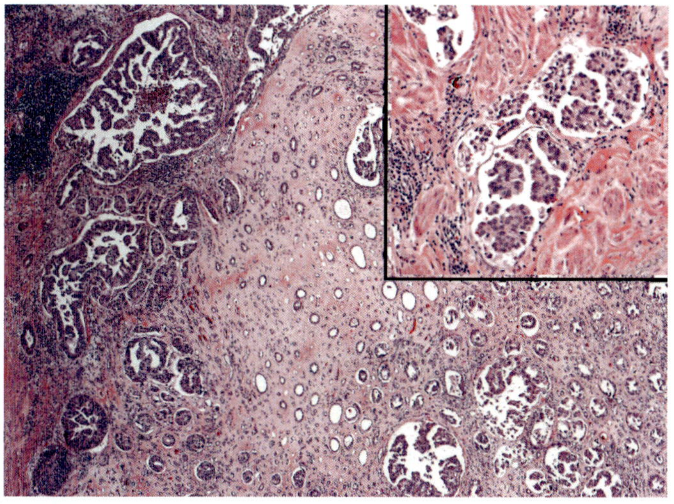

Figure 9.16 — Urothelial carcinoma of renal pelvis, histologic section. Invasive micropapillary urothelial carcinoma of the renal pelvis. This high-grade urothelial carcinoma shows invasion into the renal parenchyma as well as extension into the renal tubules. Micropapillary urothelial carcinoma is an aggressive form of the disease with early lymphatic invasion (inset) and associated lymph node metastases (H&E stain, low and medium power).

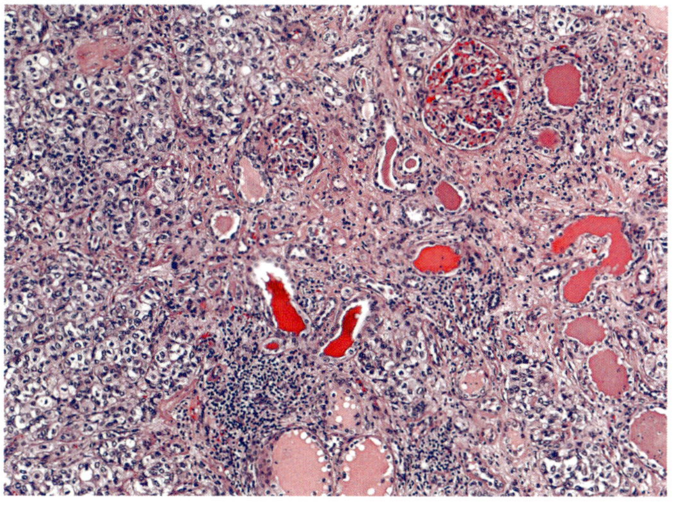

Figure 9.17 — Urothelial carcinoma of renal pelvis, histologic section. High-grade urothelial carcinoma of the pelvis invading renal parenchyma. The left side of the image shows infiltrating nests of urothelial carcinoma adjacent to renal tubules and glomeruli. Invasion of the renal parenchyma is T3 stage. Nearly 2 to 4 percent of patients with bladder cancer develop upper tract urothelial carcinoma; however, 40 percent of patients with upper tract urothelial carcinoma develop bladder cancer (H&E stain, medium power).

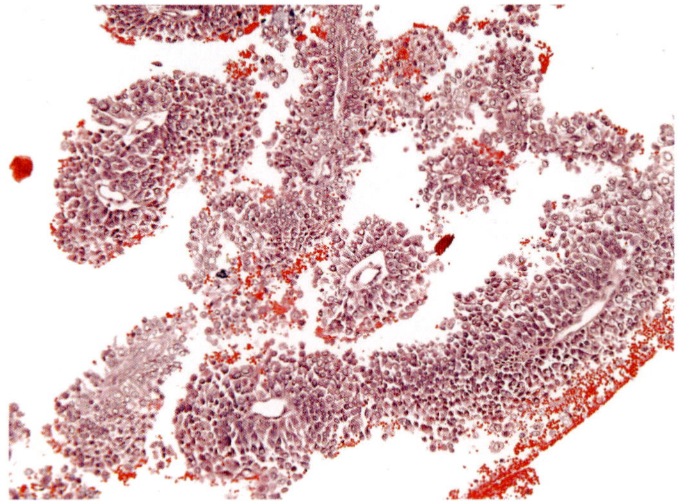

Figure 9.18 — Noninvasive, high-grade papillary urothelial carcinoma of the ureter, histologic section. Papillary ureteral tumor depicts well-formed fibrovascular cores lined by urothelial cells with pleomorphism, increased N/C ratios and loss of polarity (H&E stain, low power).

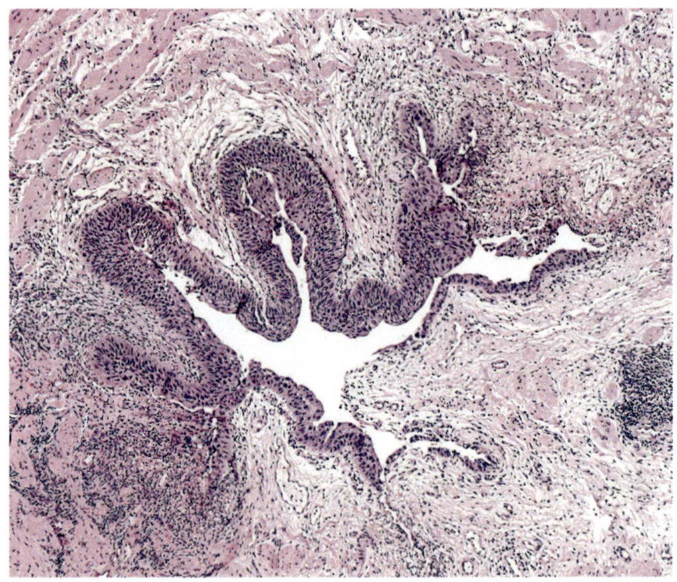

Figure 9.19 — Urothelial carcinoma of the ureter, histologic section. Ureter with flat urothelial carcinoma in situ (CIS). Treatment of upper urinary tract carcinoma is nephroureterectomy with resection of bladder cuff. The lumen of the ureter appears dilated with loss of part of the urothelium due to the dyscohesive nature of CIS cells (H&E stain, low power). [Photograph courtesy of Dr. Charles J. Sailey, University of Maryland Medical Center, Baltimore.]

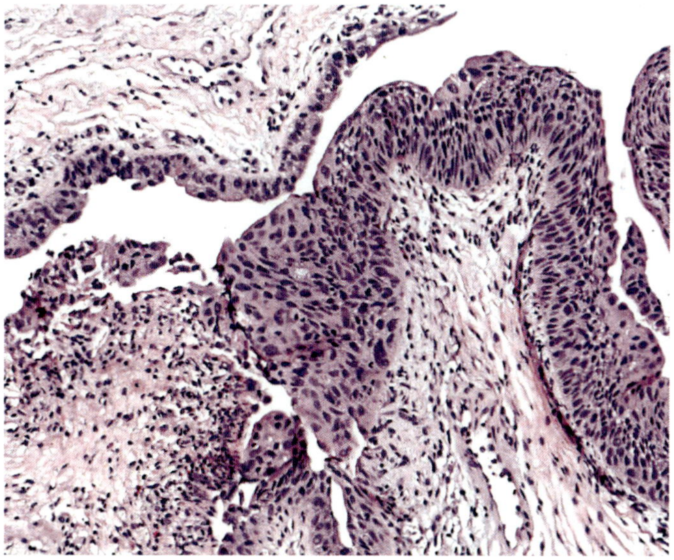

Figure 9.20 — Urothelial carcinoma of the renal pelvis, histologic section. Ureter with flat urothelial carcinoma in-situ (CIS) with enlarged hyperchromatic nuclei and nuclear membrane irregularities. There is disorderly arrangement of the cells with crowding (H&E stain, medium power). [Photograph courtesy of Dr. Charles J. Sailey, University of Maryland Medical Center, Baltimore.]

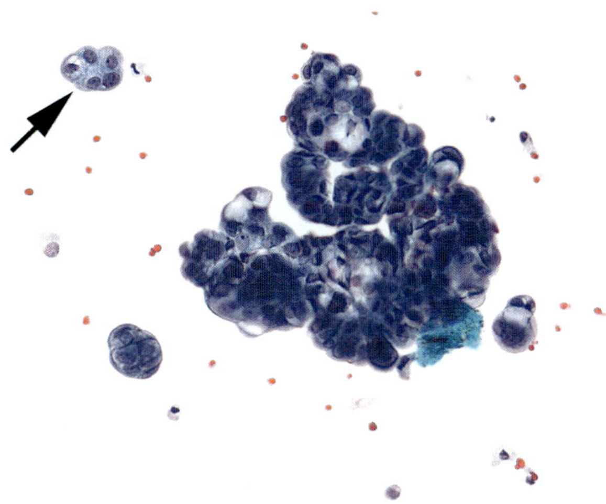

Figure 9.21 — Atypical urothelial cells of the upper urinary tract, instrumented specimen. (Follow-up: low-grade urothelial carcinoma). Vacuolization in urothelial cells is common and can produce an atypia that may mimic a glandular lesion. In this particular case, careful inspection of the nuclei and nuclear chromatin indicates deviation from the normal cells seen in the small group in the upper left hand corner (arrow). In the large fragment, nuclei are of varying size and shape but are still small enough to suspect only a low-grade lesion and not a high-grade lesion. The red blood cells in the background are fresh, and could be either a result of a papillary lesion or from instrumentation trauma (Papanicolaou stain, medium power).

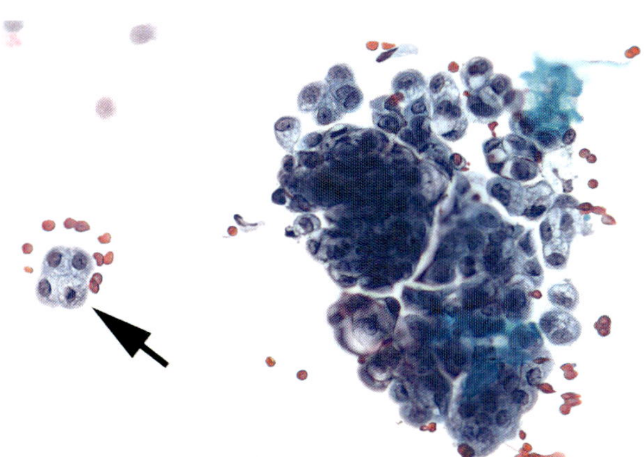

Figure 9.22 — Atypical urothelial cells of the upper urinary tract, instrumented specimen. (Follow-up: low-grade urothelial carcinoma). The small group of four cells in the left-hand field should be considered the normal internal control (arrow). Compare with the cells in the large fragment with variable size nuclei and disordered architecture. Although the cells themselves are not highly atypical, the architectural disarray is suspect for a low-grade lesion (Papanicolaou stain, medium power).

Figure 9.23 — Atypical urothelial cells of the upper urinary tract, instrumented specimen. (Follow-up: low-grade urothelial carcinoma). As in cells from the urinary bladder, the cells of a low-grade lesion are not always different from totally benign urothelial cells, as in this fragment covered by umbrella cells. Once again, this accounts for the low sensitivity of urinary cytology for detecting low-grade urothelial lesions either in the bladder or the upper urinary tract (Papanicolaou stain, high power).

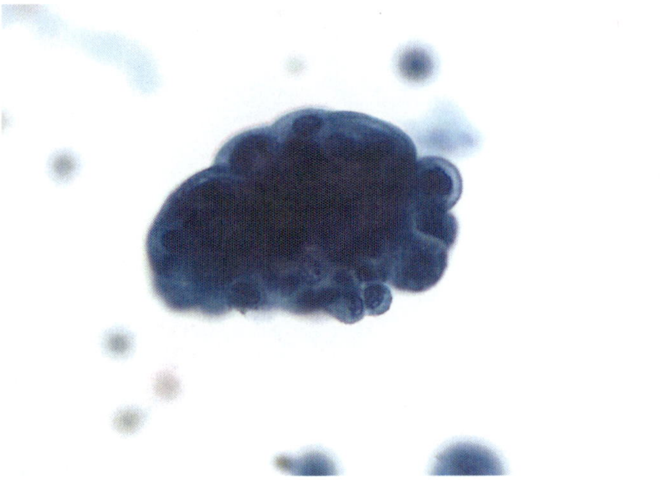

Figure 9.24 — Atypical urothelial cells of the upper urinary tract, instrumented specimen. (Follow-up: high-grade urothelial carcinoma). Within a fragment of epithelium covered by normal umbrella cells, one might observe cells suspicious for a high-grade lesion. These juxtaposed cell types are a result of instrumentation, and the worst cells in the group should be considered for the final interpretation, which in this case is "suspicious for a high-grade lesion". Fresh red blood cells in the background are of no importance, since they are probably a result of instrumentation (Papanicolaou stain, high power).

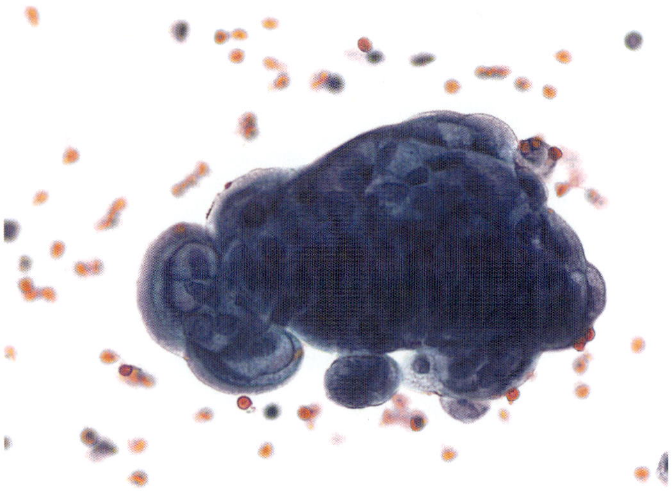

Figure 9.25 — Atypical urothelial cells of the upper urinary tract, instrumented specimen. (Follow-up: high-grade urothelial carcinoma). Although most of the cells in these three groups are small with low N/C ratios, the group to the left has a binucleate cell (arrow) with very abnormal nuclei and coarse nuclear chromatin. The ultimate diagnosis was high grade and this sample should be interpreted as suspicious for that lesion (Papanicolaou stain, high power).

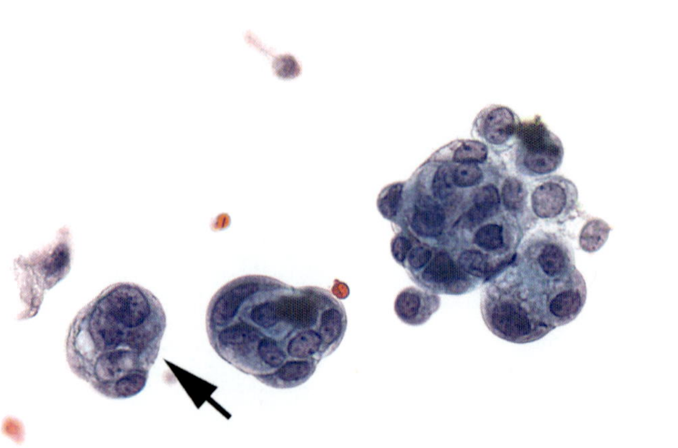

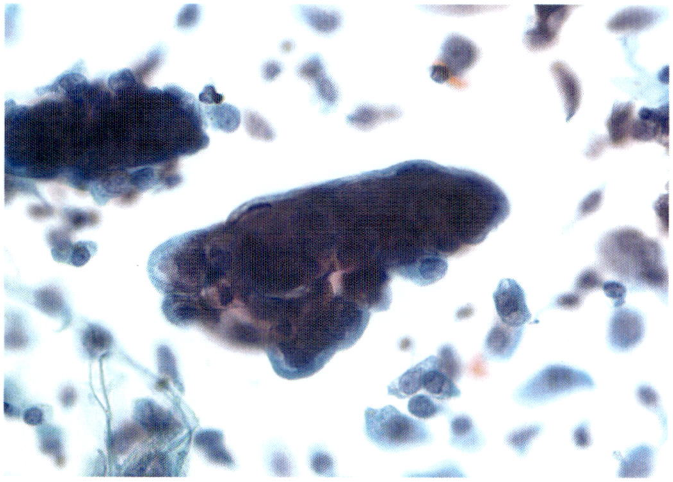

Figure 9.26 — Atypical urothelial cells of the upper urinary tract, instrumented specimen. (Follow-up: high-grade urothelial carcinoma). Although this fragment is covered by umbrella cells, the underlying cells are markedly atypical; diagnosis should indicate that a high-grade lesion is suspected (Papanicolaou stain, high power).

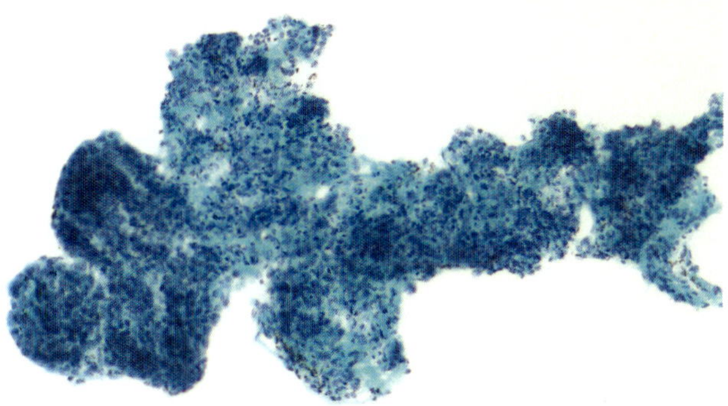

Figure 9.27 — Low-grade urothelial carcinoma of the upper urinary tract, instrumented specimen. This low-power photograph of a papillary lesion is essentially identical to a tissue biopsy. Fibrovascular cores can be identified within the tissue surrounded by uniform small urothelial cells (Papanicolaou stain, very low power).

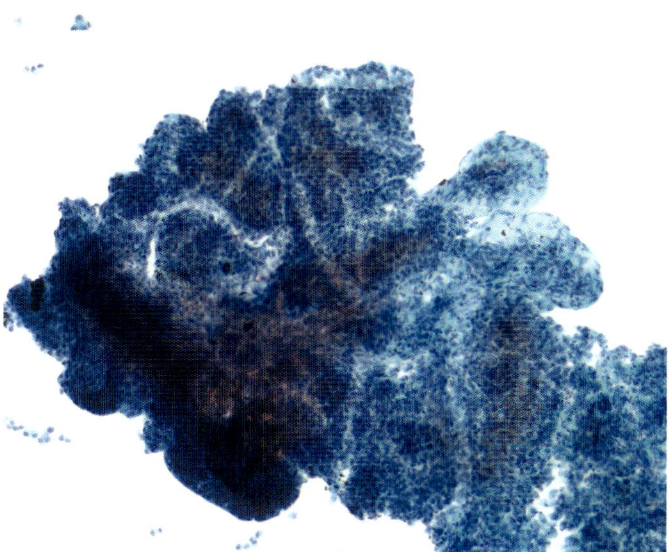

Figure 9.28 — Low-grade urothelial carcinoma of the upper urinary tract, instrumented specimen. Slightly higher power of the same lesion as in Figure 9.27 determines the uniformity of the cells within the fragments indicating a low-grade lesion. Definitive grading must be determined by higher power examination (Papanicolaou stain, medium power).

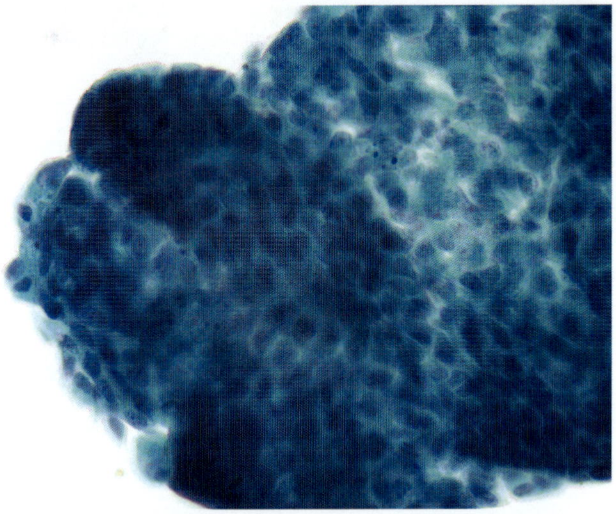

Figure 9.29 — Low-grade urothelial carcinoma of the upper urinary tract, instrumented specimen. Here, the nuclei from the preceding two photographs can be clearly visualized, seen to be small and uniform, consistent with a low-grade papillary lesion (Papanicolaou stain, high power).

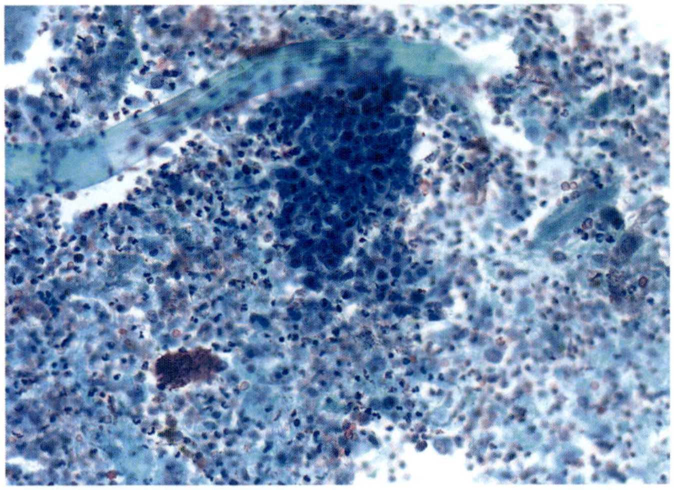

Figure 9.30 — Low-grade urothelial carcinoma of the upper urinary tract, instrumented specimen. Within a very busy visual scene, hyperchromatic crowded groups may be lurking. Careful inspection is needed to determine the grade of the cellular abnormalities (Papanicolaou stain, low power).

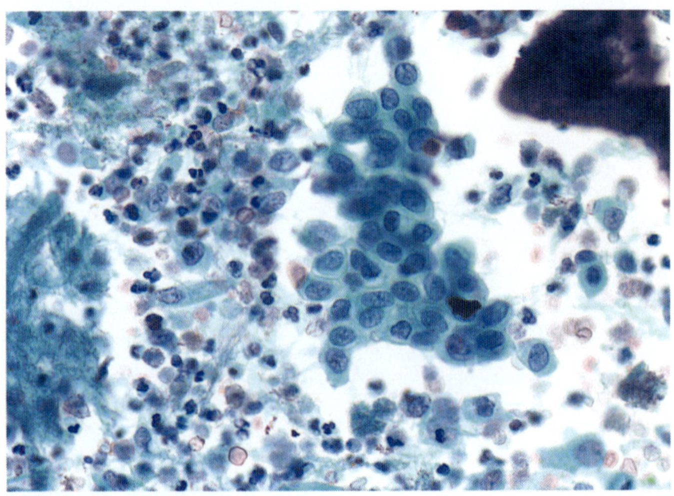

Figure 9.31 — Low-grade urothelial carcinoma of the upper urinary tract, instrumented specimen. Higher power inspection of the cells seen in Figure 9.30 reveals the nuclei to be round to oval with pale nuclear chromatin and thin nuclear membranes. The deviation from the norm, especially in a background of such acute inflammation is very minimal, and although a low-grade urothelial carcinoma was ultimately diagnosed, the cells should not be interpreted as anything other than normal. Even if originating in the neoplasm, these account for the poor sensitivity of urinary cytology in detecting low-grade neoplasms of the urinary tract (Papanicolaou stain, medium power).

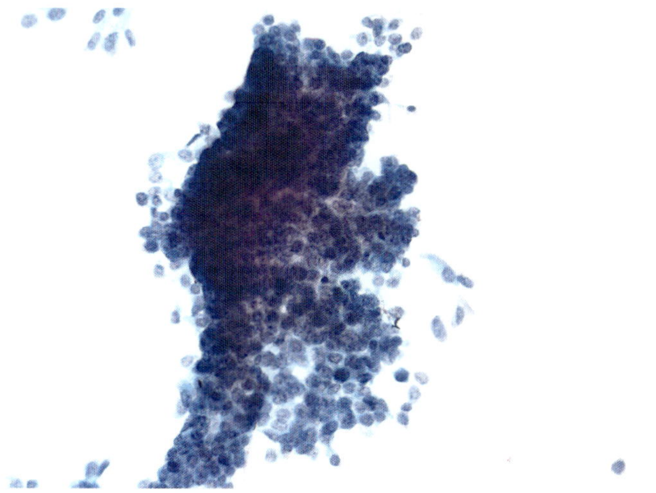

Figure 9.32 — Low-grade urothelial carcinoma of the upper urinary tract, instrumented specimen. A large fragment comprises monotonous small urothelial cells with bland nuclei and scant cytoplasm. The only truly reliable indicator of neoplasia is the disorganized architecture and crowding. Although crowding may be produced by instrumentation, careful focus through the fragments will determine the internuclear distances, which would be greater in benign lesions and less in neoplastic lesions (Papanicolaou stain, medium power).

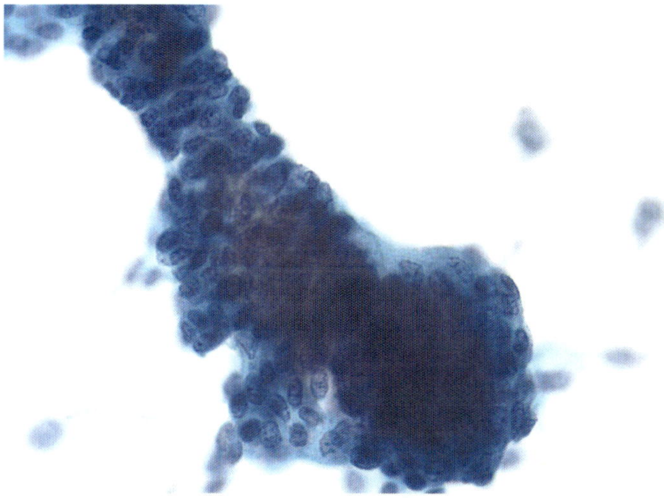

Figure 9.33 — Low-grade urothelial carcinoma of the upper urinary tract, instrumented specimen. Higher power of Figure 9.32 displays the uniform cell size and N/C ratios, but the overlapping nuclei and disorganization favor a neoplastic process (Papanicolaou stain, high power).

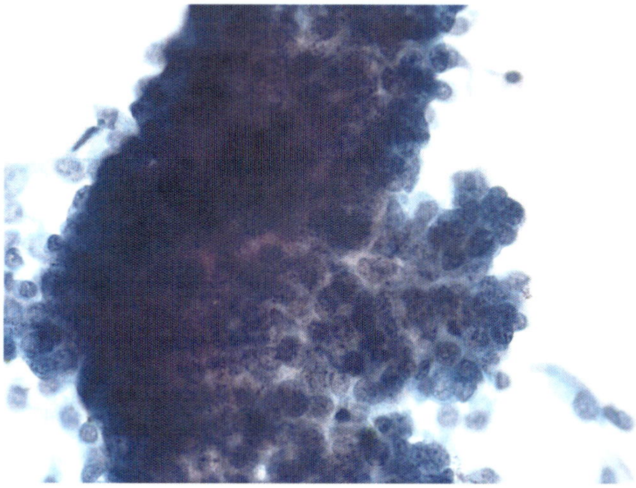

Figure 9.34 — Low-grade urothelial carcinoma of the upper urinary tract, instrumented specimen. Another view of the same lesion displays the high N/C ratio and granular chromatin of these otherwise uniform cells (Papanicolaou stain, high power).

Figure 9.35 — Low-grade urothelial carcinoma of the upper urinary tract, instrumented specimen. The cytomorphology of lesions of the upper tract is essentially the same as within the upper tract is essentially the same as within the urinary bladder. One only has to remember that instrumentation has captured these cells. Nuclear enlargement, overlapping cells, and disorganized architecture are the same throughout the urinary tract when describing low-grade urothelial neoplasia (Papanicolaou stain, high power).

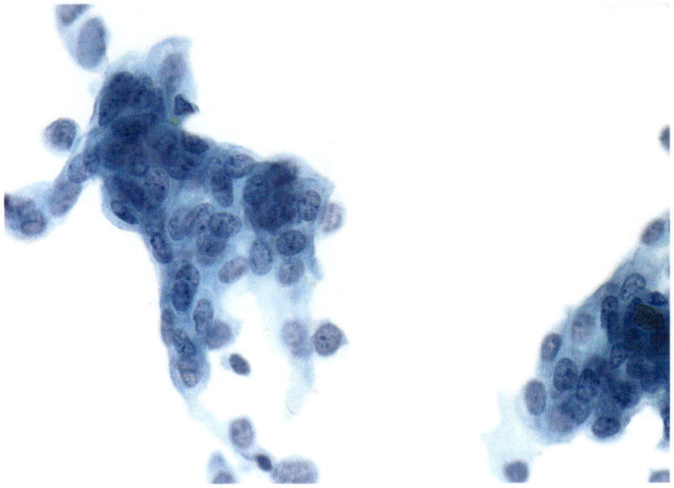

Figure 9.36 — Low-grade urothelial carcinoma of the upper urinary tract, instrumented specimen. Not every lesion can be easily compartmentalized into low or high grade. Cells pictured here have nuclei of varying size and shape with coarsened chromatin and increased N/C ratios. The lone cell at 11 o'clock (arrow) has a very high N/C ratio and is larger than the others. A high-grade lesion should be suspected, although the final diagnosis in this patient was low-grade (Papanicolaou stain, high power).

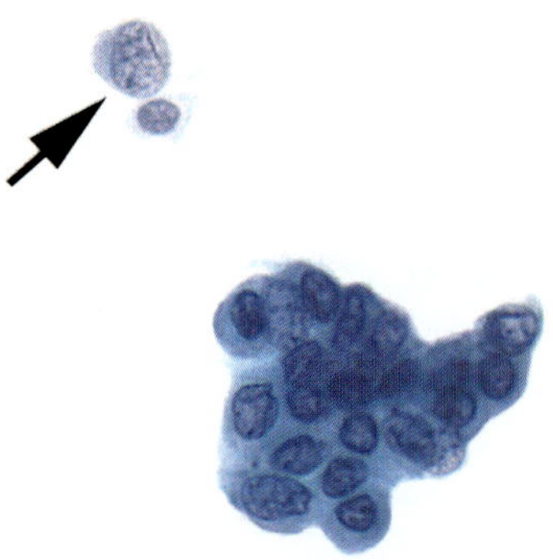

Figure 9.37 — Low-grade urothelial carcinoma of the upper urinary tract, instrumented specimen. Although the rule for high-grade urothelial carcinoma is singly shed cells, this photograph depicts cells from a low-grade lesion. Therefore, the presence of single cells in itself does not make the diagnosis high grade. The fine nuclear chromatin and thin nuclear membranes in these tumor cells are consistent with a low-grade lesion. The next figure shows a tissue fragment from this same patient (Papanicolaou stain, high power).

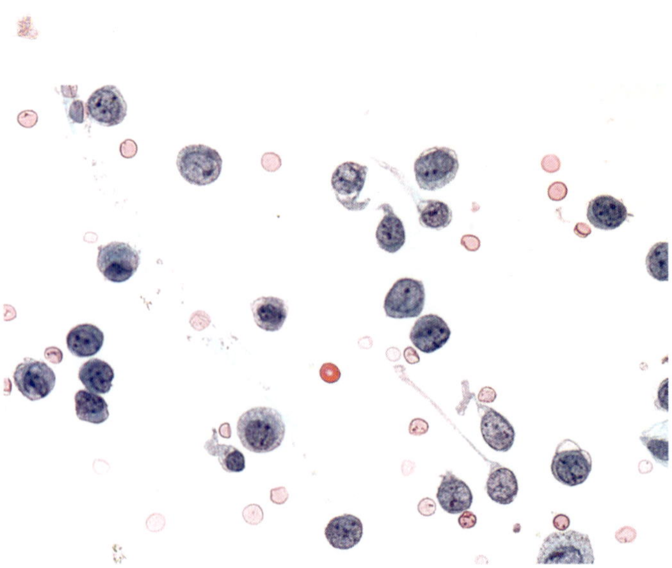

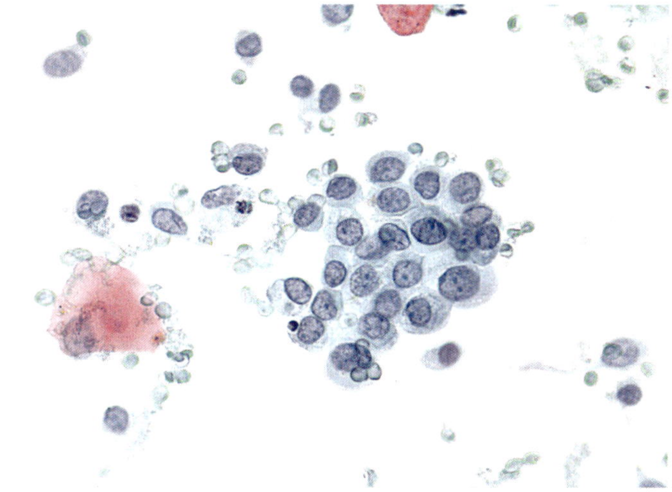

Figure 9.38 — Low-grade urothelial carcinoma of the upper urinary tract, instrumented specimen. A fragment from the patient's sample as depicted in Figure 9.37 confirms the uniformity of the cell size and nuclear chromatin as well as a relatively uniform architecture. There is some variation in the chromatin distribution as well as occasional nuclear overlapping, supporting a neoplastic diagnosis (Papanicolaou stain, high power).

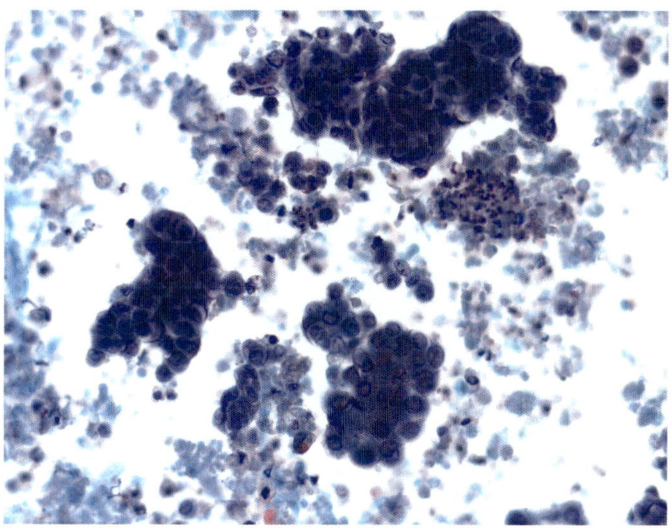

Figure 9.39 — High-grade urothelial carcinoma of the upper urinary tract, instrumented specimen. Because samples from the upper urinary tract are obtained by instrumentation, the classic pattern of a high-grade carcinoma with numerous single cells is not seen so apparently in these samples. However, in addition to the fragments are numerous single cells as well as degenerated fragments of cells (Papanicolaou stain, medium power).

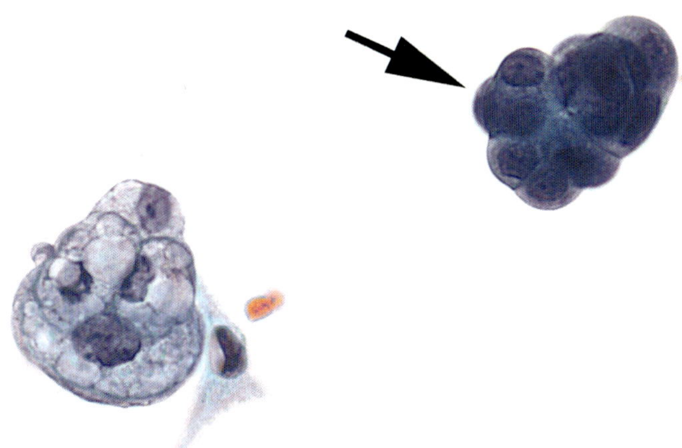

Figure 9.40 — High-grade urothelial carcinoma of the upper urinary tract, instrumented specimen. Compare the group of normal urothelial cells on the left with the group on the right (arrow). The high N/C ratios of the latter as well as the difference in nuclear chromatin indicate a high-grade lesion (Papanicolaou stain, high power).

Figure 9.41 — High-grade urothelial carcinoma of the upper urinary tract, instrumented specimen. A very large fragment of abnormal urothelium requires higher power review in order to grade the cells. However, scattered single cells surrounding the fragment suggest a high-grade lesion (Papanicolaou stain, low power).

Figure 9.42 — High-grade urothelial carcinoma of the upper urinary tract, instrumented specimen. Higher-power review of the tissue seen in Figure 9.41 discloses large cells with high N/C ratios and dark nuclear chromatin. The vacuolization is most likely cytoplasmic differentiation, although some may be residual umbrella cells. Comparison with normal umbrella cells in the rest of the sample will make the distinction (Papanicolaou stain, medium power).

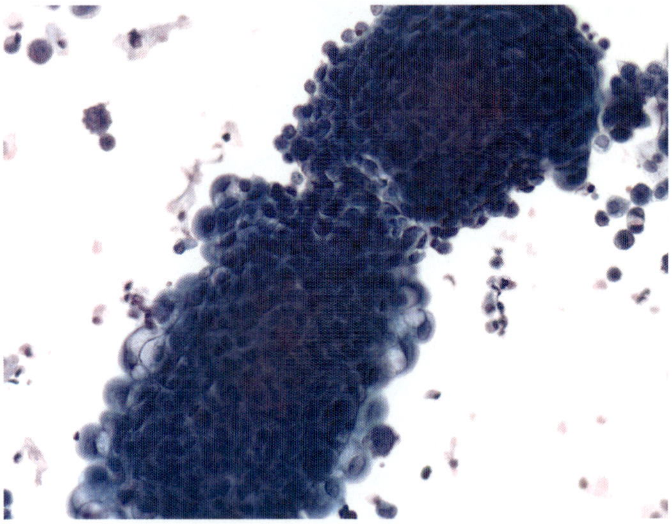

Figure 9.43 — High-grade urothelial carcinoma of the upper urinary tract, instrumented specimen. Compare the normal umbrella cells at the far left (arrow) with the rest of the cells both singly occurring and in the tissue fragment. The high N/C ratio of the latter, the coarse nuclear chromatin and the disorganized architecture within the fragment are all indicators of a high-grade lesion (Papanicolaou stain, high power).

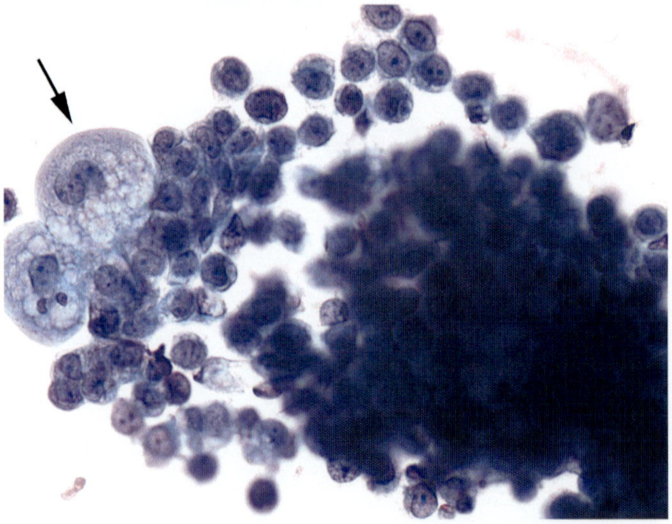

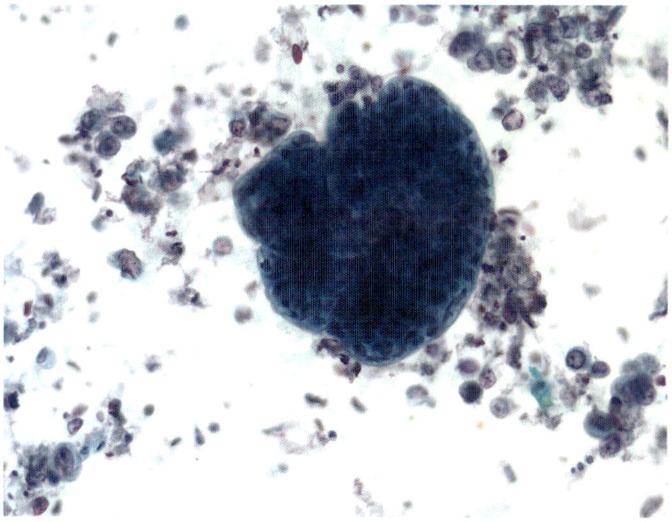

Figure 9.44 — High-grade urothelial carcinoma of the upper urinary tract, instrumented specimen. Recalling that instrumentation will dislodge fragments from the urothelium, this large fragment may not actually be from the lesion within the patient, as it appears to be covered with umbrella cells, and abundant cytoplasm can be seen in the more central portion of the fragment. Surrounding this large piece of tissue are numerous large cells with high N/C ratios and characteristics of a high-grade lesion. Higher-power review of the fragment will be needed to determine whether or not it also is neoplastic (Papanicolaou stain, medium power).

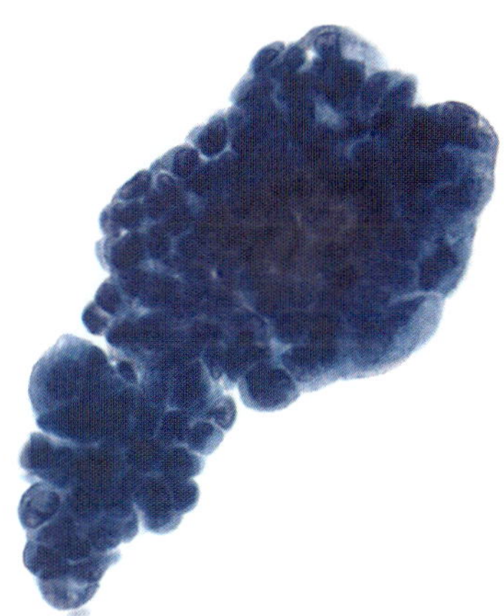

Figure 9.45 — High-grade urothelial carcinoma of the upper urinary tract, instrumented specimen. This fragment of urothelium comprises tightly packed large urothelial cells with high N/C ratios and irregular nuclear outlines. The fragment is thick with nuclei so that light transmission is impeded (Papanicolaou stain, high power).

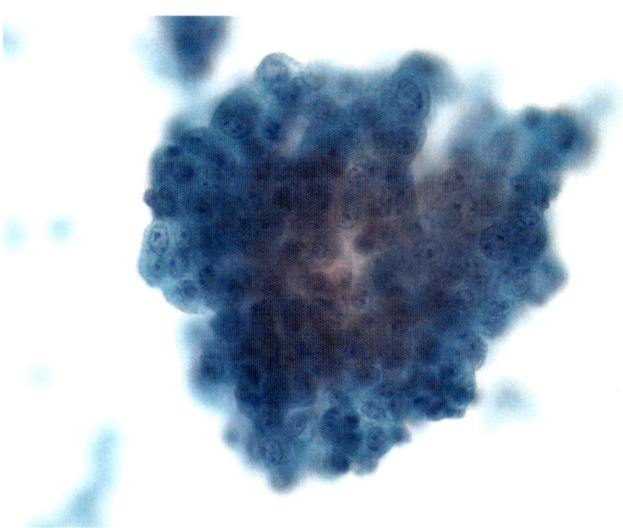

Figure 9.46 — High-grade urothelial carcinoma of the upper urinary tract, instrumented specimen. Sometimes the nuclear chromatin in high-grade lesions is not classically dark, but may appear washed out. The high N/C ratios and disorganized architecture are the clues to the grade of this kind of lesion (Papanicolaou stain, high power).

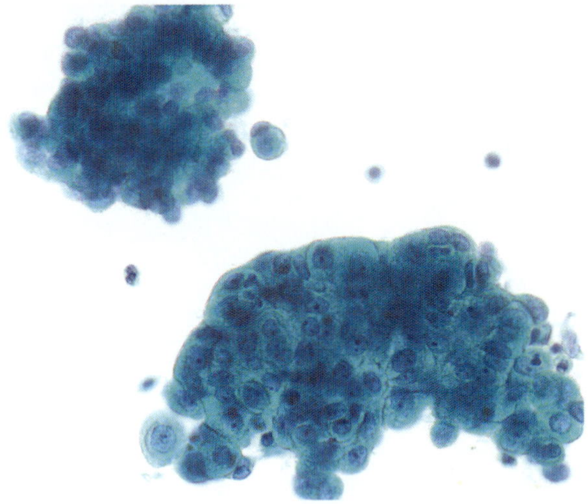

Figure 9.47 — High-grade urothelial carcinoma of the upper urinary tract, instrumented specimen. Although some high-grade urothelial carcinomas may mimic benign urothelium, careful examination of the architecture of the fragment as well as the features of each nucleus will provide an accurate diagnosis. Also, comparison with benign umbrella cells in the same sample will clarify the difference between benign and malignant cells (Papanicolaou stain, medium power).

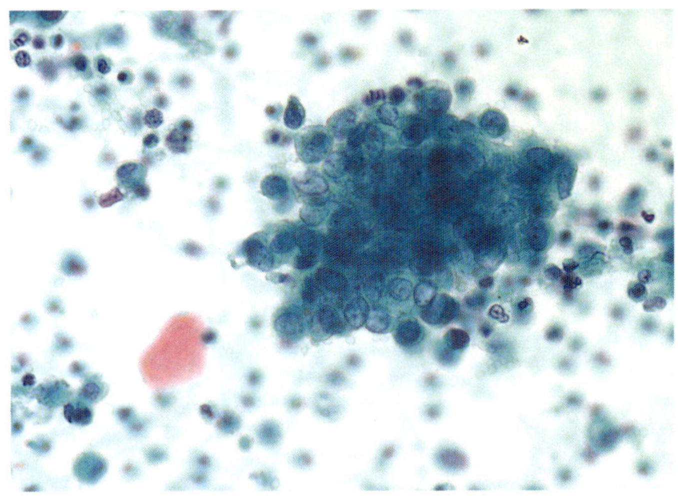

Figure 9.48 — High-grade urothelial carcinoma of the upper urinary tract, instrumented specimen. Aggregates of high-grade urothelial carcinoma can demonstrate severe degenerative changes that may mask their true identity, especially in a background of severe inflammation. Careful search for well preserved cells is important for the correct diagnosis (Papanicolaou stain, high power).

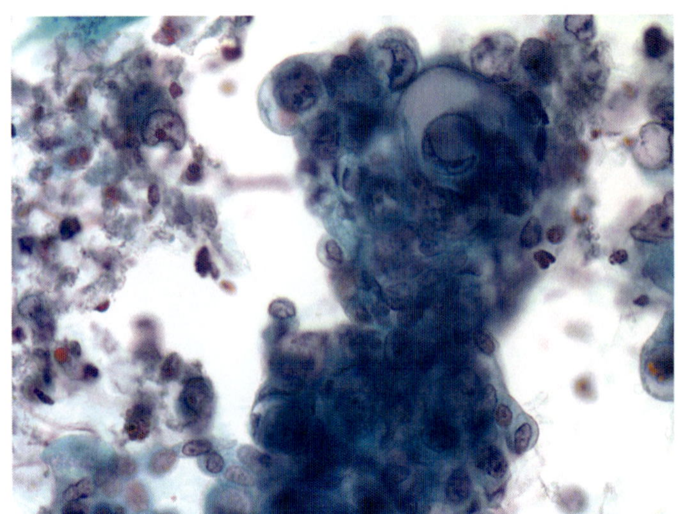

Figure 9.49 — High-grade urothelial carcinoma of the upper urinary tract, instrumented specimen. Cytoplasmic differentiation in a high-grade lesion is to be expected. Instead of the fine vacuolization seen in normal umbrella cells, a high-grade lesion will mimic an adenocarcinoma with large vacuoles and some pseudoglandular formation. Unless the entire neoplastic sample shows such differentiation, the diagnosis is considered that of a urothelial carcinoma, high grade (Papanicolaou stain, high power).

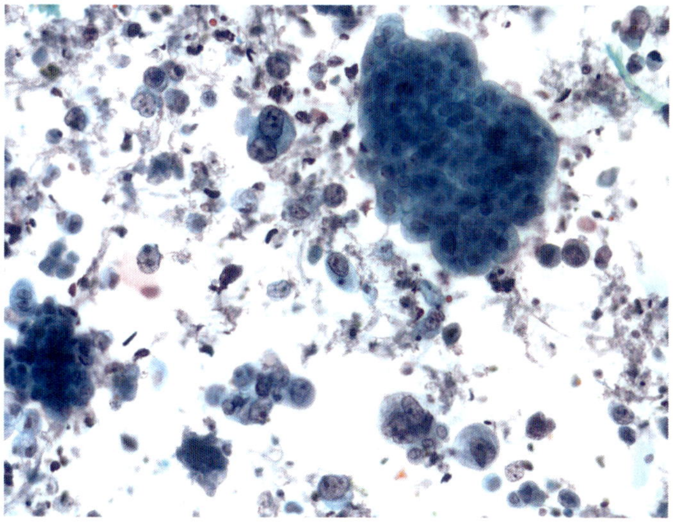

Figure 9.50 — High-grade urothelial carcinoma of the upper urinary tract, instrumented specimen. If the cellular changes within a tissue fragment are equivocal for neoplasm, careful search of the surrounding cells will usually reveal the grade of the lesion, in this case, high grade (Papanicolaou stain, medium power).

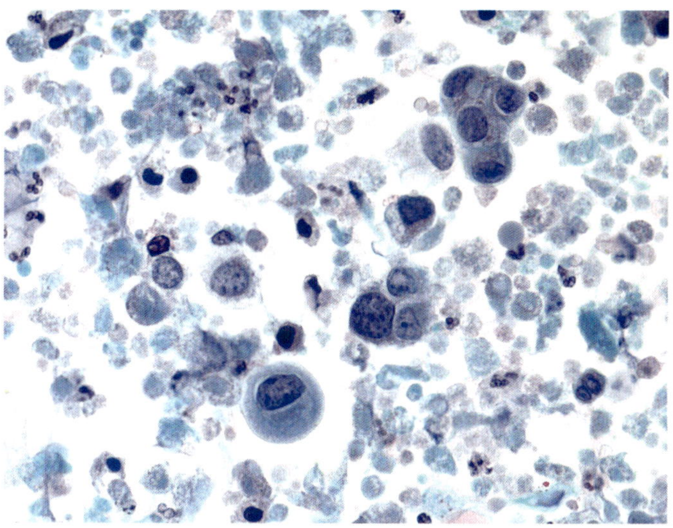

Figure 9.51 — High-grade urothelial carcinoma of the upper urinary tract, instrumented specimen. With squamous differentiation, the N/C ratio may decrease, but the large malignant nucleus will remain as the hallmark of the grade of the lesion. Since not every cell shows squamous differentiation, the typical high-grade urothelial cells with high N/C ratios in the same sample will aid in the definitive diagnosis. Note the extensive degeneration in the background (Papanicolaou stain, medium power).

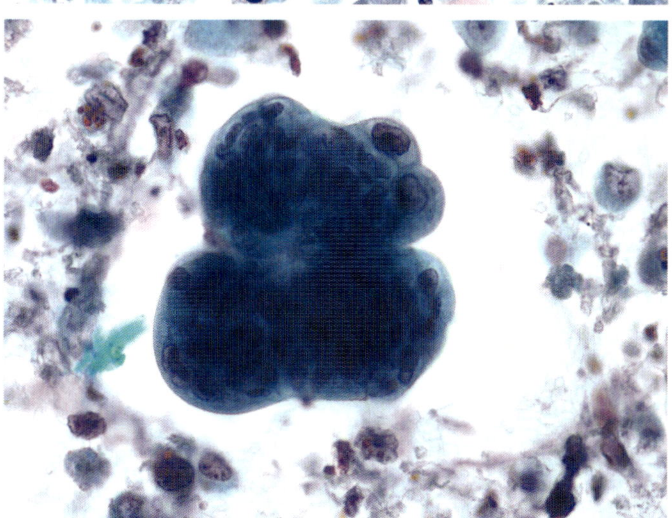

Figure 9.52 — High-grade urothelial carcinoma of the upper urinary tract, instrumented specimen. Not every dislodged fragment in a sample from the upper urinary tract is diagnostic for the putative lesion. Careful examination of the individual cells within the fragment as well as individual cells in the background is needed for proper identification (Papanicolaou stain, high power).

Figure 9.53 — High-grade urothelial carcinoma of the upper urinary tract, instrumented specimen. Individual cells in a cluster may display varying types of cytoplasmic differentiation. The overall diagnosis should be that of a urothelial lesion with nuclear features determining the grade, in this case high (Papanicolaou stain, high power).

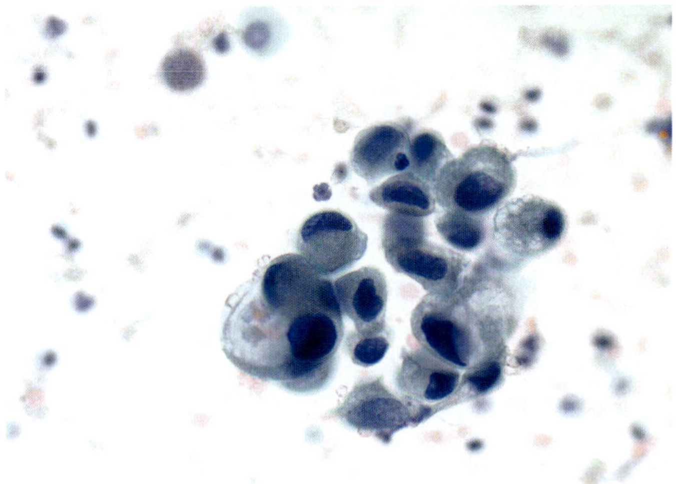

Figure 9.54 — High-grade urothelial carcinoma of the upper urinary tract, instrumented specimen. While most urothelial cells have nuclei within a certain size range, occasional megacells may be seen. This can be the result of treatment with radiation or chemotherapy, or an occasional aberration of the cell cycle with lack of nuclear division (Papanicolaou stain, high power).

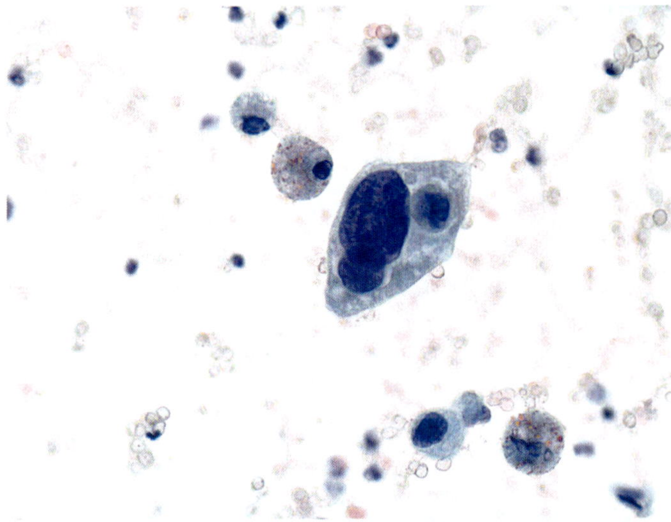

Figure 9.55 — High-grade urothelial carcinoma of the upper urinary tract, instrumented specimen. When degeneration is severe, careful search for well preserved diagnostic cells is imperative. Usually, when such degeneration is present, a high-grade lesion should be immediately suspected (Papanicolaou stain, medium power).

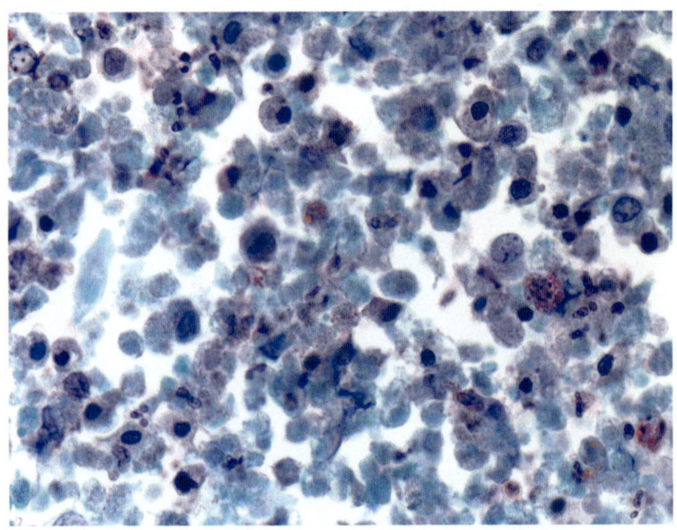

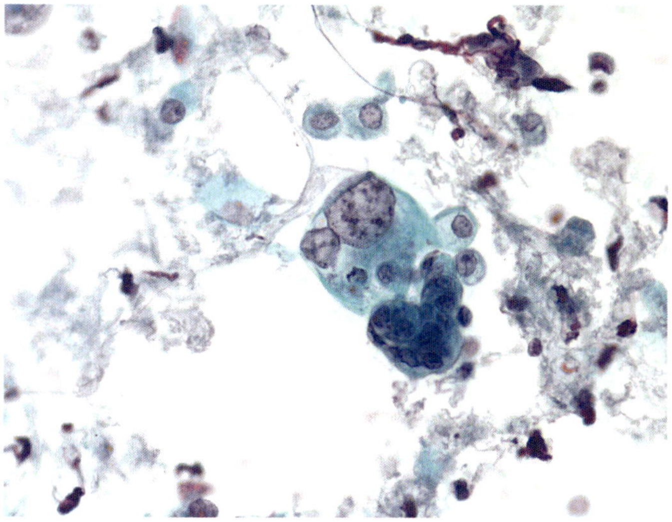

Figure 9.56 — High-grade urothelial carcinoma of the upper urinary tract, instrumented specimen. Uneven cell division is an immediate sign of neoplasia, in this case a high-grade lesion (Papanicolaou stain, high power).

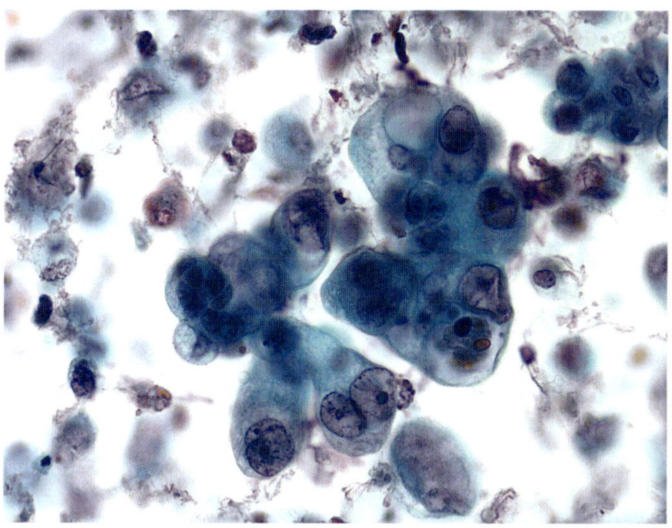

Figure 9.57 — High-grade urothelial carcinoma of the upper urinary tract, instrumented specimen. Large cytoplasmic vacuoles imply glandular differentiation, as compared with smaller vacuoles that can be a result of inflammatory change. (Papanicolaou stain, high power).

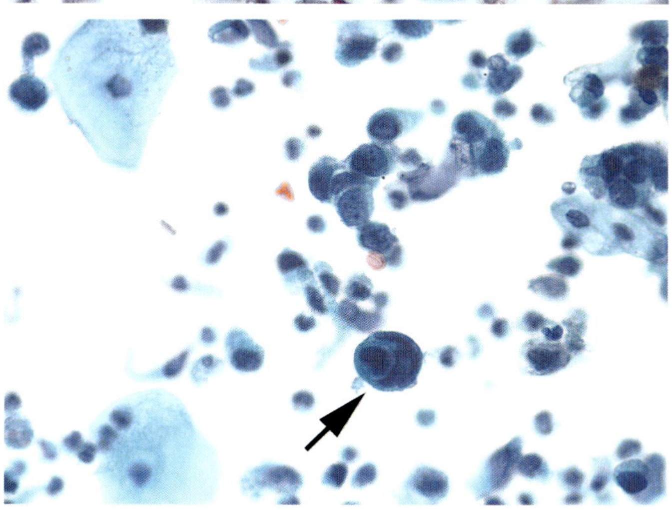

Figure 9.58 — High-grade urothelial carcinoma of the upper urinary tract, instrumented specimen. Within the same sample, both glandular and squamous differentiation may be appreciated. The cell in the bottom center has the typical ball-in-claw configuration of squamous differentiation (arrow); (Papanicolaou stain, high power).

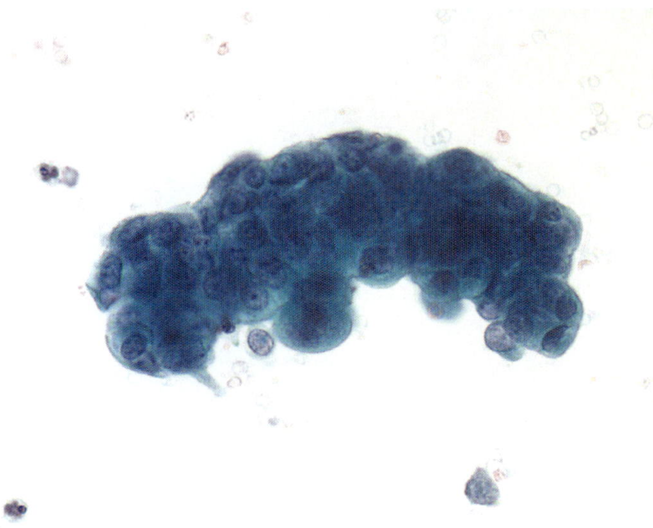

Figure 9.59 — High-grade urothelial carcinoma of the upper urinary tract, instrumented specimen. Within a single fragment of tissue are varying grades of cell change, frequently a characteristic of a high-grade lesion, that is, variable N/C ratio, nuclear size, and chromatin distribution. The architectural disorganization and nuclear variation are helpful to make the diagnosis of high grade (Papanicolaou stain, high power).

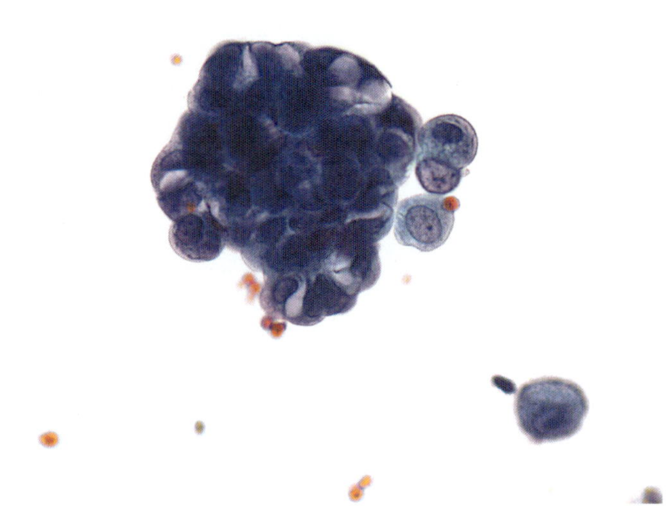

Figure 9.60 — High-grade urothelial carcinoma of the upper urinary tract, instrumented specimen. While some of these cells are vacuolated, most are typical of a high-grade lesion. Therefore, the temptation to consider glandular differentiation should be curtailed unless many other cells in the sample display vacuolization (Papanicolaou stain, high power).

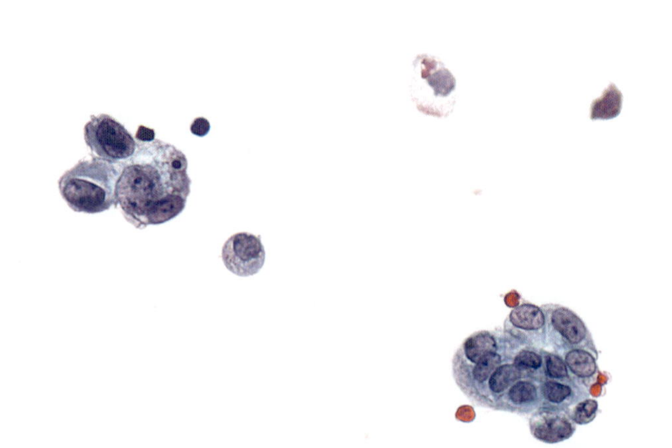

Figure 9.61 — High-grade urothelial carcinoma of the upper urinary tract, instrumented specimen. Comparing the group in the right corner of the photograph with the left group provides the immediate appreciation of enormous variation in nuclear size, shape, and chromatin pattern. This variation is typical of a high-grade lesion, and all of these cells should be considered from the same high-grade neoplasm (Papanicolaou stain, high power).

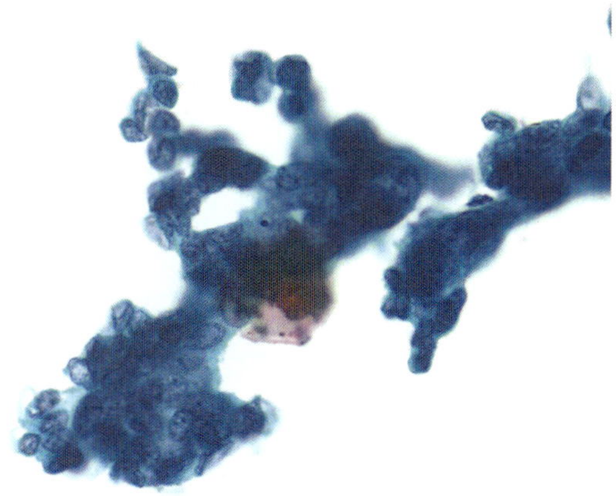

Figure 9.62 — High-grade urothelial carcinoma of the upper urinary tract, instrumented specimen. Severe architectural disorganization, even in a lesion in which the cells are relatively uniform, should persuade the diagnosis of high grade, as in this case (Papanicolaou stain, medium power).

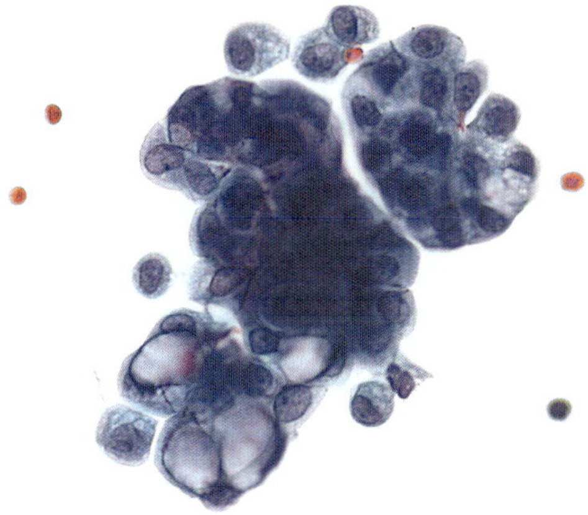

Figure 9.63 — High-grade urothelial carcinoma of the upper urinary tract, instrumented specimen. The difference between large vacuoles of glandular differentiation and the typical vacuoles seen in benign urothelial cells is very evident in this photograph (Papanicolaou stain, high power).

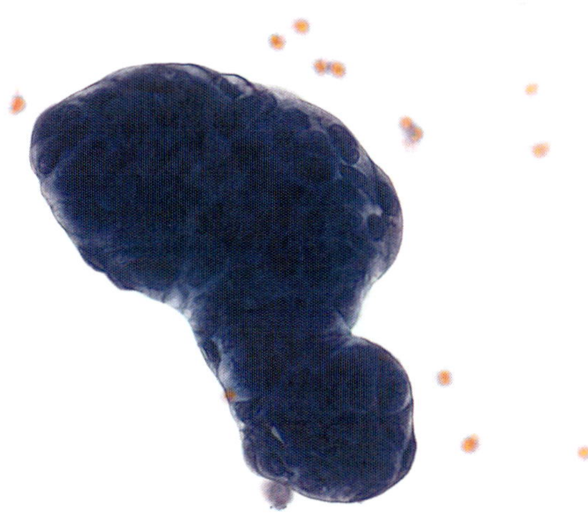

Figure 9.64 — High-grade urothelial carcinoma of the upper urinary tract, instrumented specimen. When outlines of a fragment of tissue are as smooth as this, a papillary lesion should be considered. Once the light is able to penetrate through such a thick fragment, the architectural disorganization and variation in nuclear size and N/C ratio will become evident (Papanicolaou stain, high power).

Figure 9.65 — High-grade urothelial carcinoma of the upper urinary tract, instrumented specimen. Within this fragment are large and small cells, some having glandular differentiation and others being of approximately the size of a normal urothelial cell. The most abnormal grade should be the distinguishing criterion for the diagnosis (Papanicolaou stain, high power).

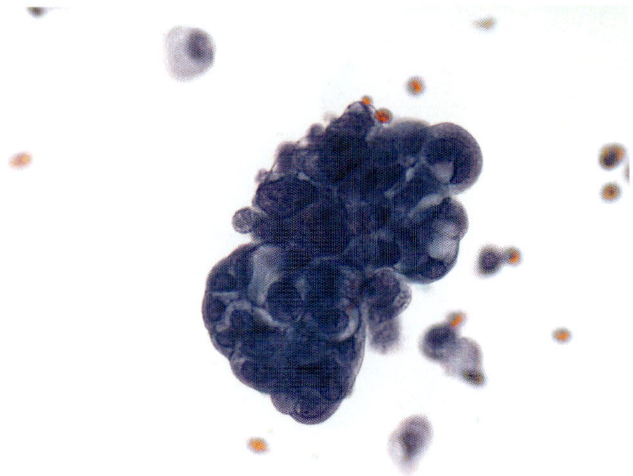

Figure 9.66 — High-grade urothelial carcinoma of the upper urinary tract, instrumented specimen. The most significant feature of this fragment is the architectural disorganization. Most of the individual cells have abundant cytoplasm and small nuclei, with only occasional ones having the criteria of a high-grade urothelial carcinoma. Overall, however, all of these features combined place the lesion in a high-grade category (Papanicolaou stain, high power).

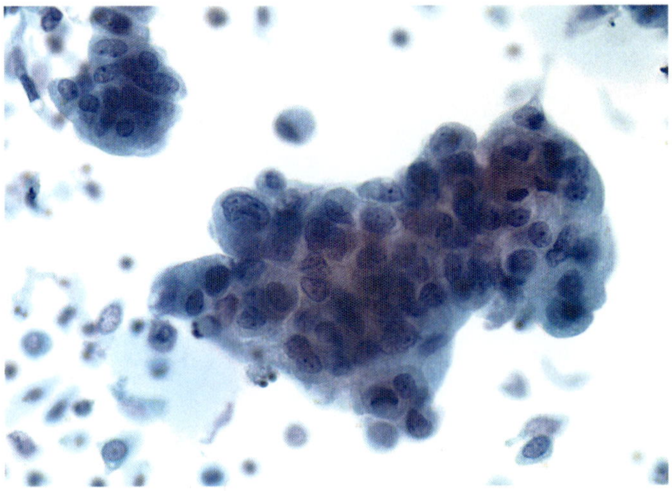

Figure 9.67 — High-grade urothelial carcinoma of the upper urinary tract, instrumented specimen. Although cellular monotony is considered the hallmark of a low-grade lesion, some of the high-grade lesions comprise nothing but high-grade, large urothelial cells with high N/C ratios, as in this case (Papanicolaou stain, high power).

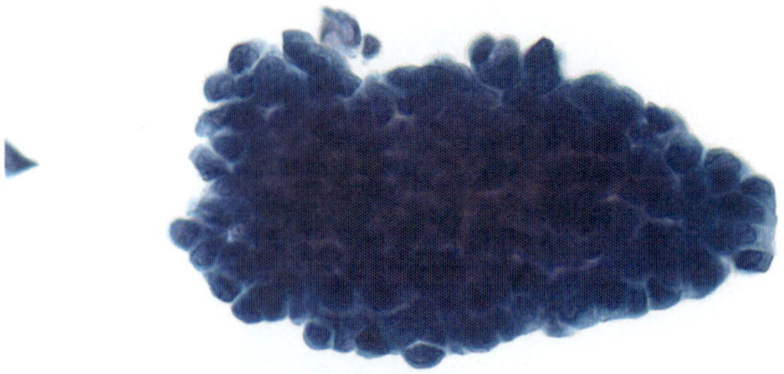

10

Metastatic and Secondary Cancers

- Locally Invasive Cancers
- Lympho-hematologic Neoplasms
- Metastatic Cancers

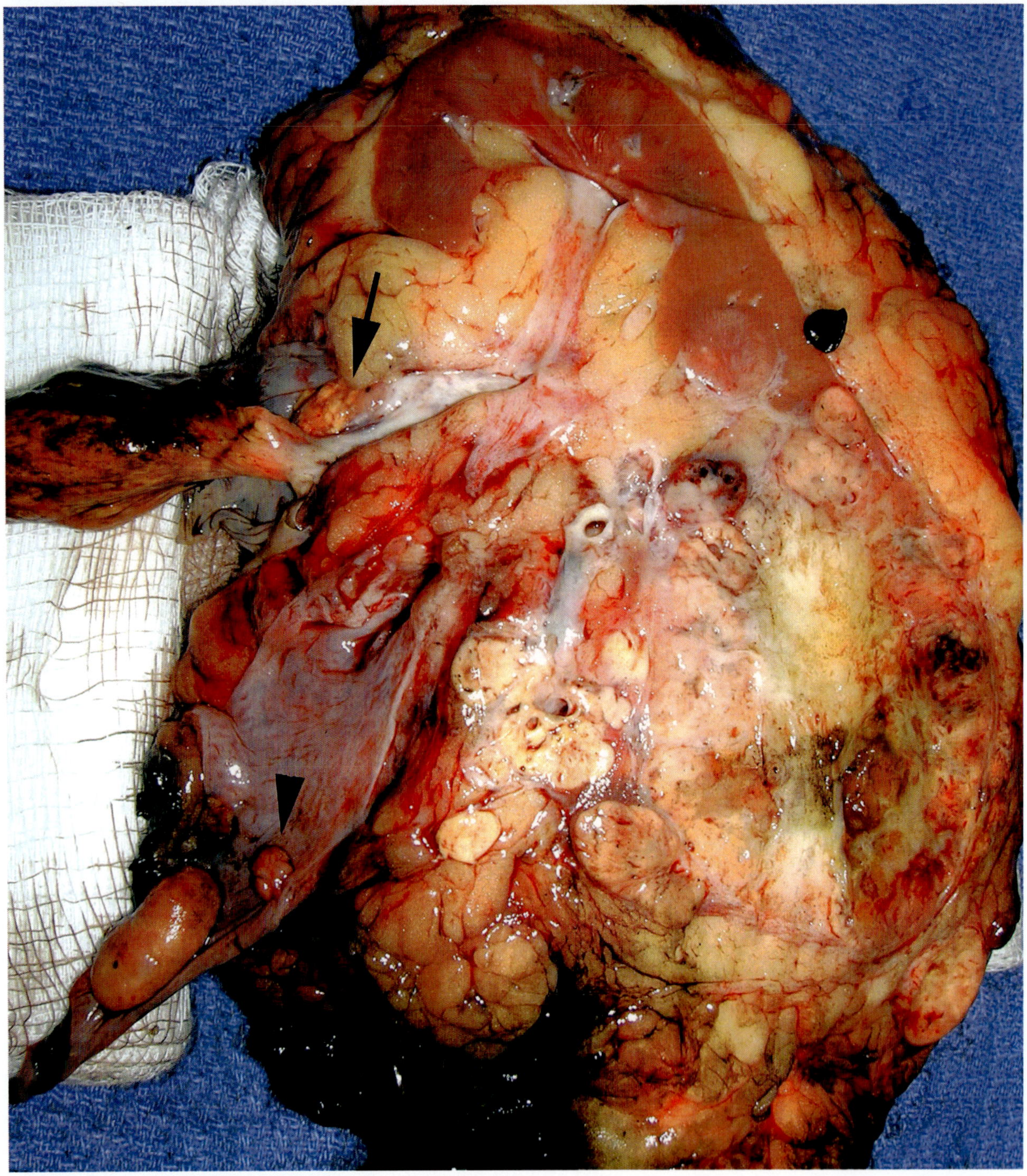

Figure 10.1 — Renal cell carcinoma involving ureter, gross specimen. Lower pole and part of the mid-pole of this kidney are replaced by a large multilobular, tan-yellow, clear-cell renal cell carcinoma that extends into the perinephric and hilar adipose tissue. Typical area of hyalinization is seen within the tumor. There is extension into the opened renal vein (arrow), and drop metastases in the longitudinally opened ureter (arrow head). Metastasis from renal cell carcinoma can also occur to the urinary bladder. These metastases can appear in urinary cytology.

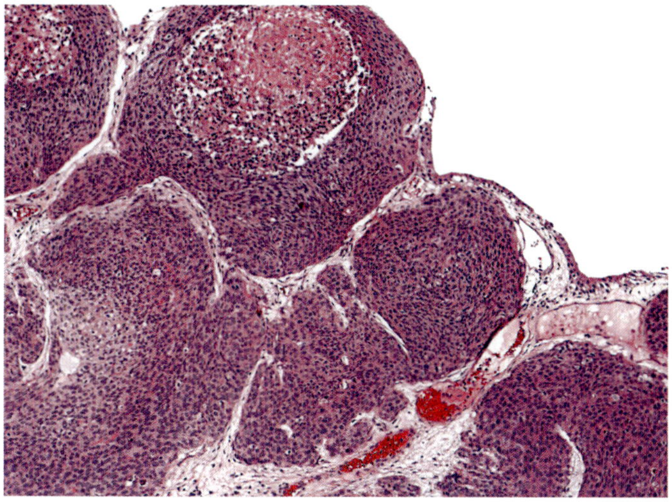

Figure 10.2 — Uterine cervical squamous cell carcinoma involving bladder, histologic section. Nonkeratinizing squamous cell carcinoma of the cervix can invade into the bladder. The morphology might be identical to urothelial carcinoma as seen in this image. Note the benign surface urothelium that the squamous carcinoma is undermining. Areas of central necrosis are present. Clinical history and imaging would be imperative for accurate diagnosis. Lack of a mucosal lesion and tumor predominantly involving the muscle layer are helpful clues. Very few immunohistochemical stains would prove useful. Urothelial carcinomas are CK7 and quite often CK20 positive, while cervical squamous cell carcinoma would not stain with CK20 but would be CK7 positive as well. Whereas p16 can also be seen in both, in situ hybridization for HPV is helpful as urothelial carcinomas are not related to HPV (H&E stain, low power).

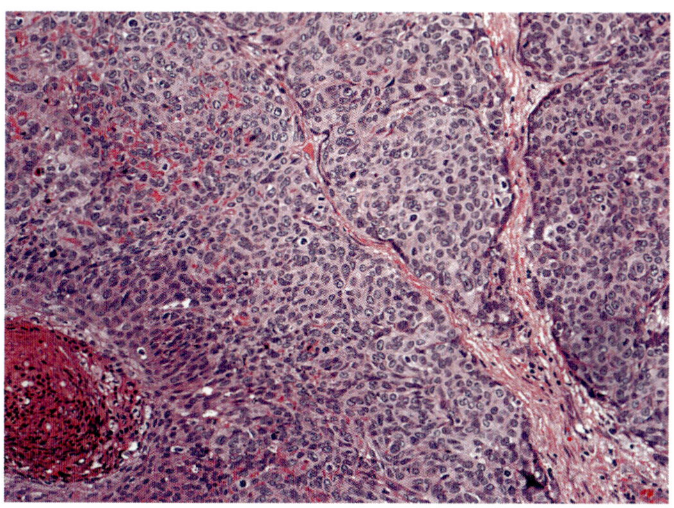

Figure 10.3 — Uterine cervical squamous cell carcinoma involving bladder, histologic section. This cervical carcinoma is showing less pleomorphism than the usual urothelial carcinoma; scattered mitoses are present. Focal necrosis is also present in the lower left corner (H&E stain, medium power).

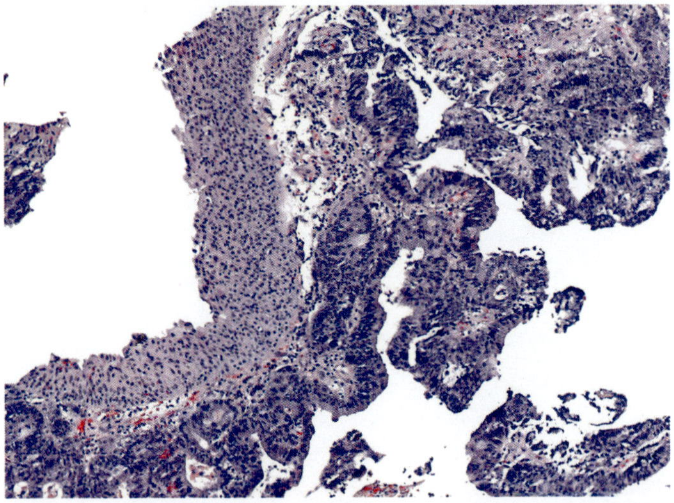

Figure 10.4 — Colorectal adenocarcinoma involving bladder, histologic section. This transurethral resection of bladder tumor specimen shows an intact, benign surface urothelium undermined by rectal adenocarcinoma directly invading the bladder wall. Quite frequently tumors invading the bladder reach up to the surface and colonize the mucosa, which could be mistaken for an in situ lesion (H&E stain, low power).

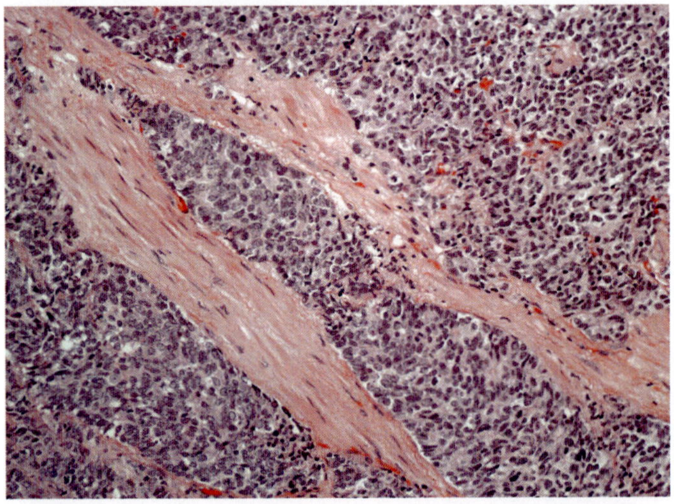

Figure 10.5 — Prostatic adenocarcinoma involving bladder, histologic section. Prostate adenocarcinoma can be in the differential diagnosis of urothelial carcinoma. Some morphologic features favoring prostate cancer include monomorphic nuclear appearance, prominent central nucleoli and areas of cribriform architecture. This image shows high-grade prostate cancer dissecting the muscularis propria layer of the bladder wall (H&E stain, medium power).

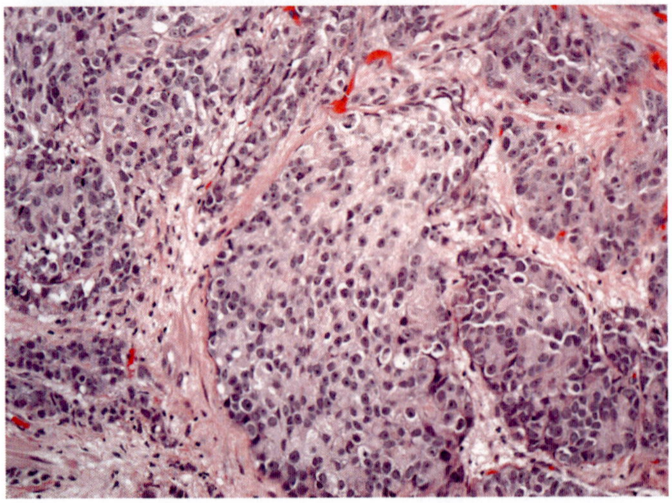

Figure 10.6 — Prostatic adenocarcinoma involving bladder, histologic section. Note the prominent central nucleoli and uniform nuclear appearance of the invading prostate adenocarcinoma. In difficult cases immunohistochemistry can be utilized (PSA, PSMA, and prostein (P501S) for prostate cancer and high molecular weight cytokeratin, thrombomodulin, and p63 for urothelial carcinoma; H&E stain, medium power).

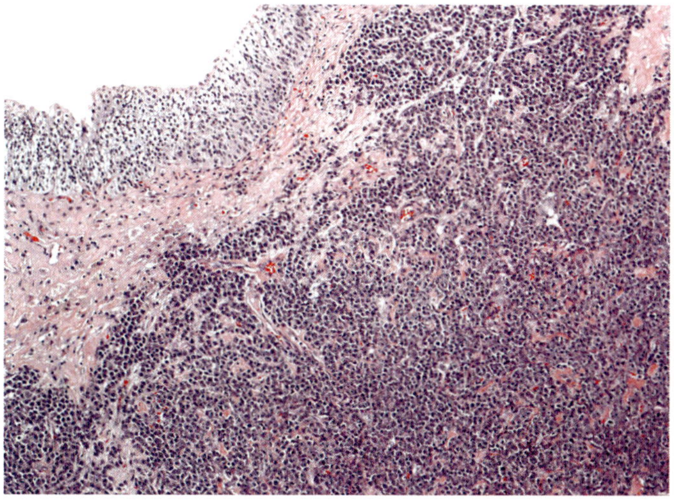

Figure 10.7 — Plasmacytoma of the bladder, histologic section. Primary plasmacytoma of the urinary bladder is rare. Patients may present with irritative symptoms and hematuria. These can form exophytic intraluminal masses. An important differential diagnosis is from urothelial carcinoma with plasmacytoid features. Urothelial carcinoma would be cytokeratin positive, while plasmacytoma would be positive for leukocyte-common antigen, kappa or lambda light chain. Intact benign urothelium is seen overlying the tumor. A pitfall is that plasmacytoid urothelial carcinoma is CD138 positive (H&E stain, low power).

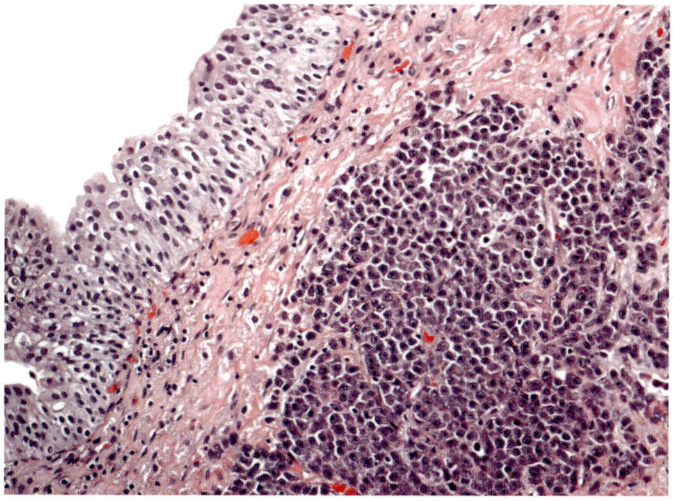

Figure 10.8 — Plasmacytoma of the bladder, histologic section. Malignant plasma cells have a rounded eccentric typical "clock face" nucleus with eosinophilic cytoplasm. They are arranged in a sheet like architecture. Intact urothelium is present (H&E stain, medium power).

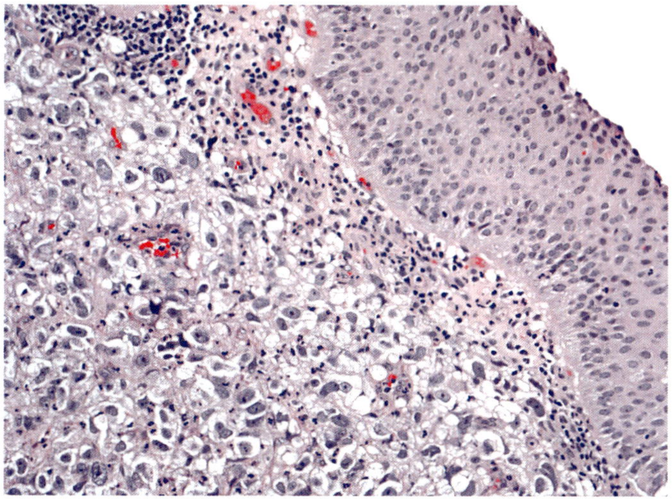

Figure 10.9 — Metastatic malignant melanoma involving bladder, histologic section. Undermining the benign surface urothelium are melanoma cells in a sheet-like arrangement. Prominent nucleoli are seen. A metastasis should be suspected when there is no surface urothelial lesion identified, for example, a flat urothelial carcinoma in situ or adenocarcinoma in situ or when there are unusual histologic features such as clear cytoplasm, uniform nuclei with prominent nucleoli, and so forth (H&E stain, medium power).

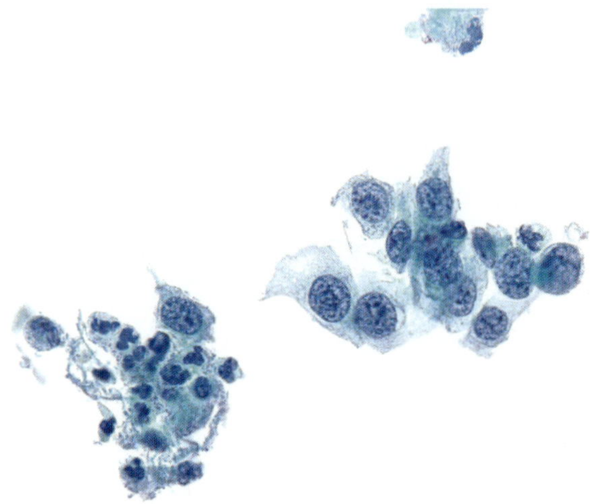

Figure 10.10 — Locally invasive, uterine cervical squamous cell carcinoma, voided urine. Cancers adjacent to the bladder may invade as in this case of carcinoma from the uterine cervix. This could be mistaken for a primary bladder cancer and emphasizes the need for complete clinical history. Malignant characteristics are present, and differential diagnoses include urothelial, squamous, and undifferentiated carcinoma (Papanicolaou stain, high power).

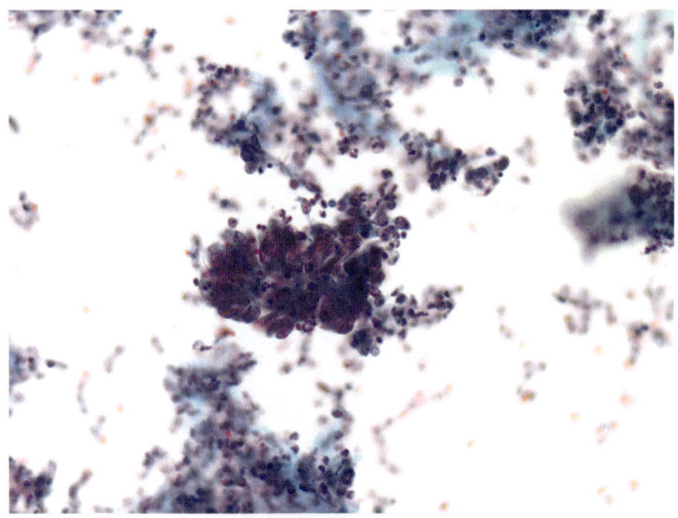

Figure 10.11 — Locally invasive, colonic adenocarcinoma, voided urine. When carcinoma of the colon metastasizes or locally invades, it commonly retains its characteristic appearance, complete with a picket fence arrangement of carrot-shaped cells (Papanicolaou stain, medium power).

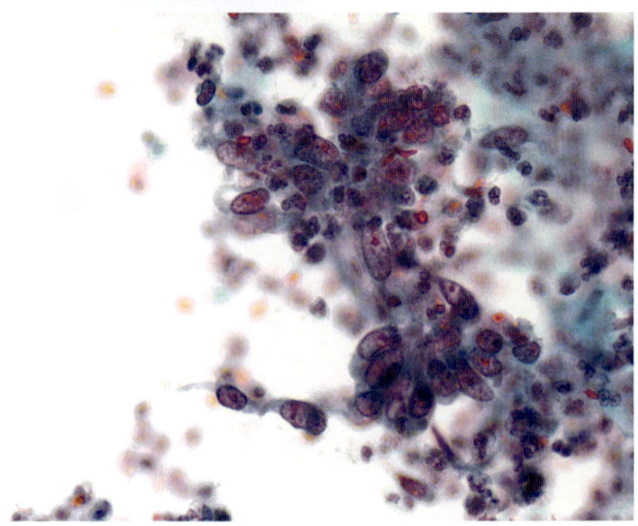

Figure 10.12 — Locally invasive, colonic adenocarcinoma, voided urine. Higher power of the preceding photograph displays the classical carrot-shaped nuclei of colon cancer (Papanicolaou stain, high power).

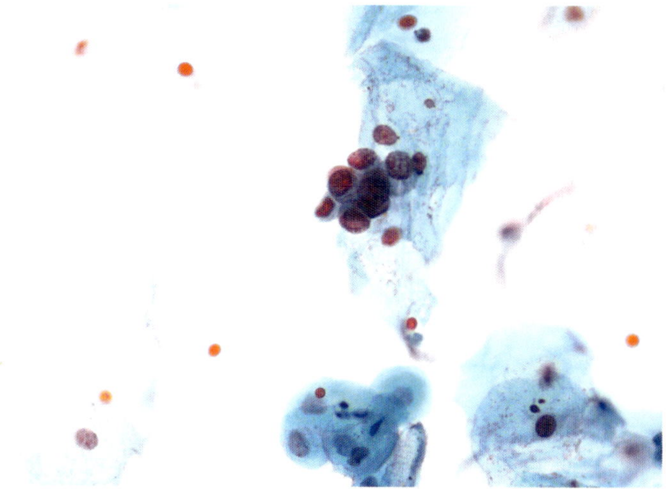

Figure 10.13 — Locally invasive, endometrial adenocarcinoma, voided urine. Endometrial carcinoma uncommonly invades the bladder but more commonly will be captured in a voided urine from a female, washed down from the vaginal tract in voiding. Characteristics of an adenocarcinoma may be present, but the organ of origin is not immediately appreciated (Papanicolaou stain, medium power).

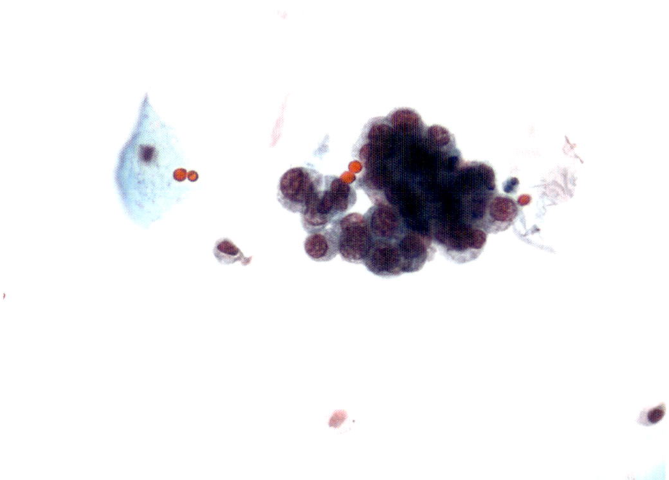

Figure 10.14 — Locally invasive, endometrial adenocarcinoma, voided urine. Distinction between invasion of the bladder by endometrial carcinoma and simple shedding into a voided urine can best be made by a catheterized specimen. Distinguishing features of an endometrial carcinoma are not apparent here, and simply a diagnosis of adenocarcinoma is appropriate (Papanicolaou stain, high power).

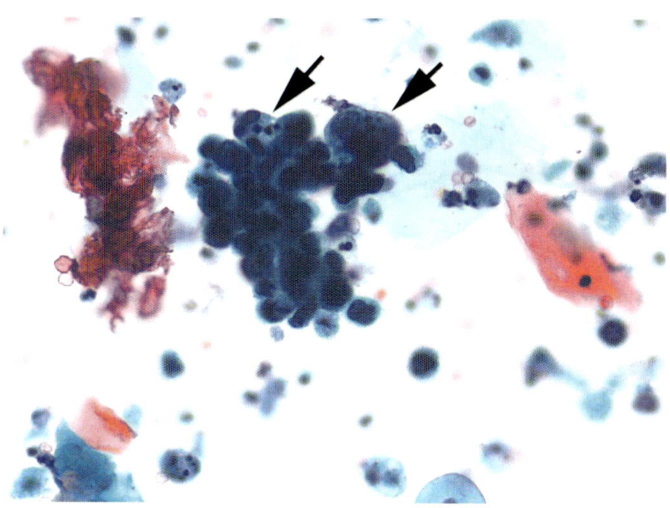

Figure 10.15 — Locally invasive, endometrial adenocarcinoma, voided urine. Sometimes the cytoplasmic inclusions of neutrophils (arrows) will provide the clue to origin in the endometrium (Papanicolaou stain, high power).

Figure 10.16 — Locally invasive, endometrial adenocarcinoma, voided urine. In addition to vacuolated cytoplasm, the neutrophils within the cytoplasmic vacuoles (arrow) are a definite clue to origin in the endometrium (Papanicolaou stain, medium power).

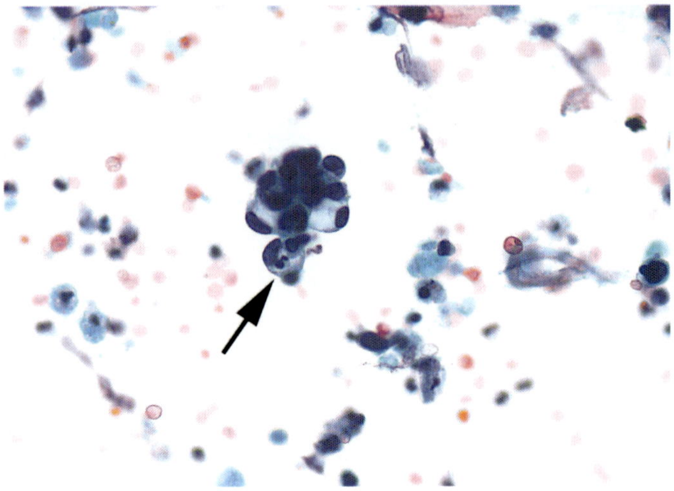

Figure 10.17 — Locally invasive, uterine malignant mixed mesodermal tumor (MMMT), voided urine. This biphasic tumor usually presents with adenocarcinoma in invasion or metastases, as in this instance. The neutrophils within the cytoplasm could convince one that the origin is in the endometrium. Biopsy is needed for definitive diagnosis (Papanicolaou stain, high power).

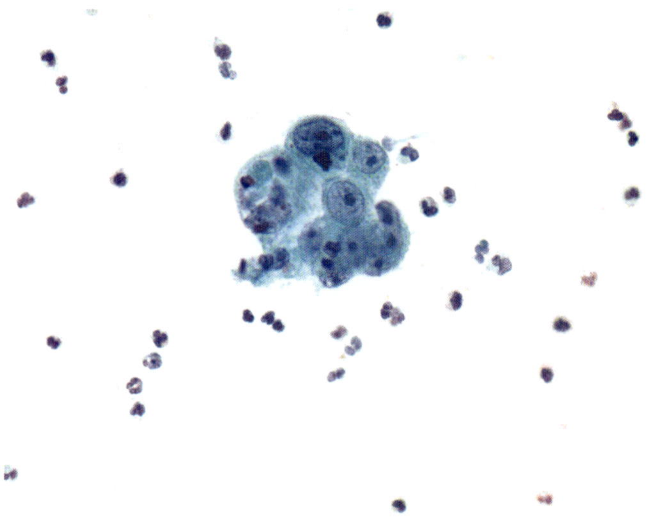

Figure 10.18 — Locally invasive, prostatic adenocarcinoma, voided urine. Prostatic carcinoma may invade directly into the bladder and will present either in glandular clusters or in poorly differentiated sheets, as in this photograph. Complete clinical history is important to decide the origin of these malignant cells (Papanicolaou stain, high power).

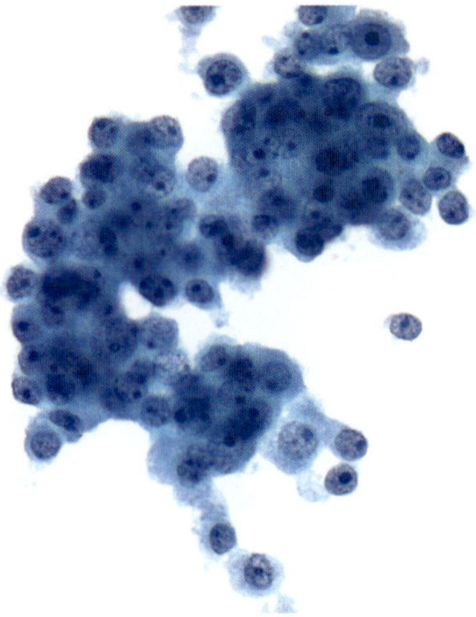

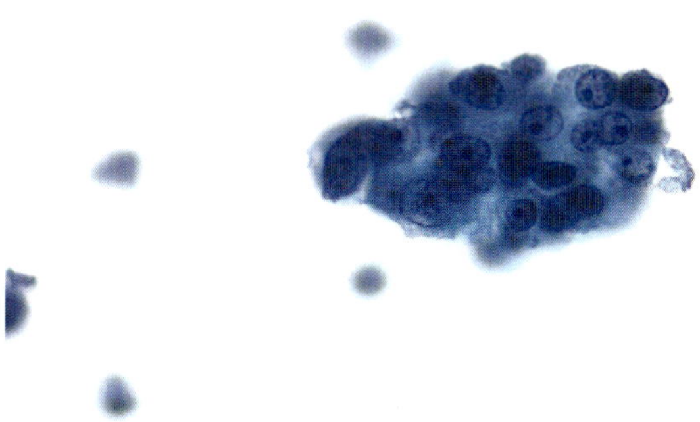

Figure 10.19 — Locally invasive, prostatic adenocarcinoma, voided urine. Glandular cells from a prostatic carcinoma are not distinct from an adenocarcinoma either originating in the bladder or from a distant site. Biomarkers are helpful as well as a clinical history (Papanicolaou stain, high power).

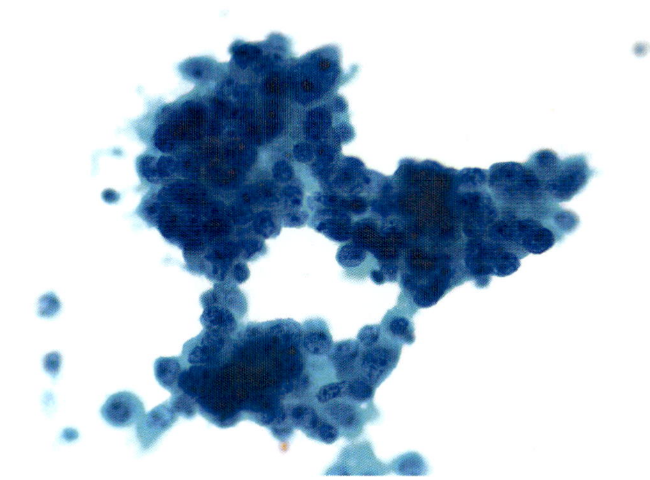

Figure 10.20 — Locally invasive, prostatic adenocarcinoma, voided urine. The less differentiated the tumor, the more difficult it is to establish the organ of origin. Some glandular formation is evident in the sheets of tumor. Appropriate clinical history is necessary (Papanicolaou stain, high power).

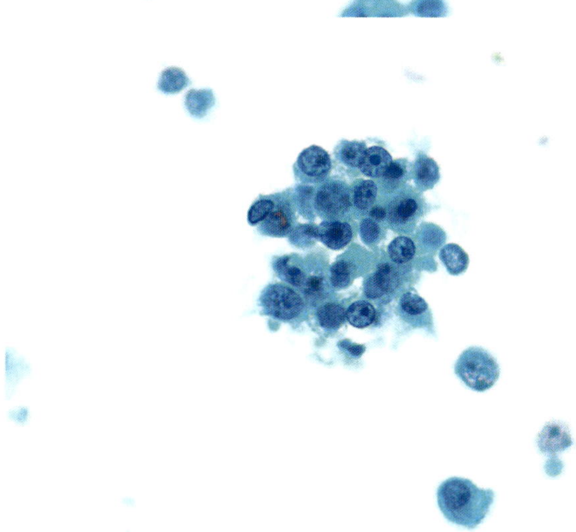

Figure 10.21 — Locally invasive, prostatic adenocarcinoma, voided urine. Prominent nucleoli and gland formation imply a moderately well-differentiated carcinoma of the prostate. Accurate Gleason grading is not appropriate for a cytologic sample such as this (Papanicolaou stain, high power).

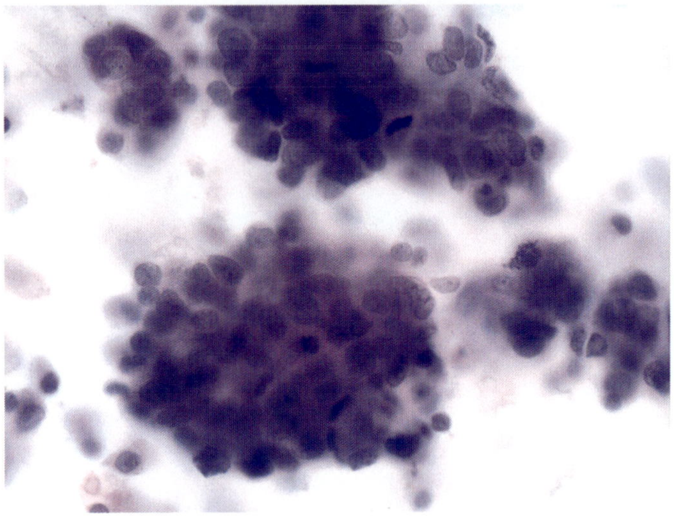

Figure 10.22 — Locally invasive, prostatic small-cell carcinoma, voided urine. Prostatic carcinomas may be mixtures of glandular and small-cell undifferentiated carcinoma or pure small-cell carcinoma. When such a component is present, the characteristics are identical to small-cell carcinoma elsewhere in the body (Papanicolaou stain, high power).

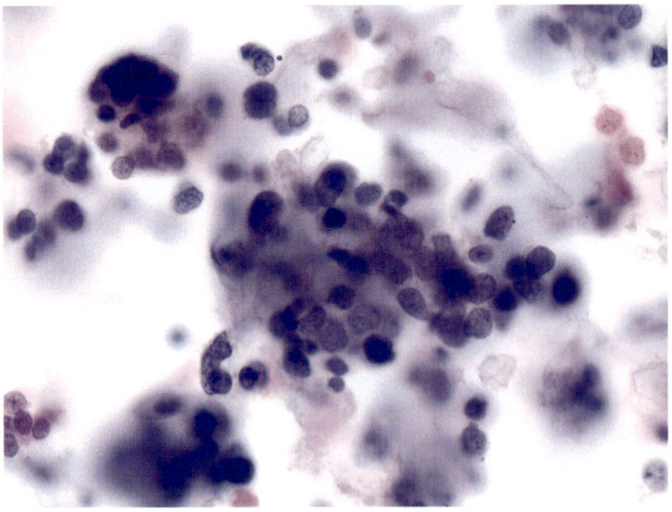

Figure 10.23 — Locally invasive, prostatic small-cell carcinoma, voided urine. Homogeneous chromatin, indistinct nucleoli, high N/C ratios, and nuclear molding can be seen within these cells, originating in the bladder or elsewhere (Papanicolaou stain, high power).

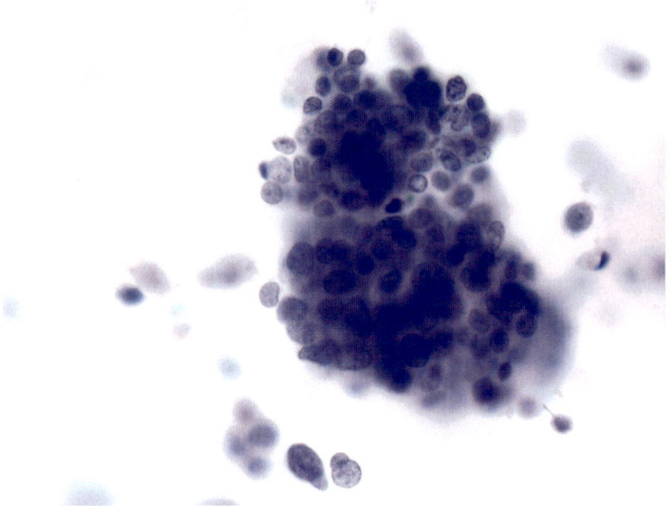

Figure 10.24 — Locally invasive, prostatic small-cell carcinoma, voided urine. When such groups float in liquid, they can assume a three-dimensional appearance, making the focal plane difficult to establish. Rosette formation should not be confused with gland formation, with the final diagnosis resting on the characteristic nuclear chromatin (Papanicolaou stain, medium power).

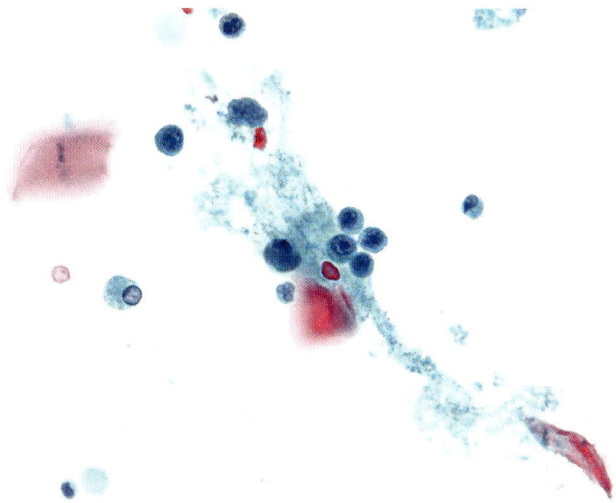

Figure 10.25 — Multiple myeloma involving bladder, voided urine. Nonepithelial tumors may involve the urinary bladder. Fortunately, most patients present with a strong clinical history, and involvement by the established tumor in the urinary tract is the clinical question. This case of multiple myeloma fortunately did not present as an unknown. Characteristics of plasma cells can be seen within the nuclei. Comparison with the original tumor should be made whenever possible (Papanicolaou stain, high power).

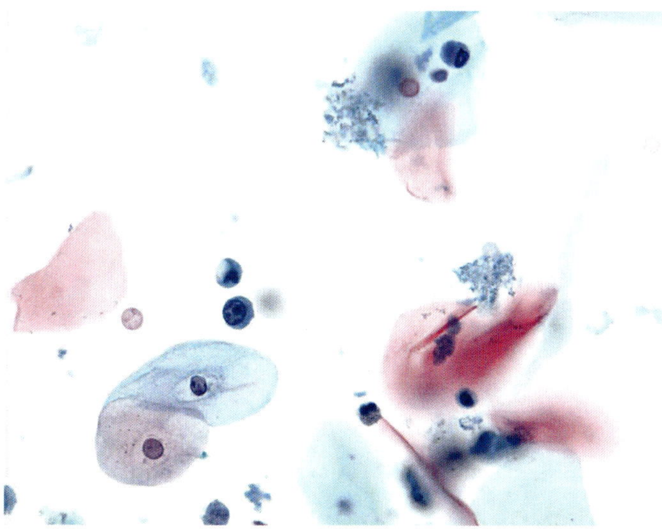

Figure 10.26 — Multiple myeloma involving bladder, voided urine. Most hematopoietic tumors involving the bladder present as rare cellular events. This makes the screening task difficult, emphasizing the importance of clinical history (Papanicolaou stain, high power).

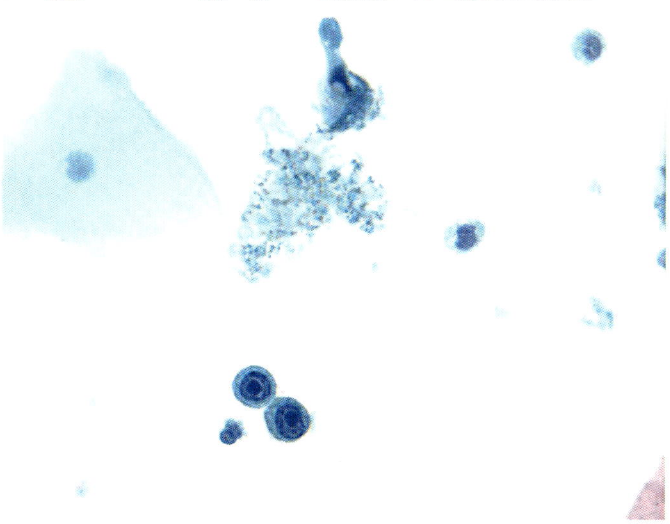

Figure 10.27 — Multiple myeloma involving bladder, voided urine. These malignant plasma cells might be mistaken for epithelial cells but the nuclear characteristics will persuade differently (Papanicolaou stain, high power).

Figure 10.28 — Multiple myeloma involving bladder, CD138 immunolabeling, voided urine. Immunohistochemistry may be successfully applied to cytologic samples, but meticulous attention to processing is essential for success. If a test is negative, this may be due to a processing fault and not actually representative of the lesion (CD138 immunostain, high power).

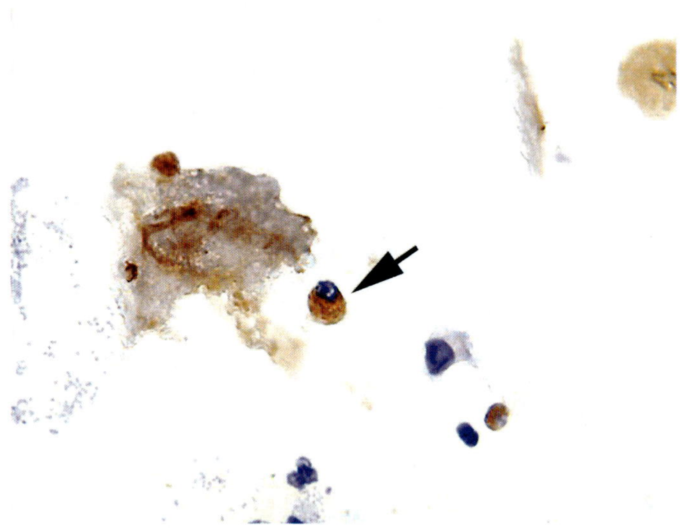

Figure 10.29 — Non-Hodgkin lymphoma involving bladder, filter prep, voided urine. Non-Hodgkin lymphomas may also involve the bladder and present in a urinary sample. Once again, complete clinical history is essential for an accurate assessment of the cells in question (Papanicolaou stain, medium power).

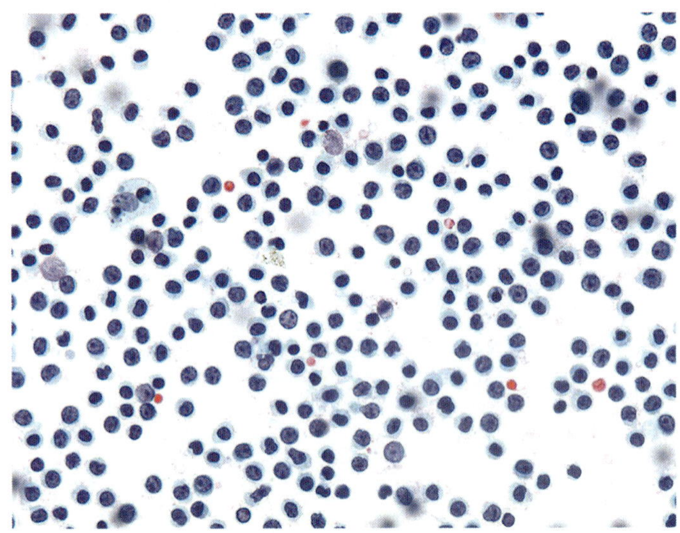

Figure 10.30 — Metastatic breast adenocarcinoma involving bladder, voided urine. (Papanicolaou stain, medium power).

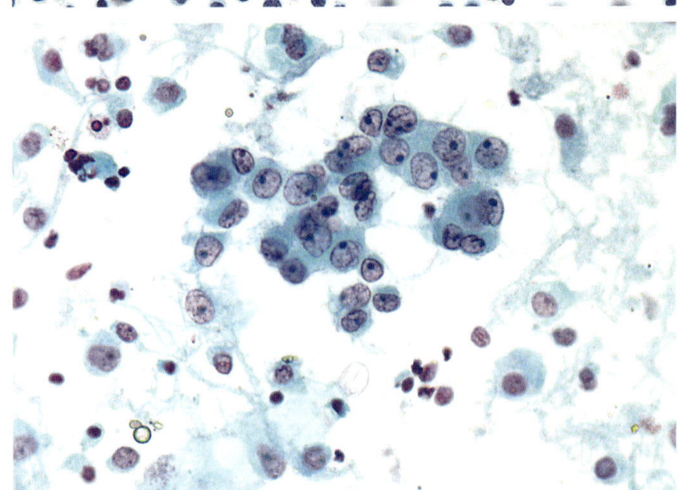

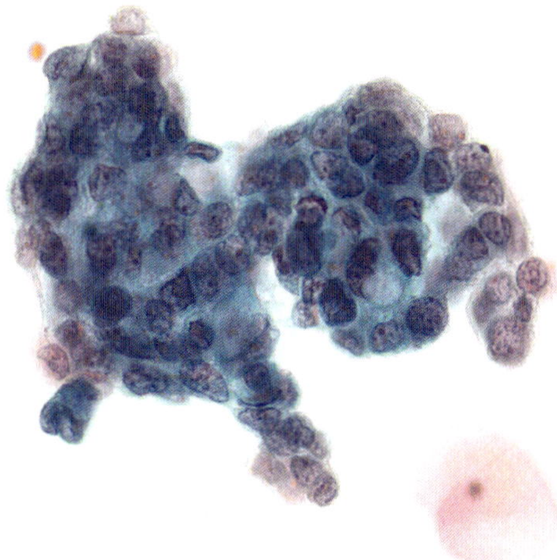

Figure 10.31 — Metastatic breast adenocarcinoma involving bladder, voided urine. (Papanicolaou stain, medium power).

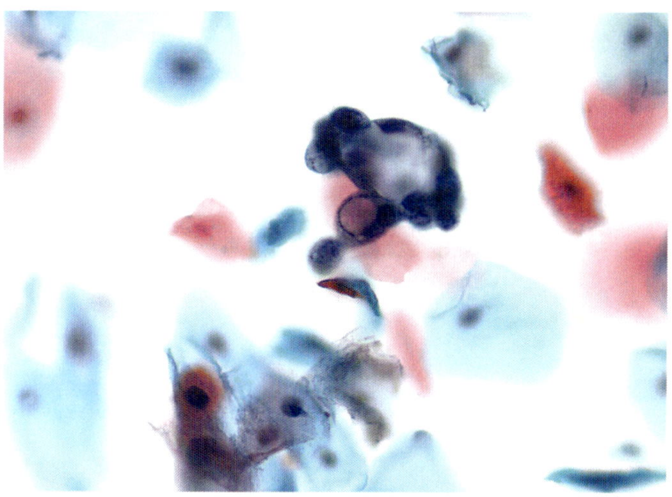

Figure 10.32 — Metastatic esophageal adenocarcinoma involving bladder, voided urine. (Papanicolaou stain, high power).

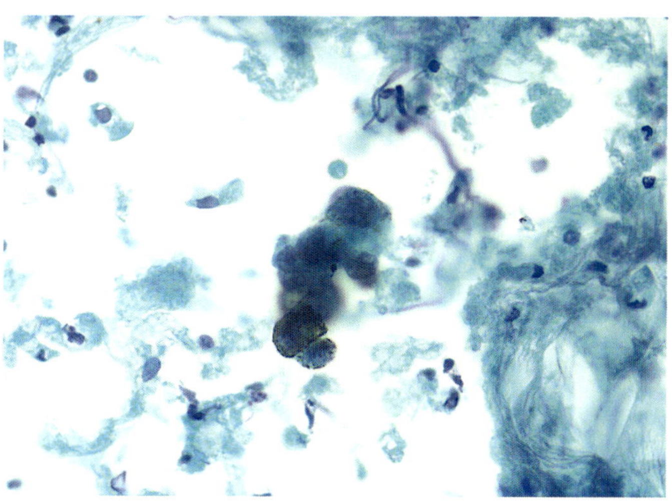

Figure 10.33 — Metastatic malignant melanoma involving bladder, voided urine. (Papanicolaou stain, medium power).

Figure 10.34 — Metastatic malignant melanoma involving bladder, voided urine. (Papanicolaou stain, high power).

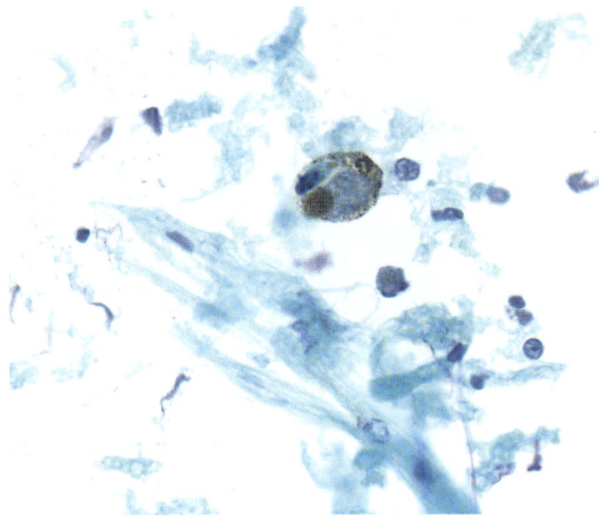

Figure 10.35 — Metastatic malignant melanoma involving bladder, voided urine. (Papanicolaou stain, high power).

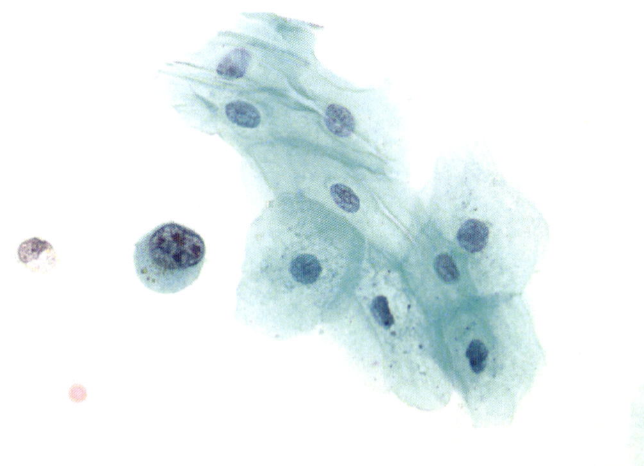

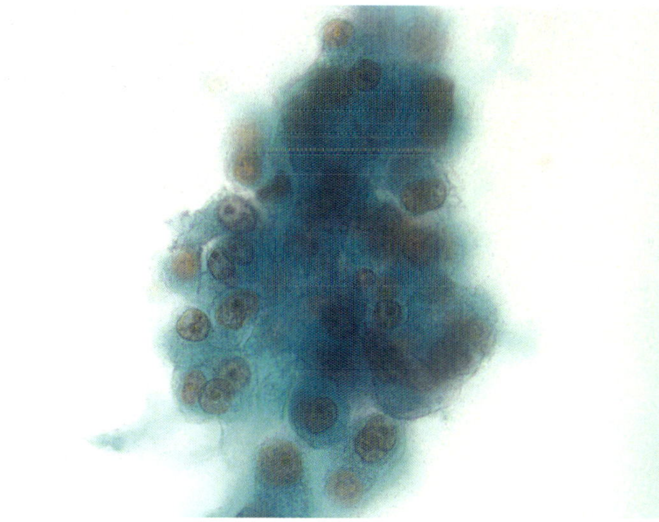

Figure 10.36 — Renal cell carcinoma, exfoliation in voided urine. (Papanicolaou stain, medium power).

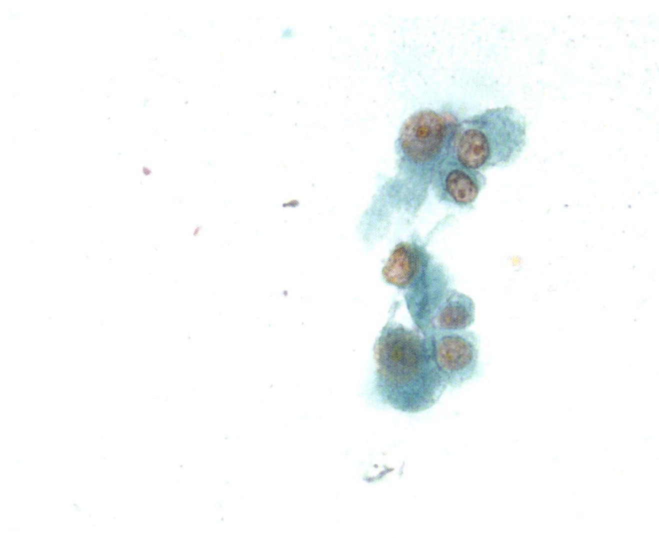

Figure 10.37 — Renal cell carcinoma, exfoliation in voided urine. (Papanicolaou stain, high power).

Index

Note: Page locaters followed by f *indicate figures. Page locators followed by* ff *indicate multiple figures on the indicated page.*